Culinary Quickies Cookbook
© Mel Alafaci 2023

First printed August 2023 by Ingram Spark

All rights reserved. Except as permitted under the Australian Copyright Act 1968 (for example, a fair dealing for the purposes of study, research, criticism or review), no part of this book may be reproduced, stored in a retrieval system, communicated or transmitted in any form or by any means without prior written permission.

Creator: Mel Alafaci (Author)
Title: Culinary Quickies Cookbook
ISBN: 9780645808476 (Paperback)
Subjects: Cook Book

Typesetting by Chloe Reynolds - Social Chloe

Chef Mel is taking on the WORLD!

With a smile that can light up a room, Chef Mel Alafaci has become a globally recognised chef and food educator. Her recent success in the USA means she's Australia's hottest rising culinary personality. Born in Zimbabwe, Chef Mel lived in South Africa before moving to Australia and starting her reign in the global foodie market.

She has an unwavering passion for cooking, eating, and teaching. And her intoxicating enthusiasm, authenticity, and unique culinary lingo will have you hungry to flex your muscles in the kitchen. Chef Mel is brilliant at adding humour, shortcuts, tricks, and hacks to all those tedious tasks, as well as making the scary ones simple and easy to accomplish.

CHEF MEL THE HAPPY CHEF | **@CHEFMEL_HAPPYCHEF** | **WWW.CHEFMEL.ME**

ABOUT MEL

Mel Alafaci has been passionate about food her whole life. She's the founder of Vanilla Zulu Cooking School, one of Australia's leading cooking schools, and has more than 28 years of professional cooking experience.

People battle to say her surname... so to make it easy she calls herself CHEF MEL.

WILD ABOUT FOOD!

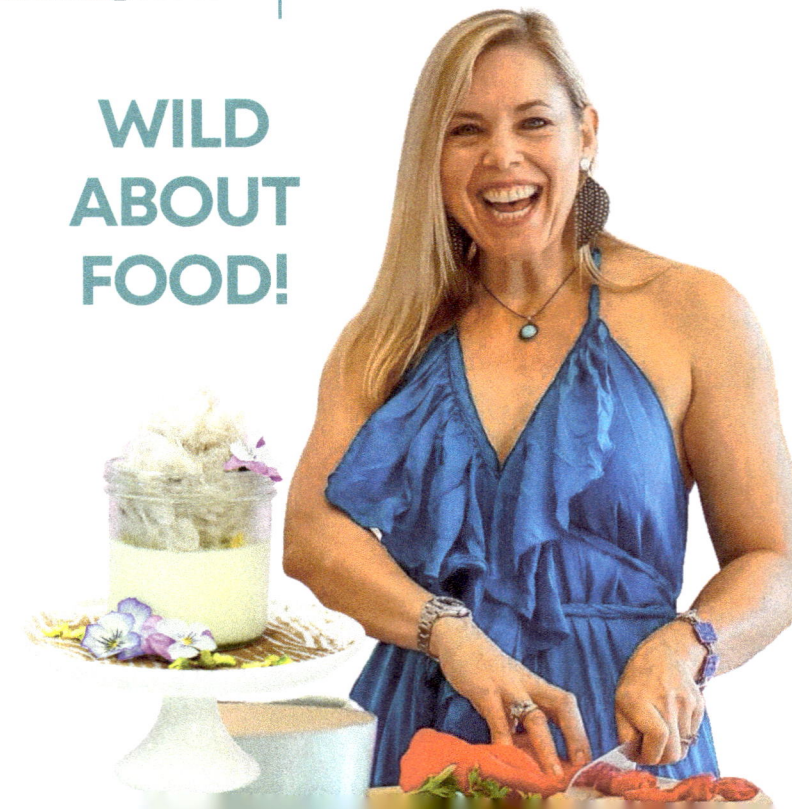

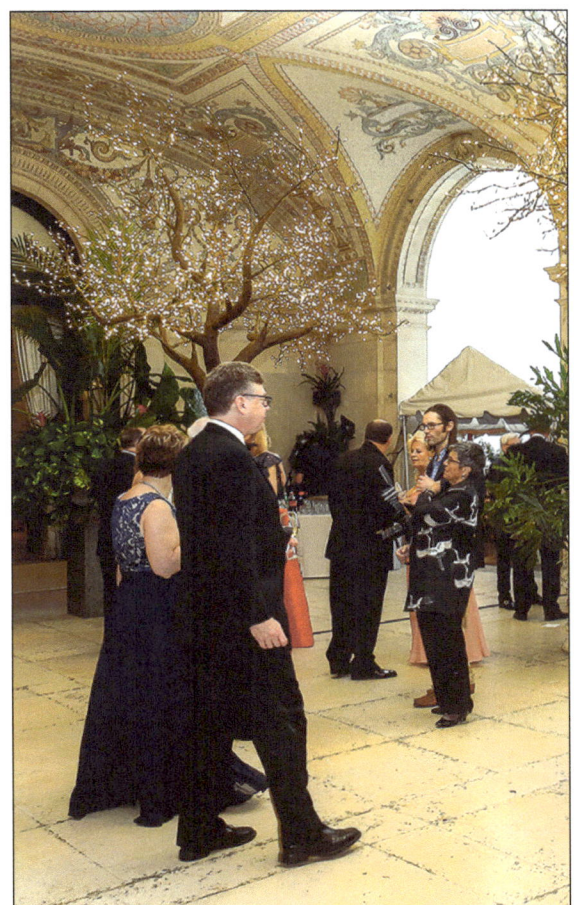
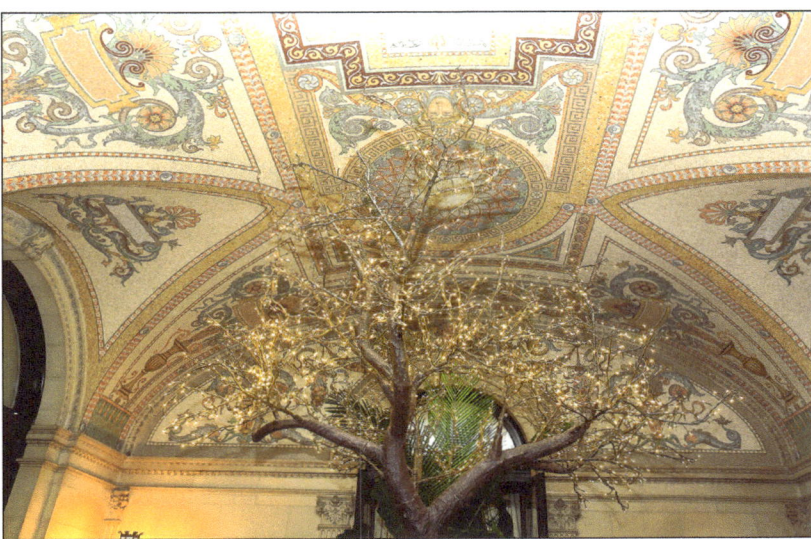
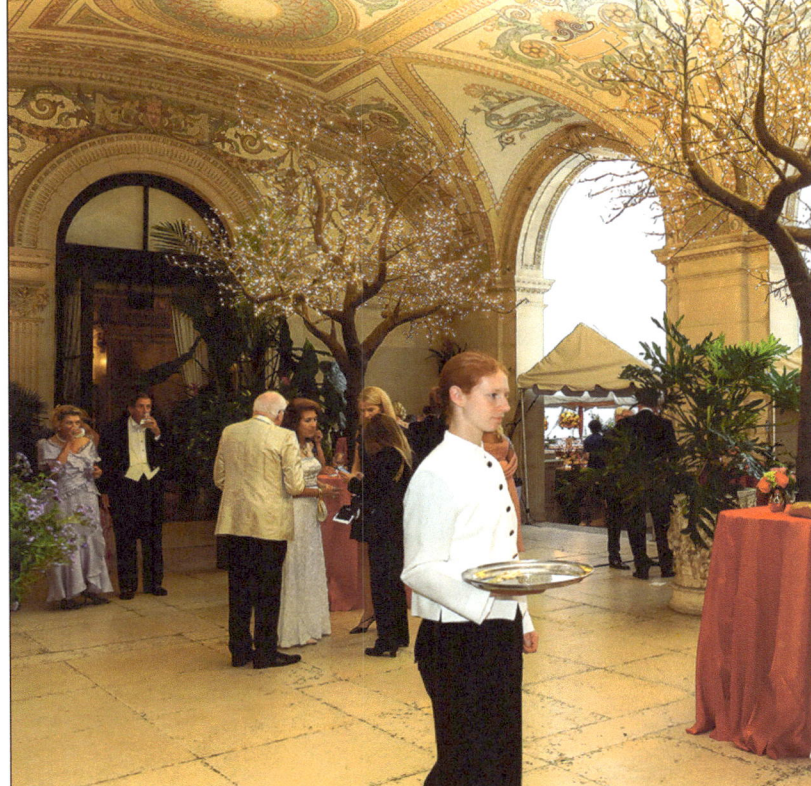
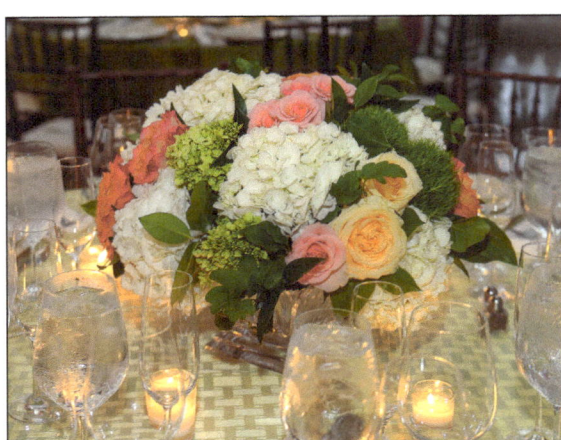

Newport Coaching Weekend

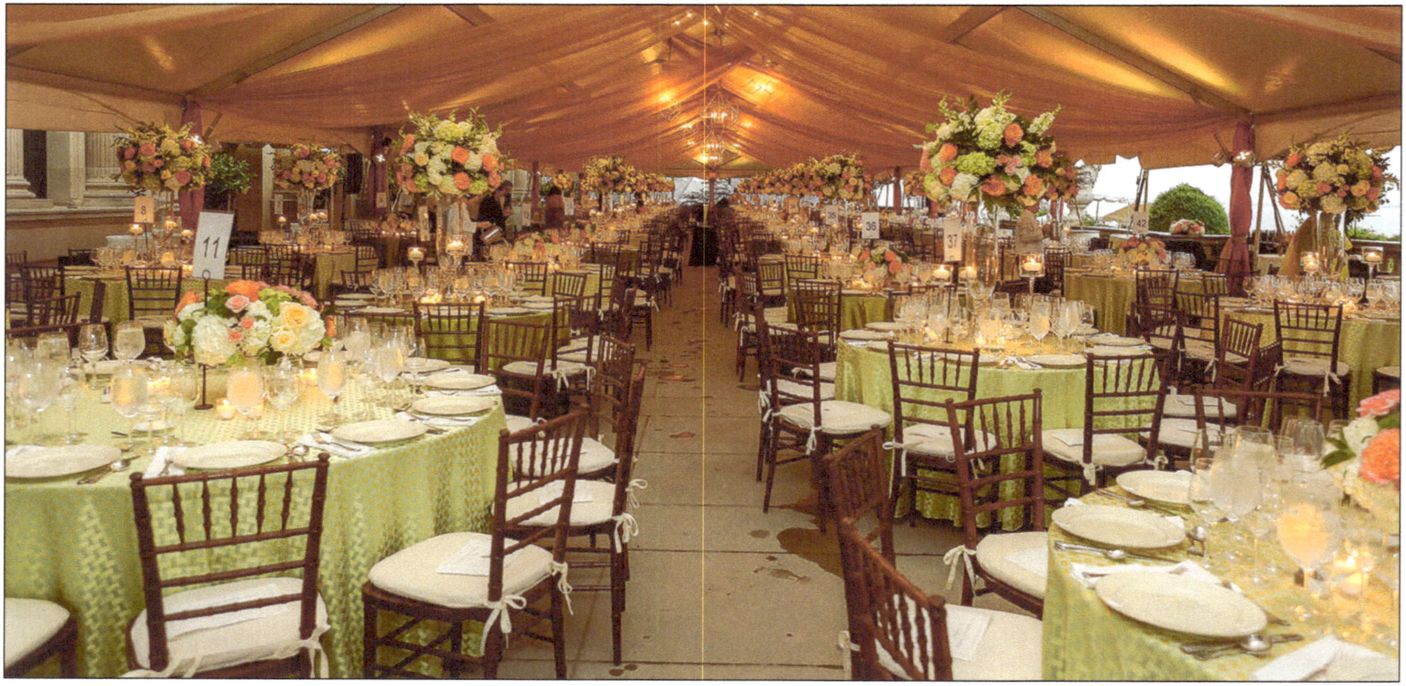

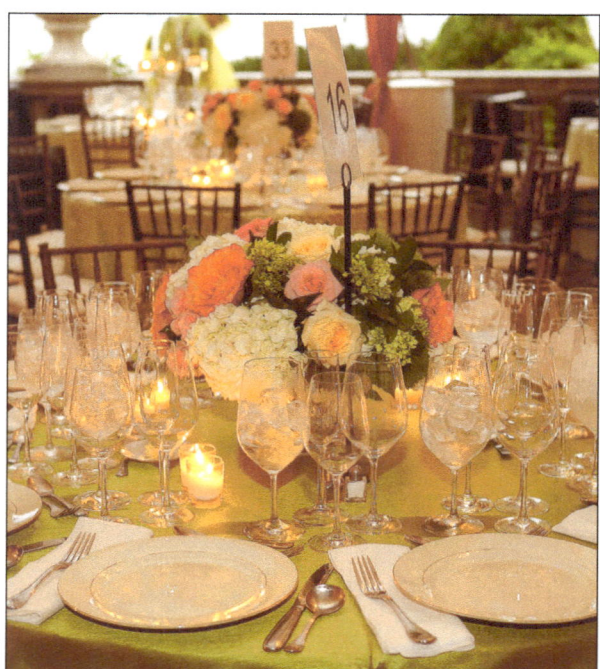
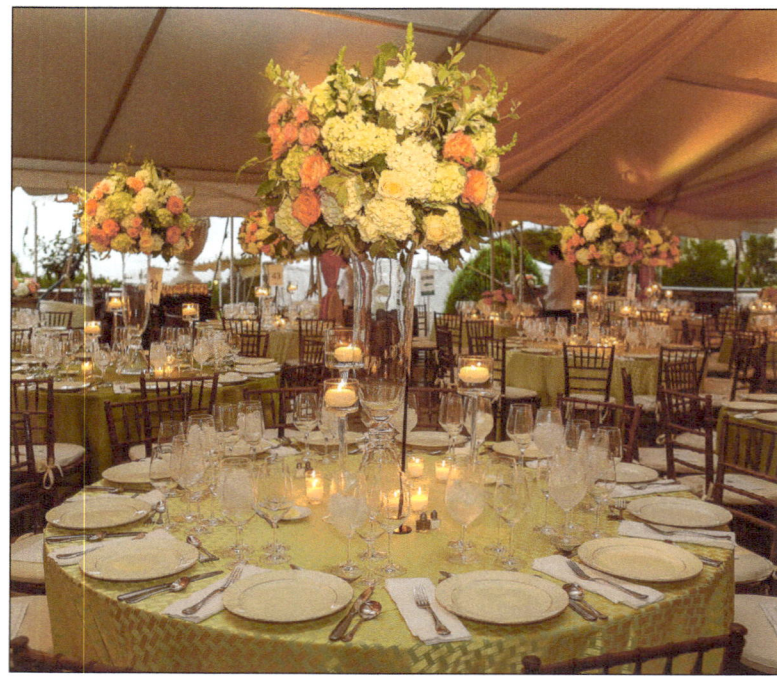

Newport Coaching Weekend

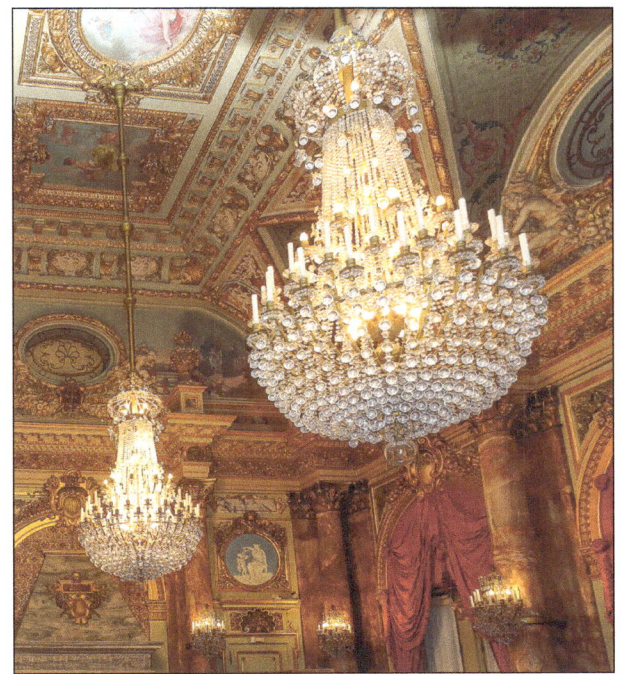
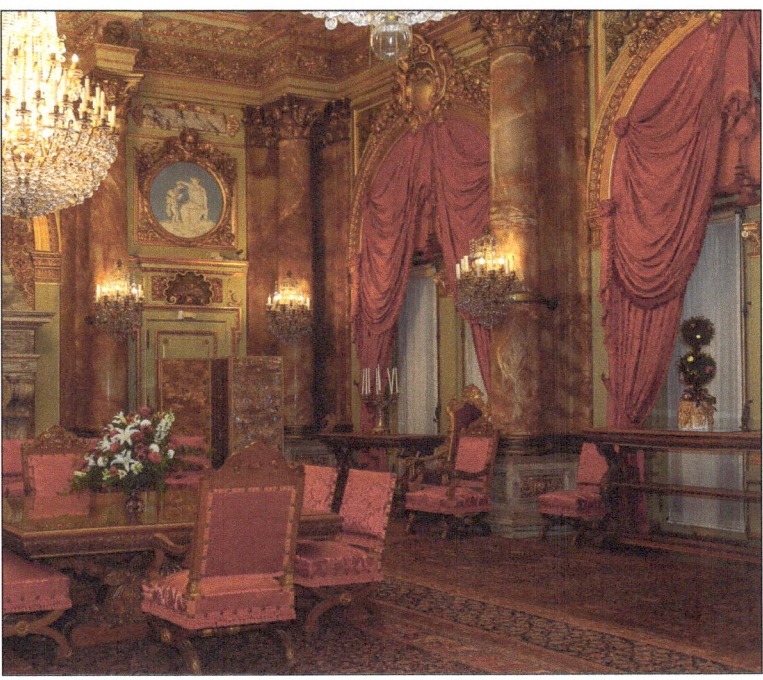
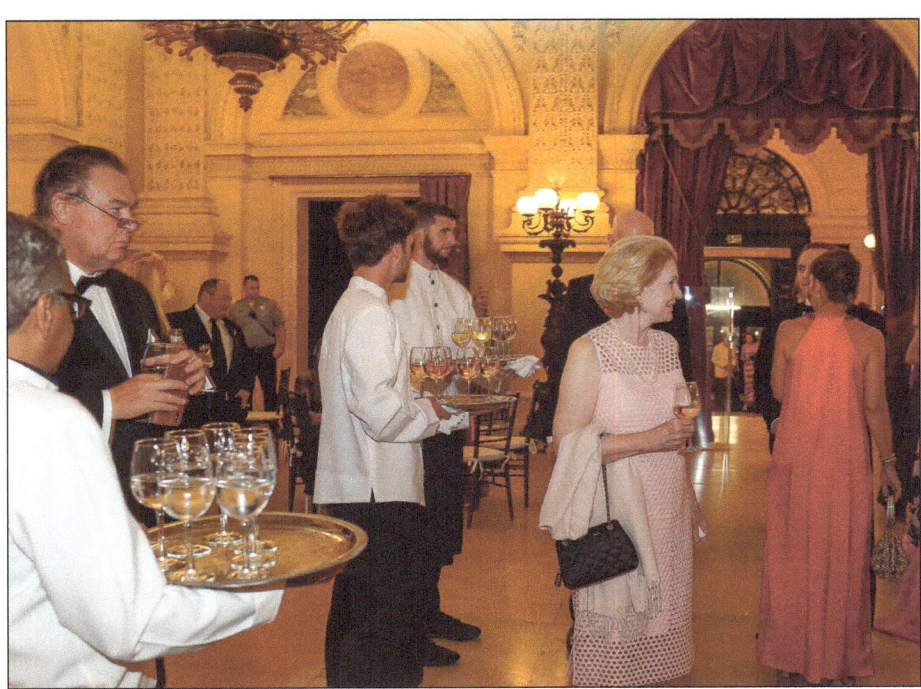
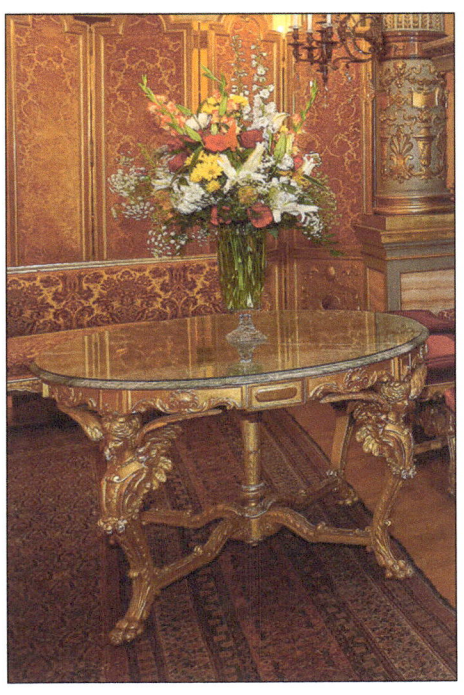

Newport Coaching Weekend

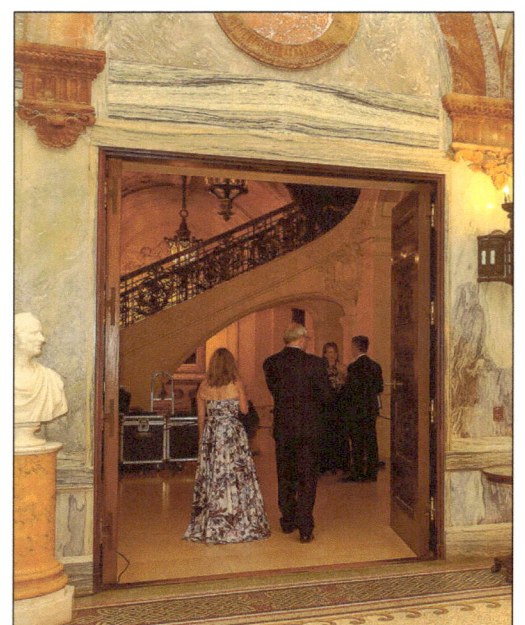
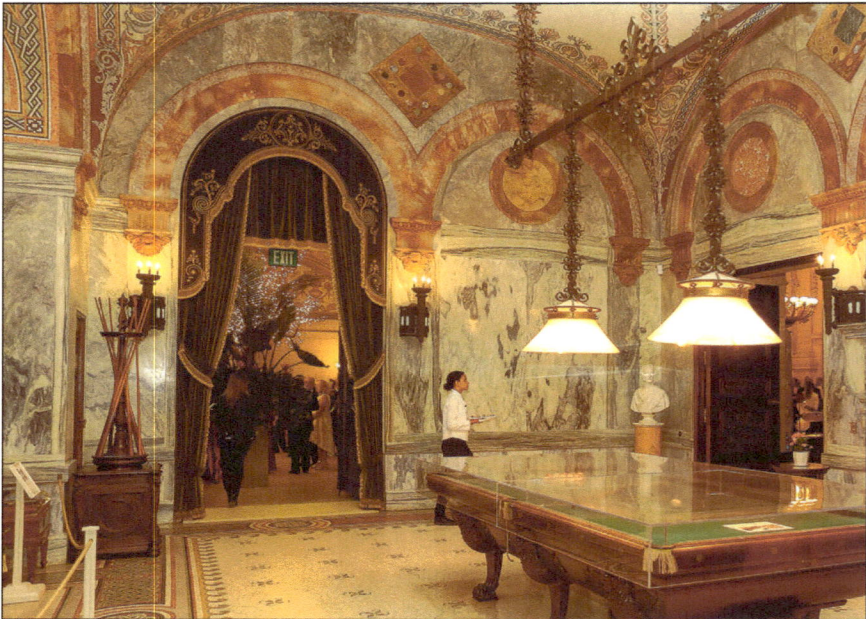

Newport Coaching Weekend

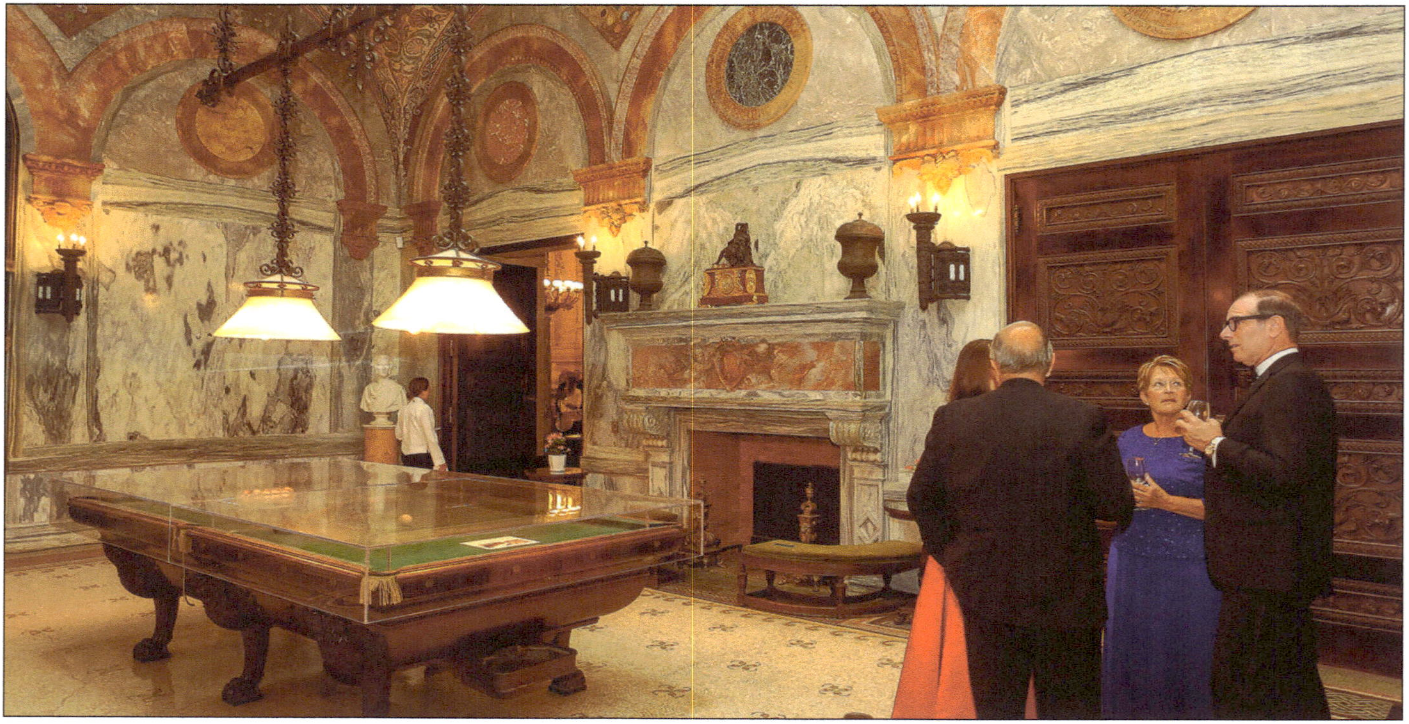

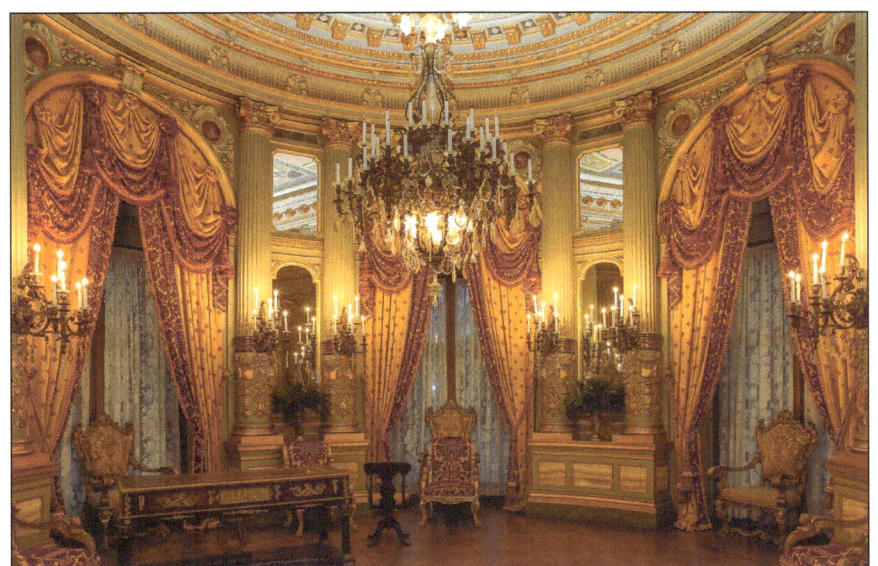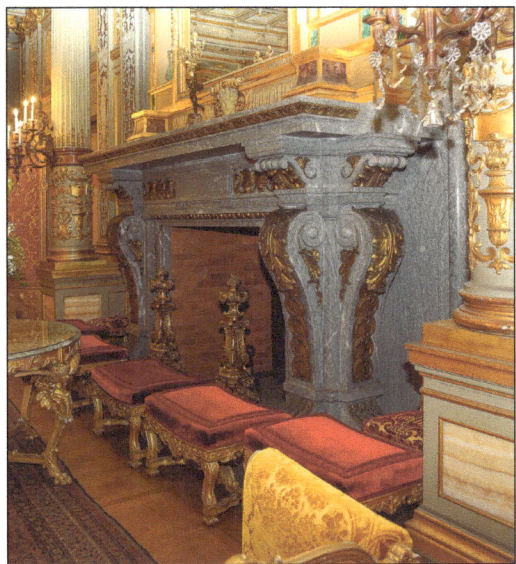

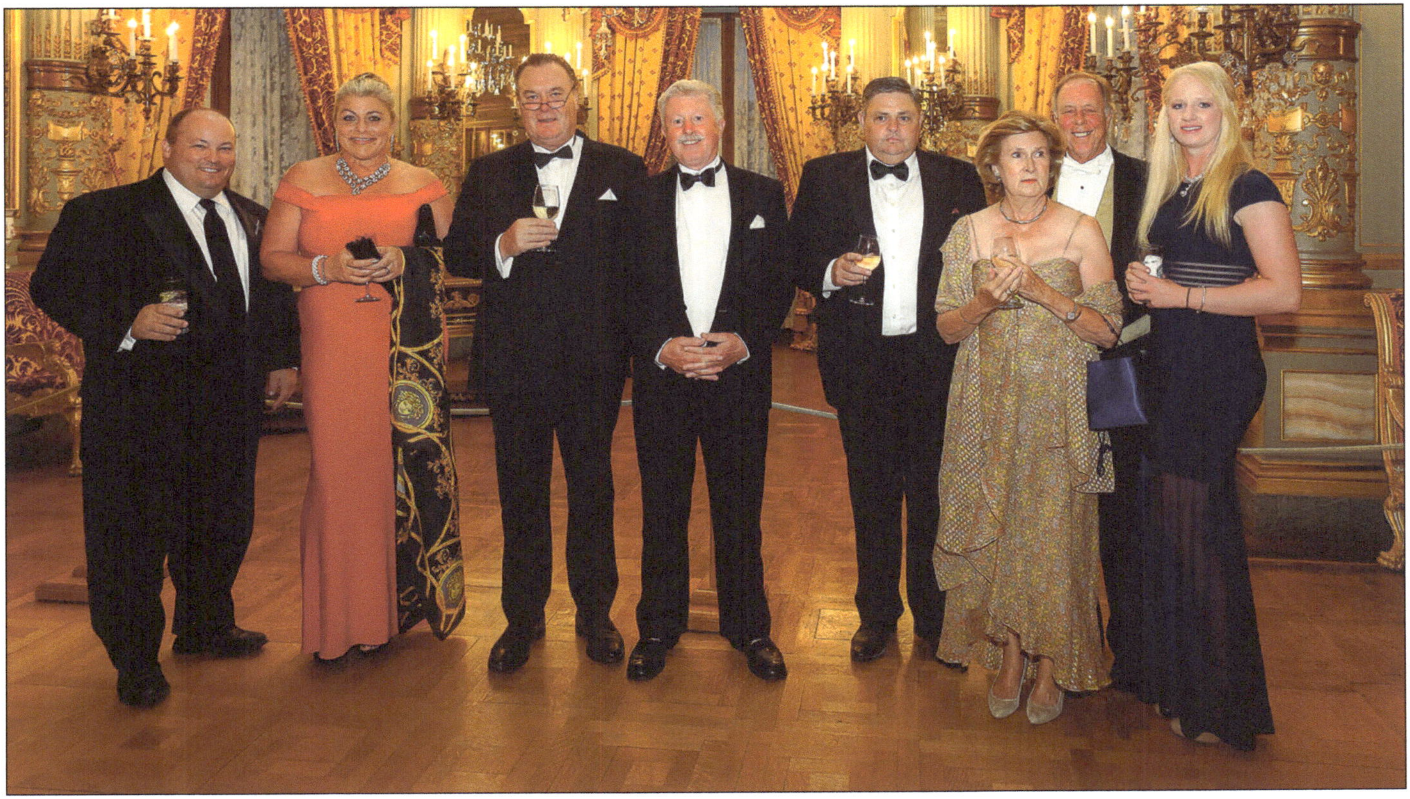

Newport Coaching Weekend

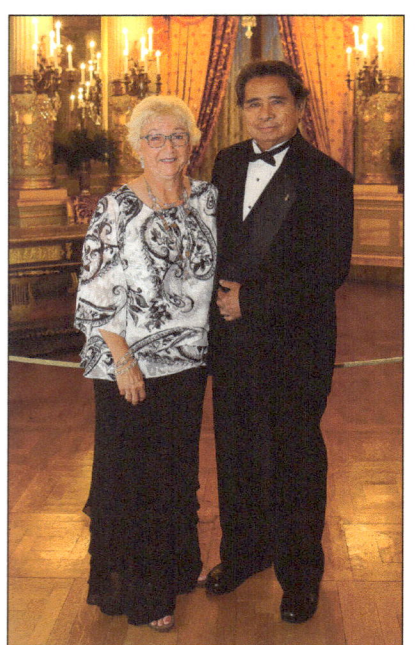 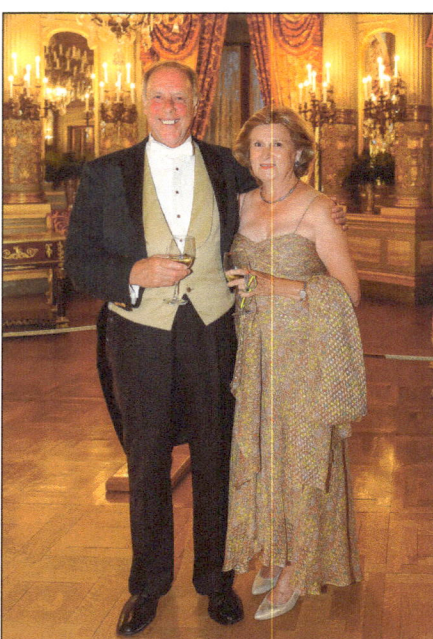 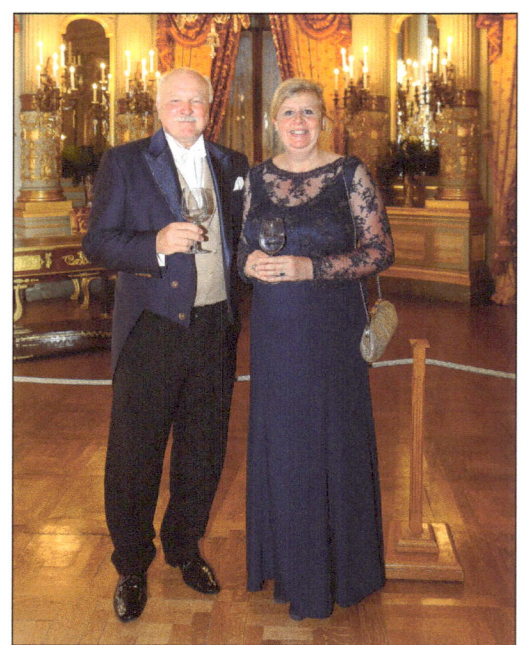

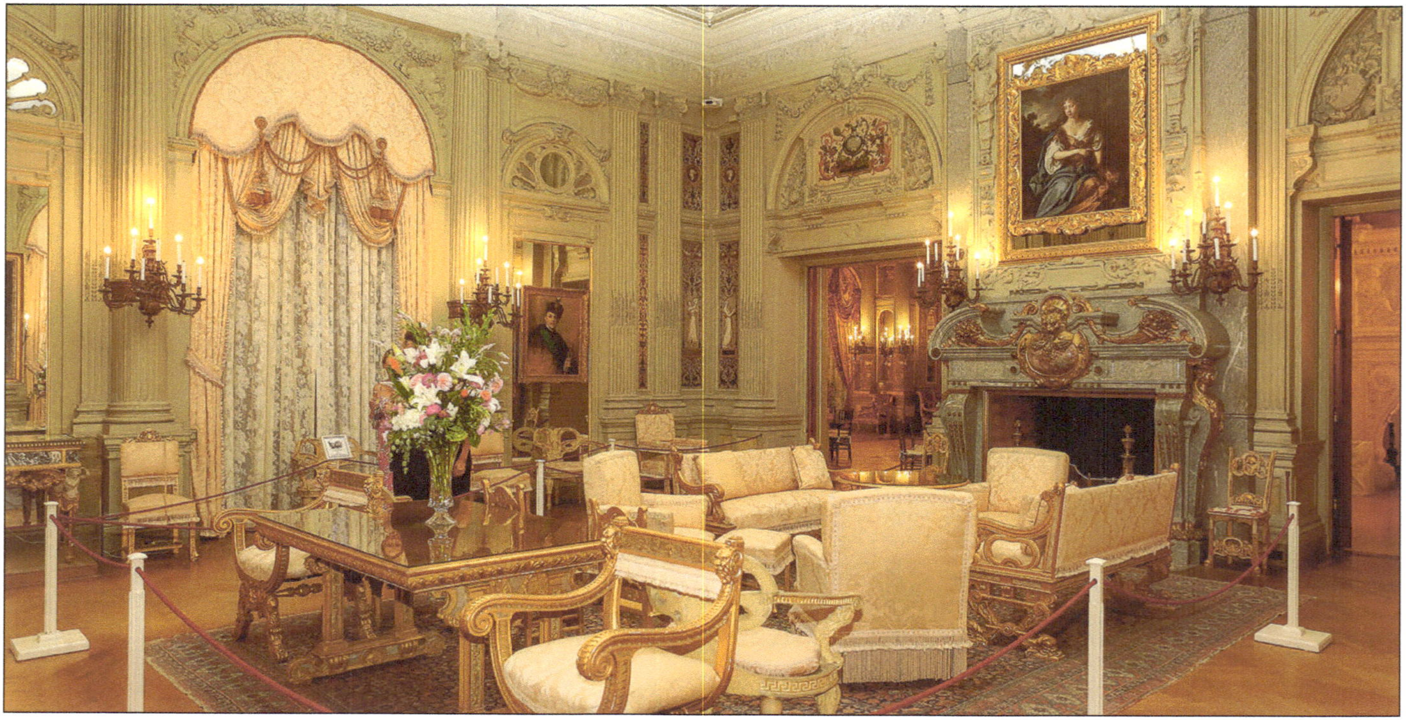

Newport Coaching Weekend

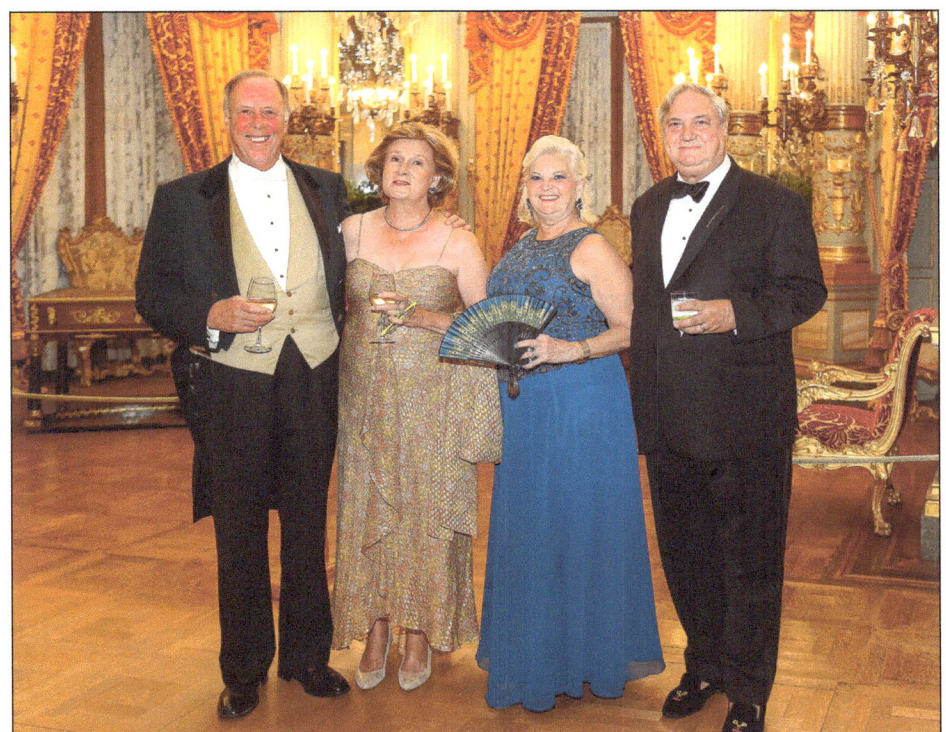
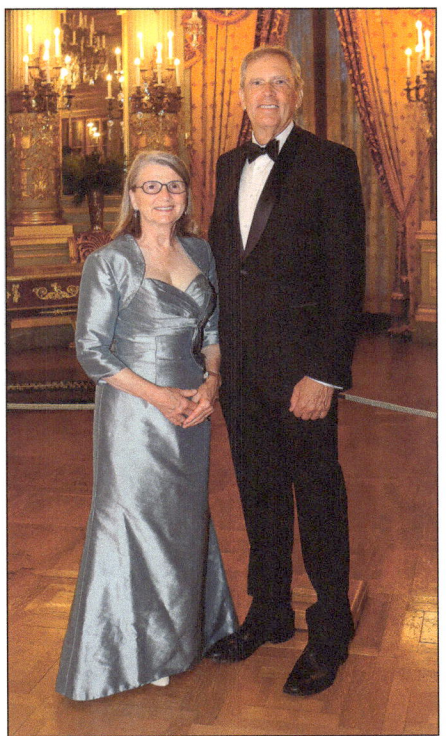
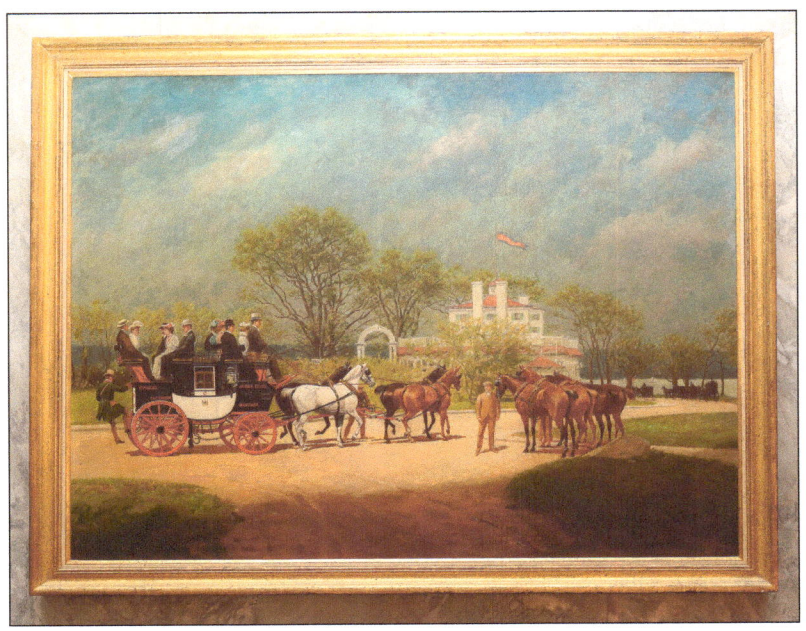
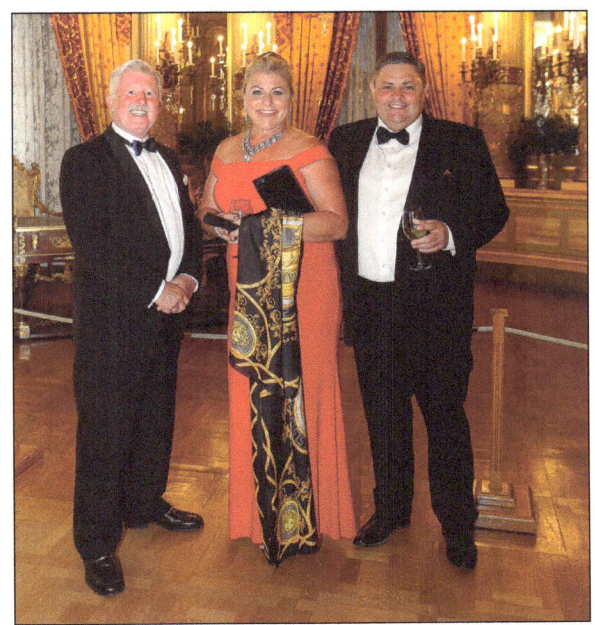

Newport Coaching Weekend

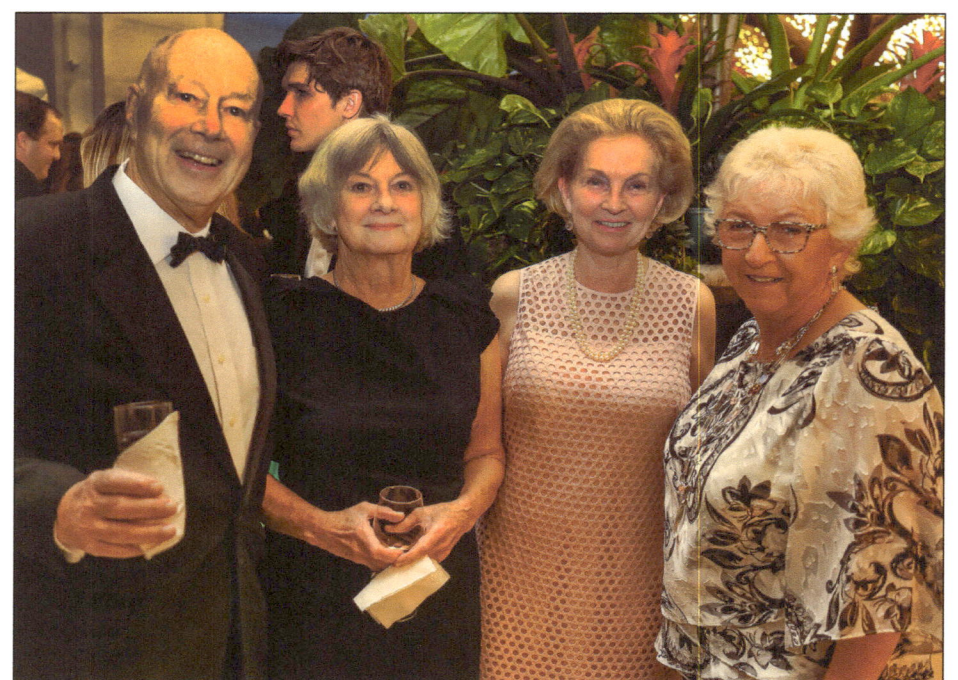
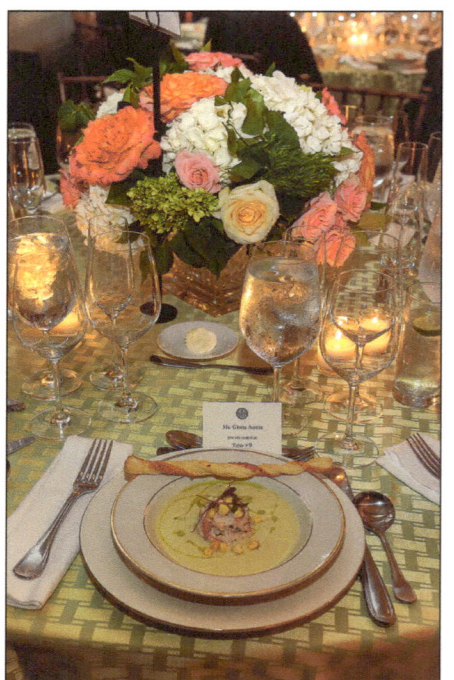

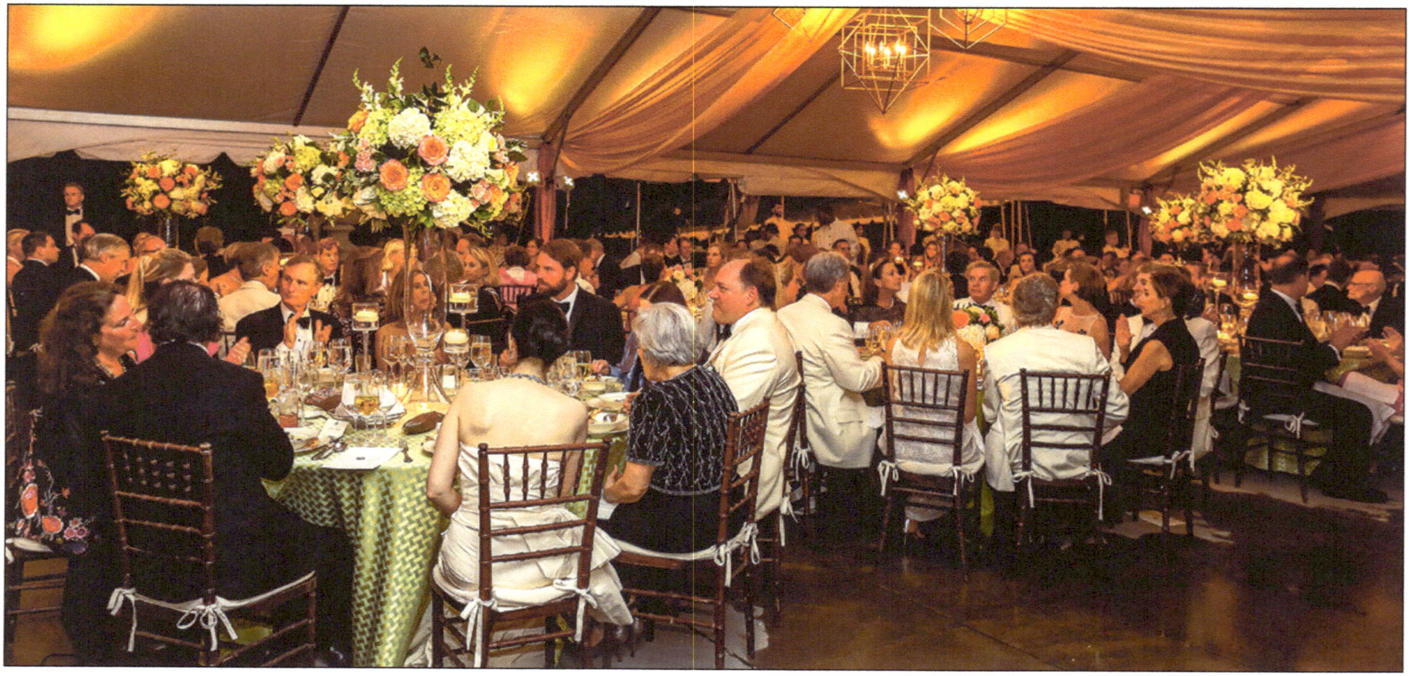

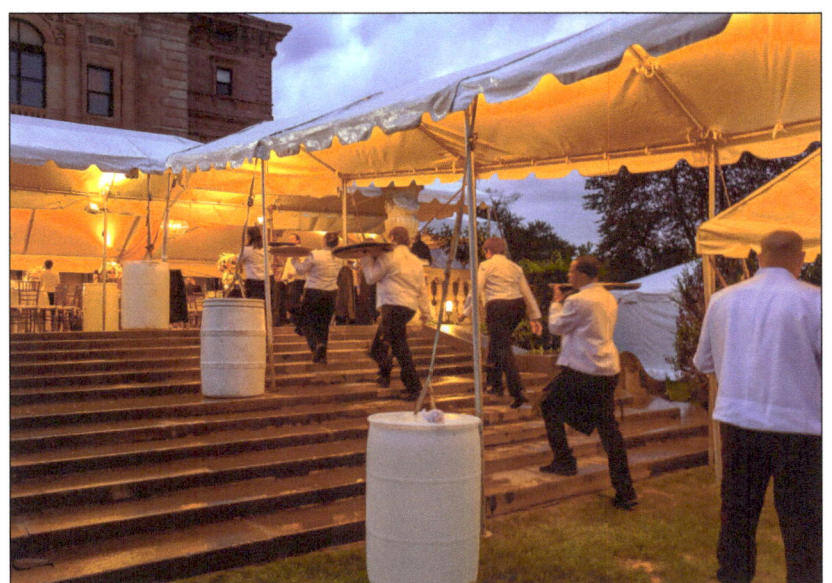
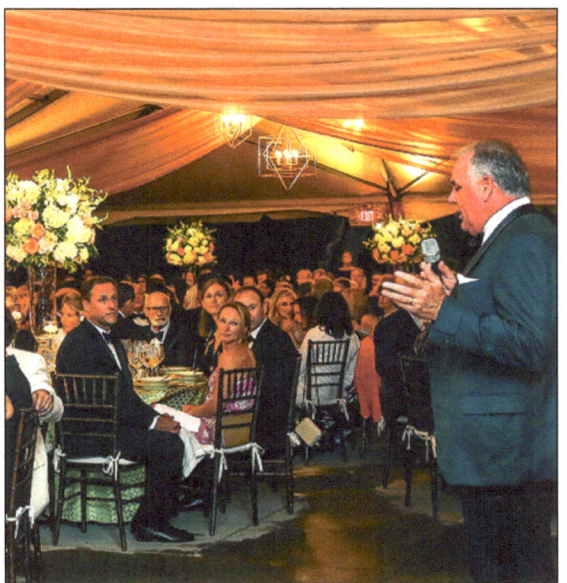

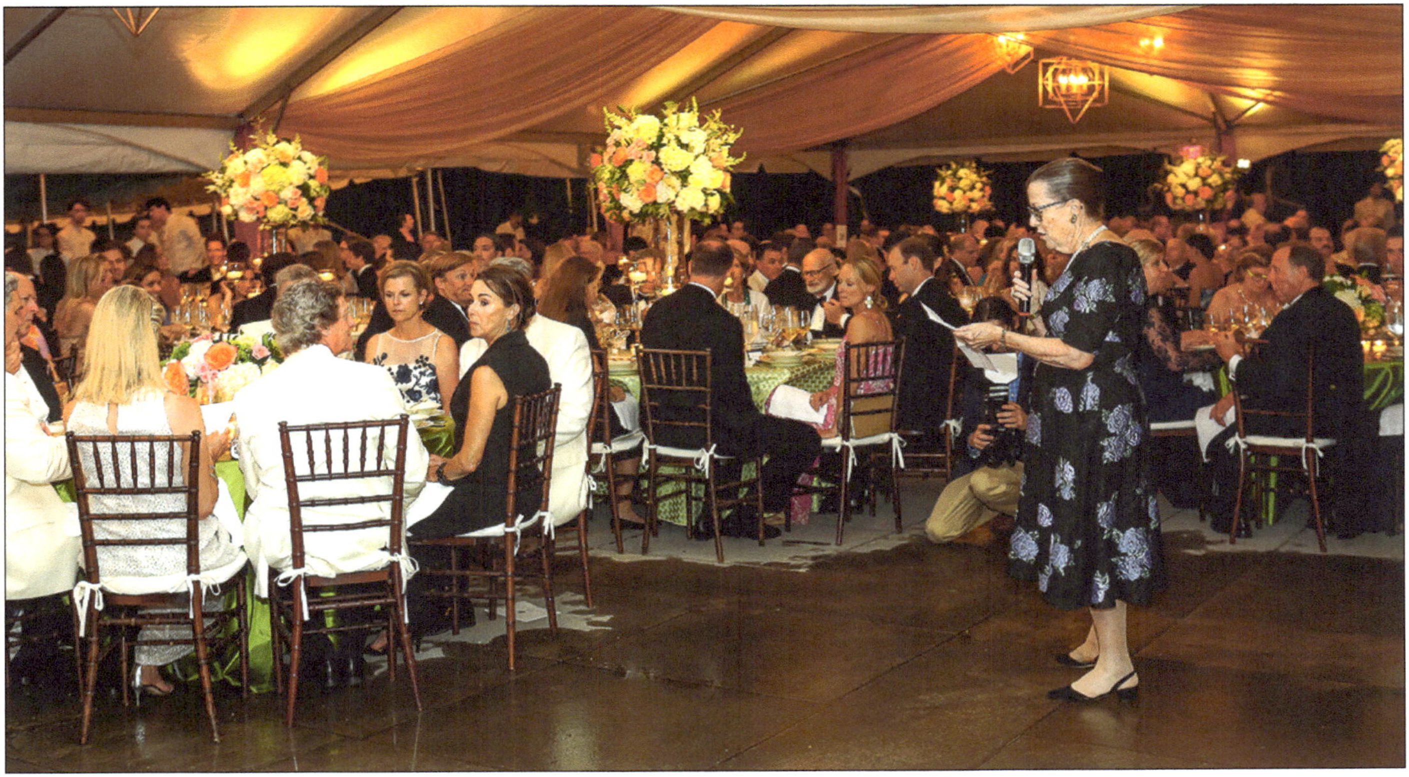

Newport Coaching Weekend

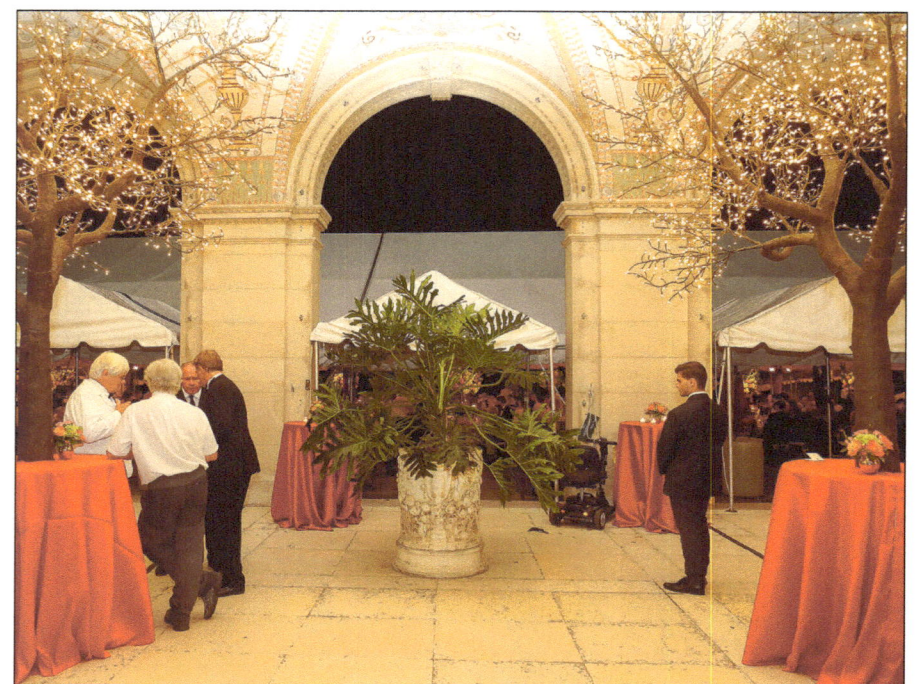

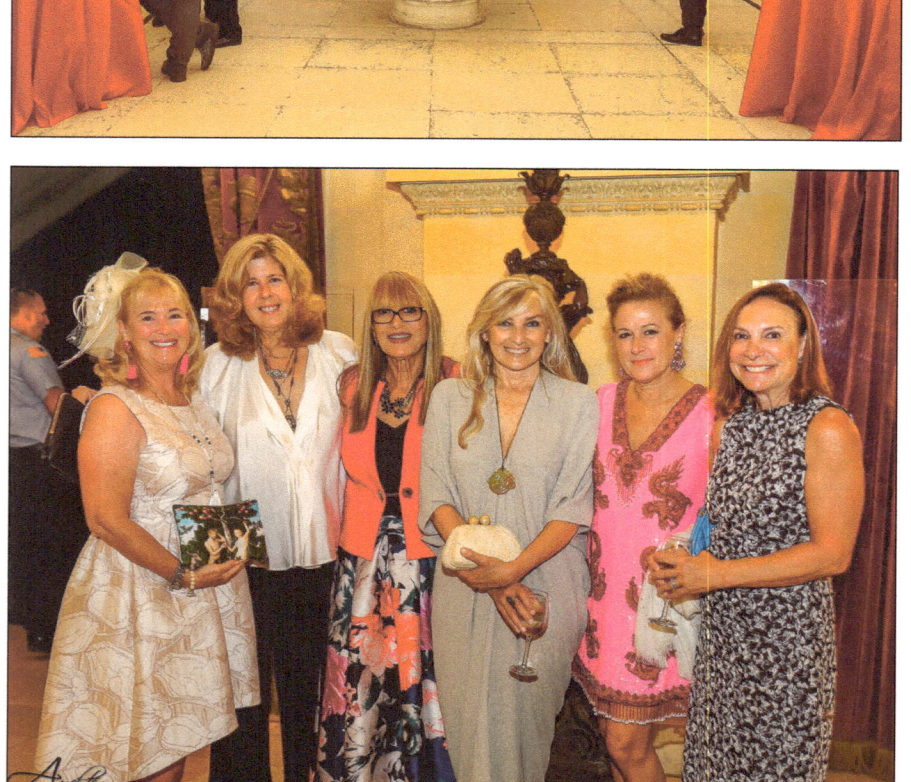
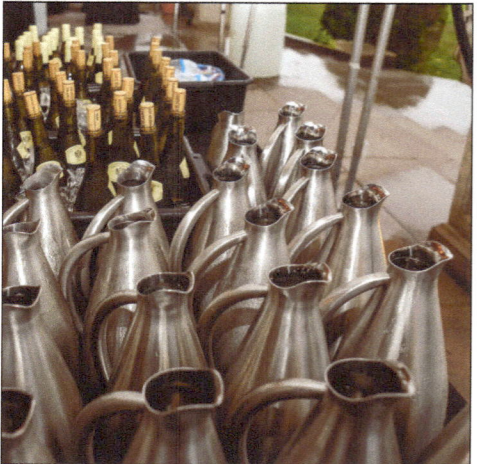

Newport Coaching Weekend

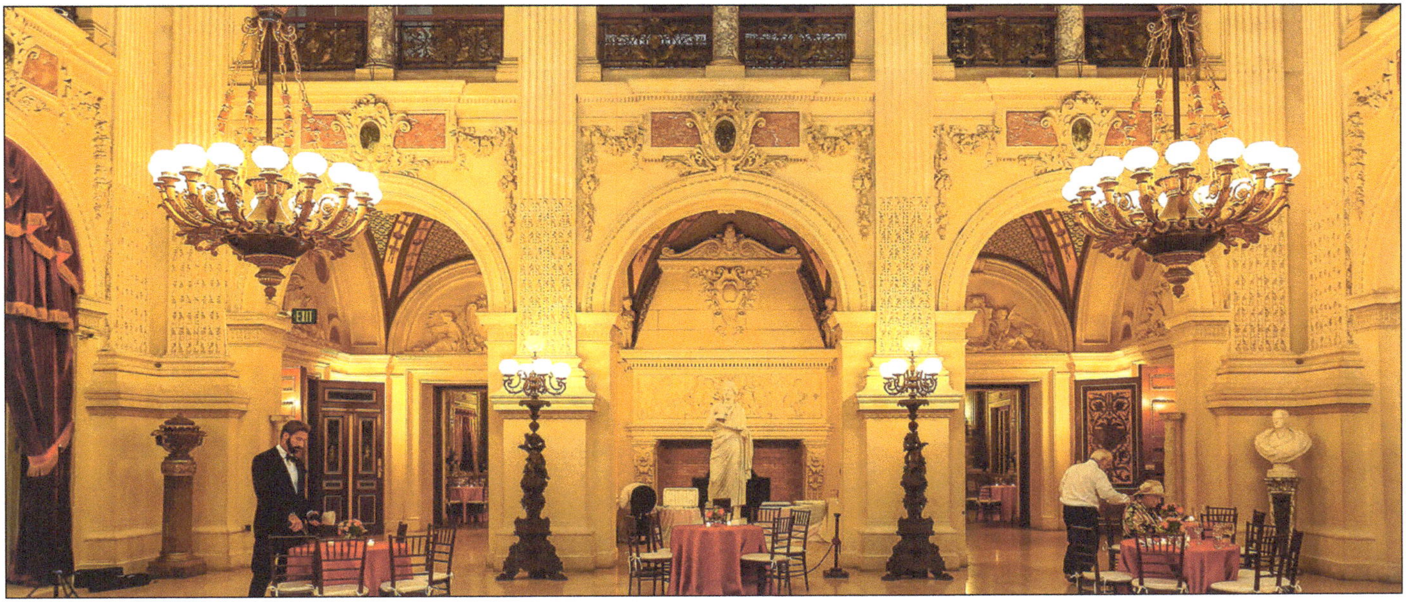

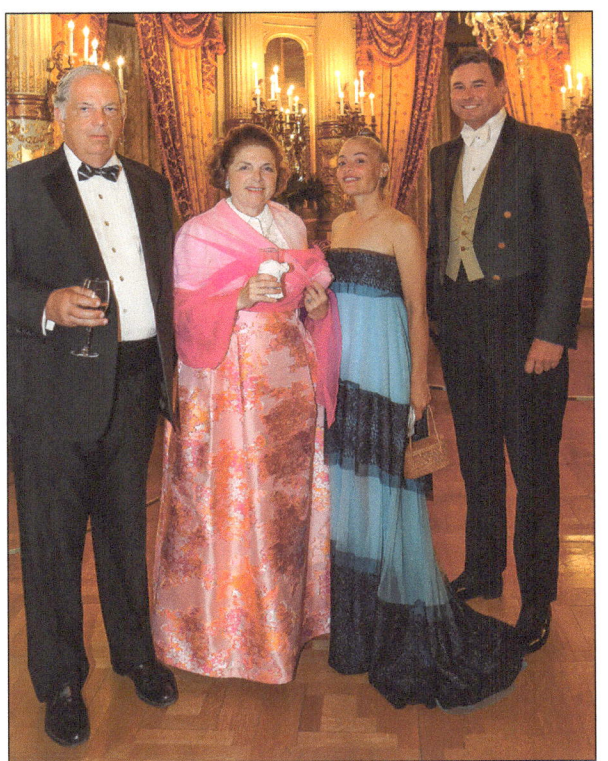
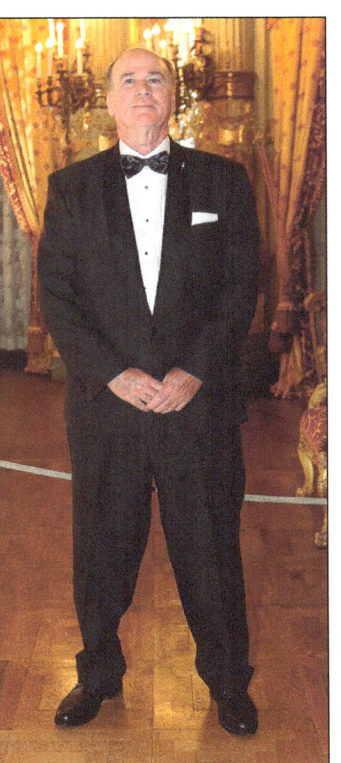
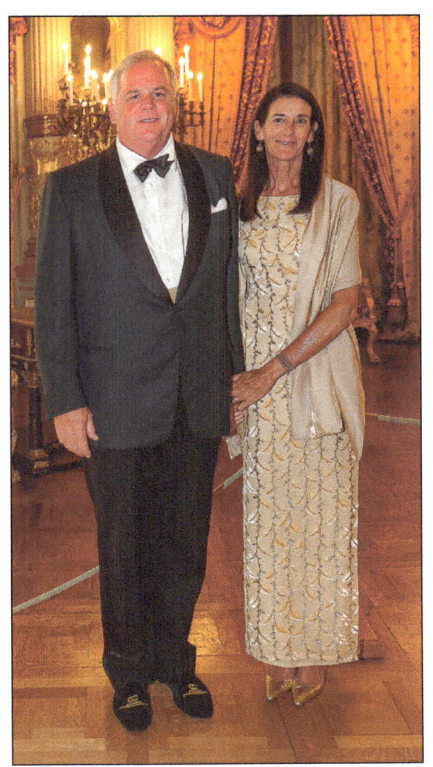

Newport Coaching Weekend

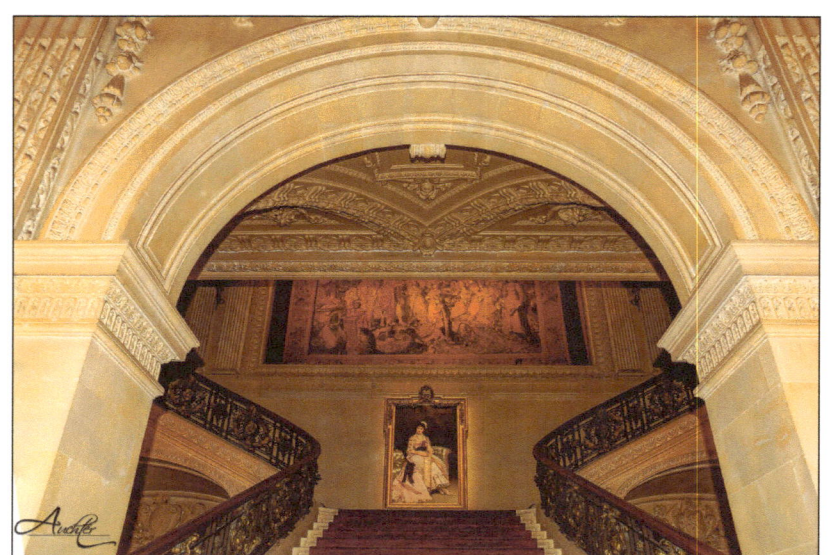
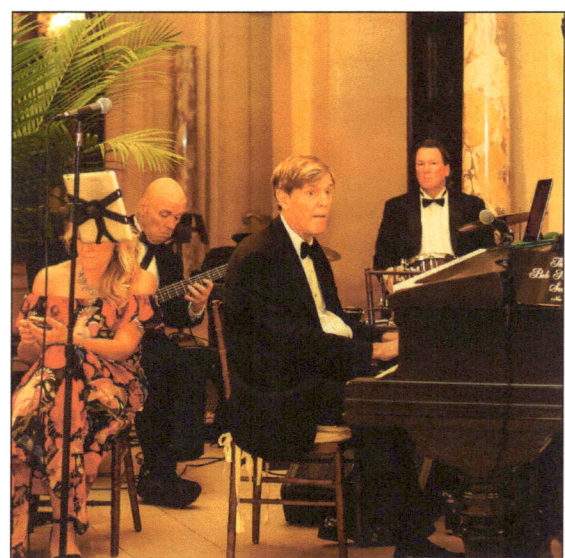
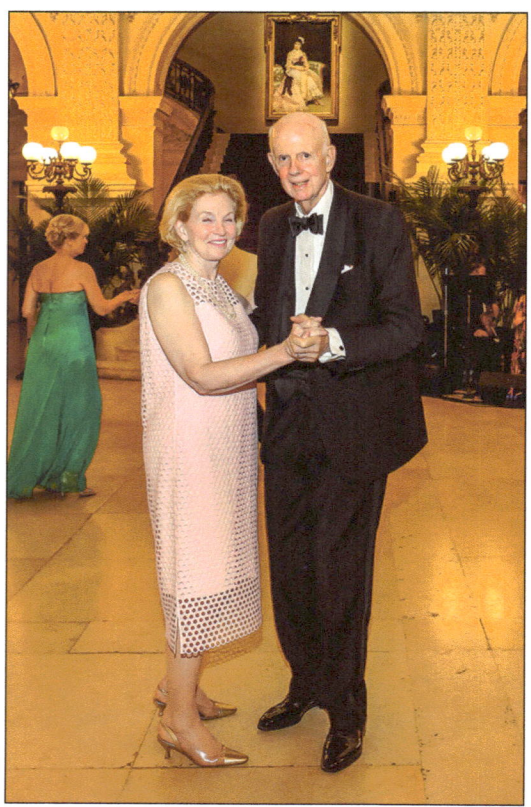
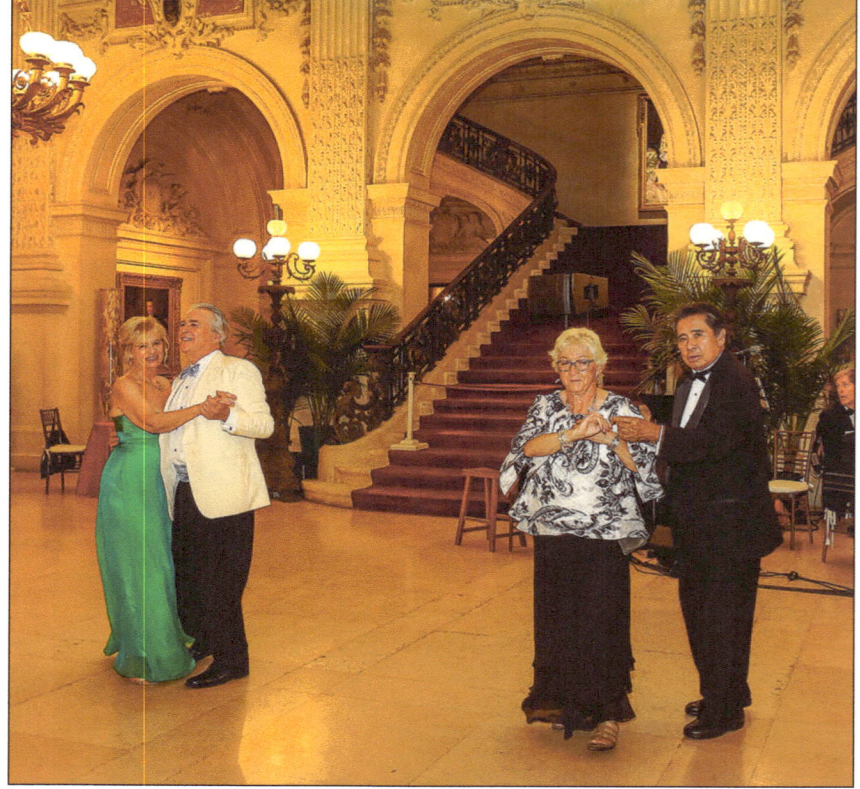

Newport Coaching Weekend

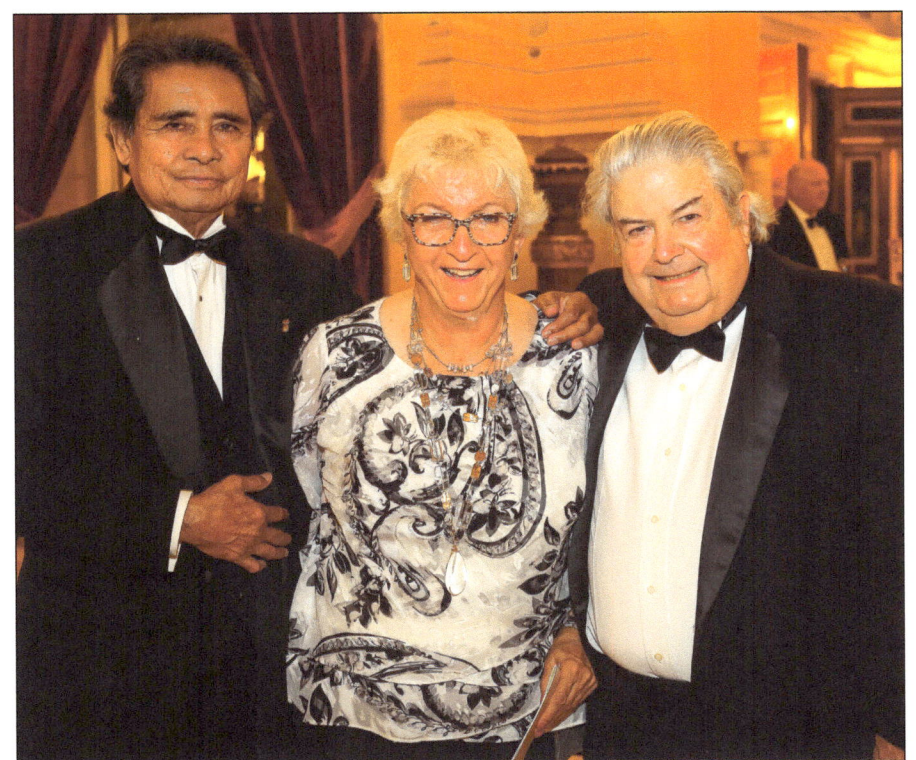
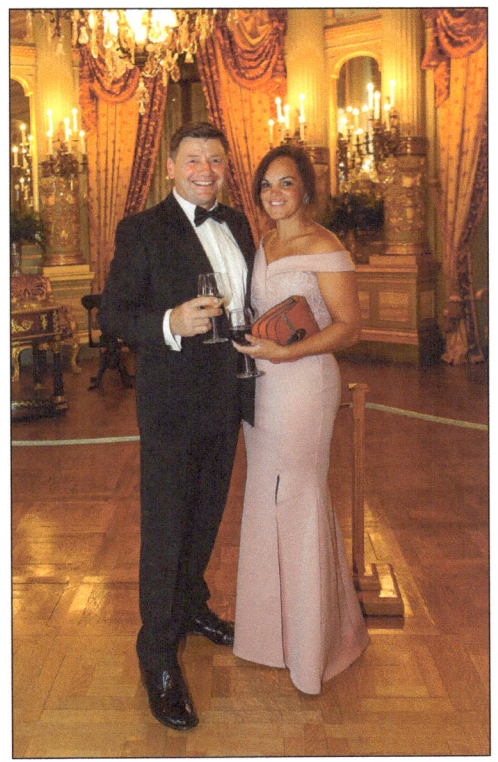
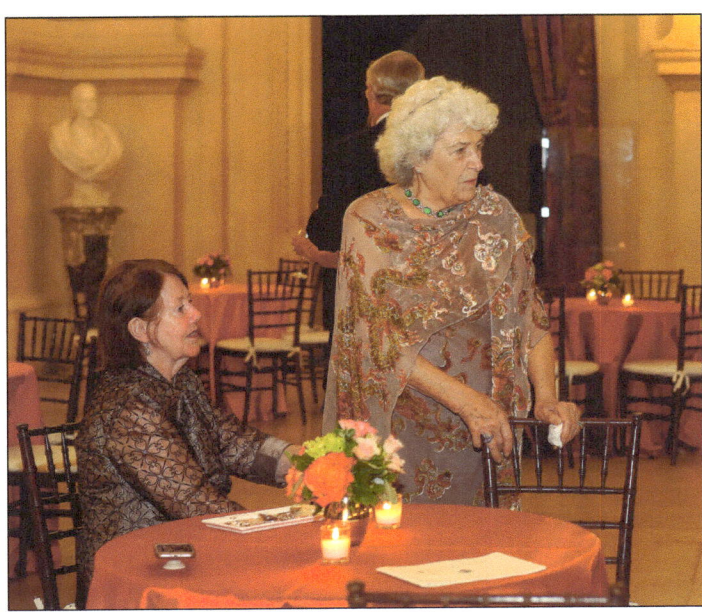
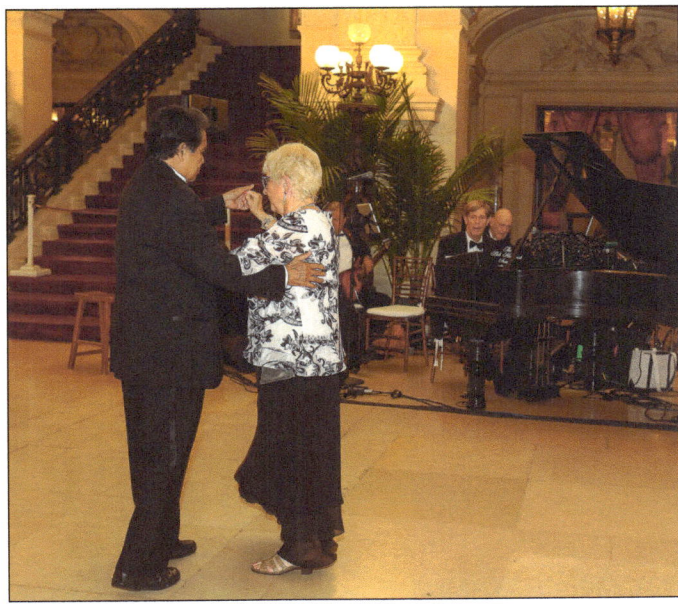

Newport Coaching Weekend · 193

SUNDAY

August 19, 2018
❶ 10:15 am Breakers Stables Departs
   10:30 am Picture at Chateau-sur-Mer
   10:45 am All depart from Chateau-sur-Mer
   11:50 am Commonwealth Ave Stop (Private)
    1:00 pm Marble House Luncheon

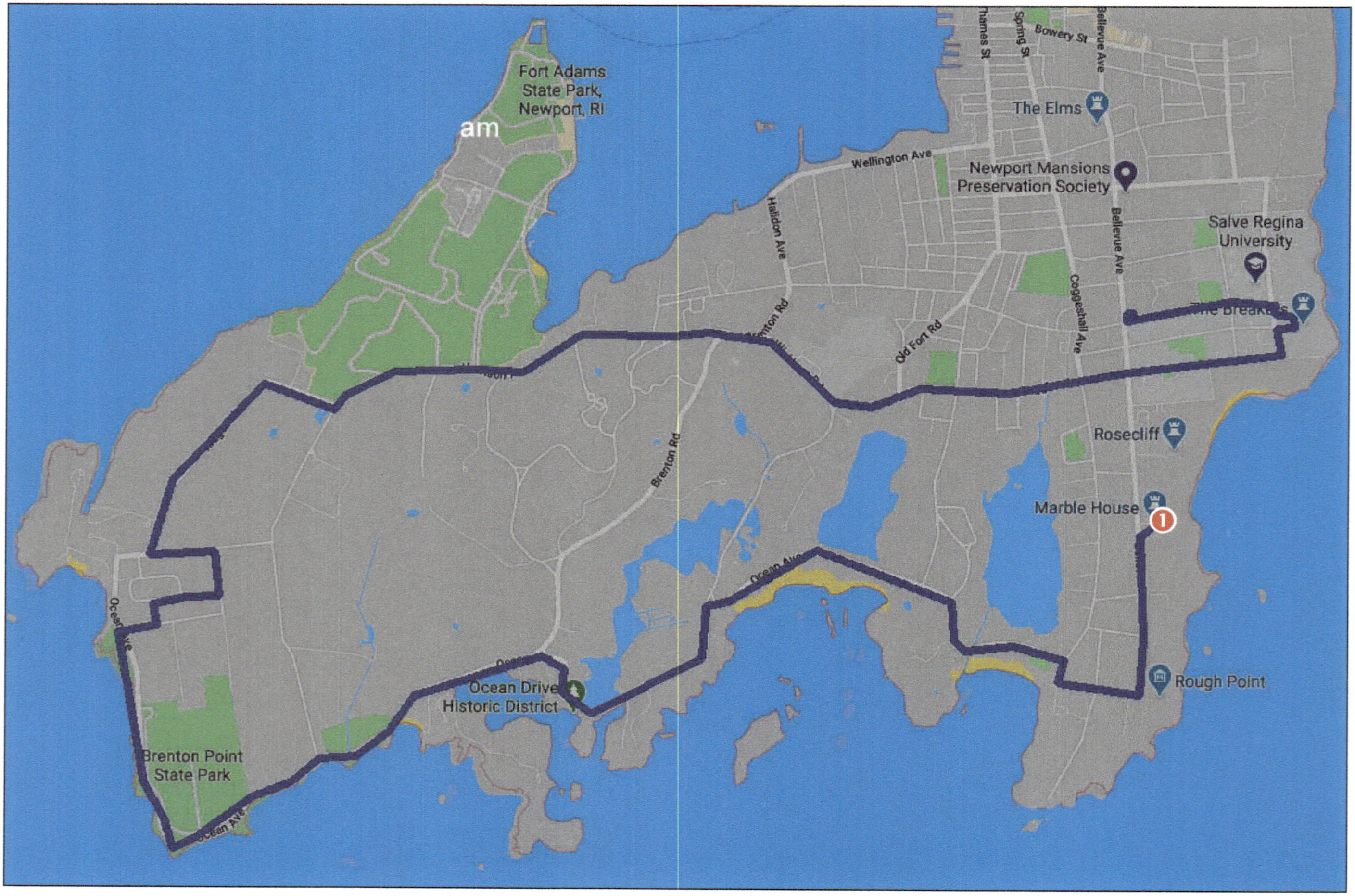

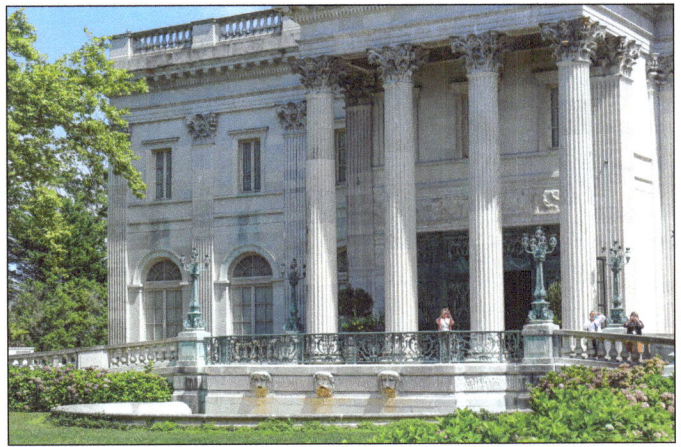

❶ Drive to Marble House Luncheon

The farewell luncheon was held on the terrace of Marble House. The president of the Coaching Club spoke to the attendees and toasts were made. Gloria Austin thanked the organizers of the weekend and the president of the Coaching Club for the opportunity and honor to drive as a woman at the Newport Coaching Weekend. The luncheon ended as all raised their glasses and proclaimed, "To the Road!".

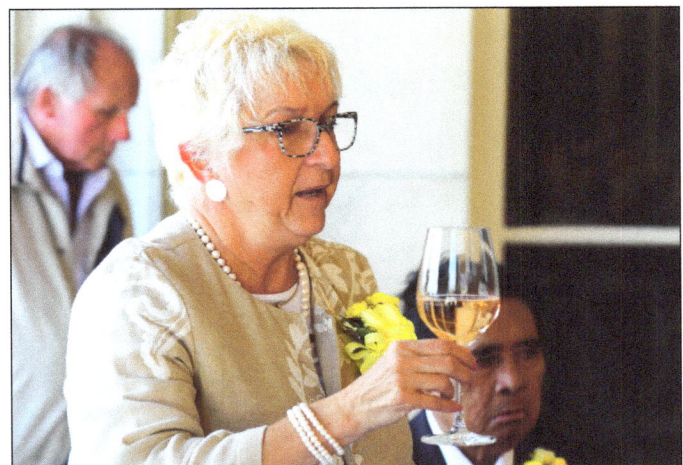

A Nod To The Past: "A quick change of clothes for the picnickers and time to start off from their stables again to the drive to the closing event of the memorable three days - High Tea and Cocktails at Bailey's Beach. Again 12 different turnouts drove through Newport streets and along the ocean to the Beach Club, leaving vehicles in the car parking lot for a last chance to talk to each other and their Preservation Society hosts.

Almost reluctantly carriages were ordered for the final drive back to the stables, while the stalwart carriage watchers stood waving along the streets, calling out "Come back again. "

At the Breakers' Stable, sun slanted high overhead from windows above the stalls as dust, confusion and nostalgia combined in the late afternoon scene. Clusters of Newporters watched as horses were led back to the stalls and carriages rolled under cover.

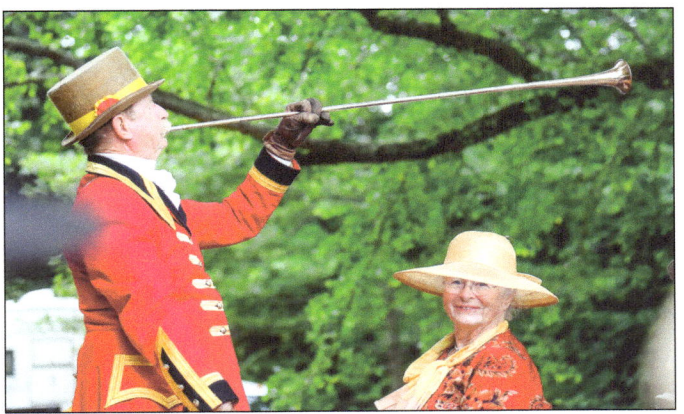

Suddenly a Coach horn sounded again. standing in the doorway, the red-coated figure of Dr. Bancroft, Mr. Ferguson's volunteer Guard, sounded the solemn notes of taps, and even the grooms fell silent back in the stable. Tomorrow the stable would be a museum again." (cited. The Carriage Journal , Vol 6. No 2. Autumn 1968. The Newport Conference of The Carriage Association of America, Inc.)

Drive to Marble House Luncheon

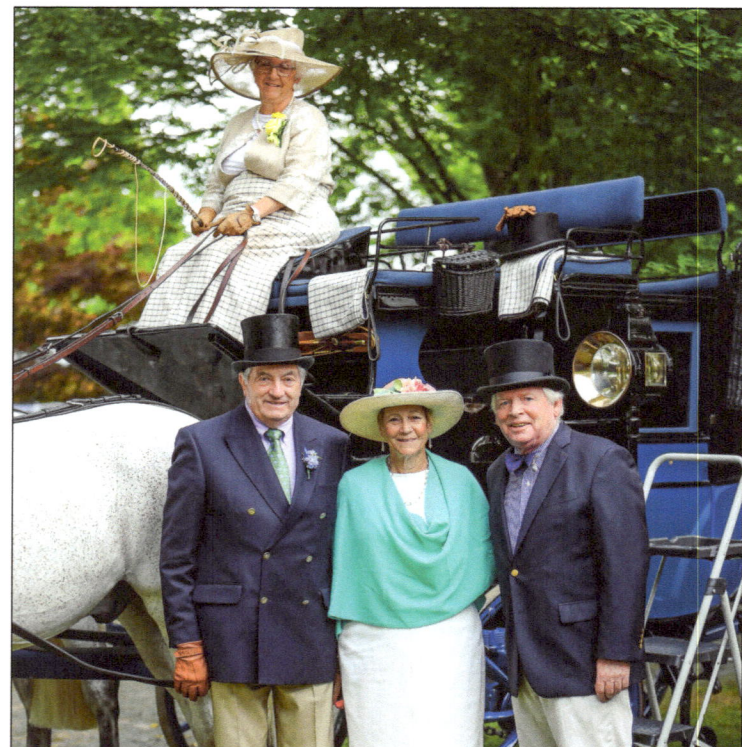
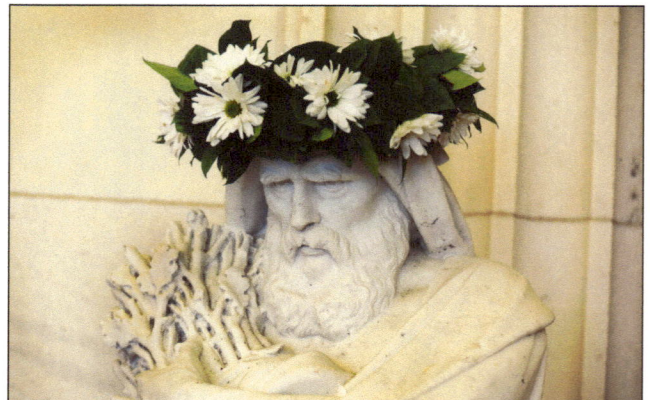
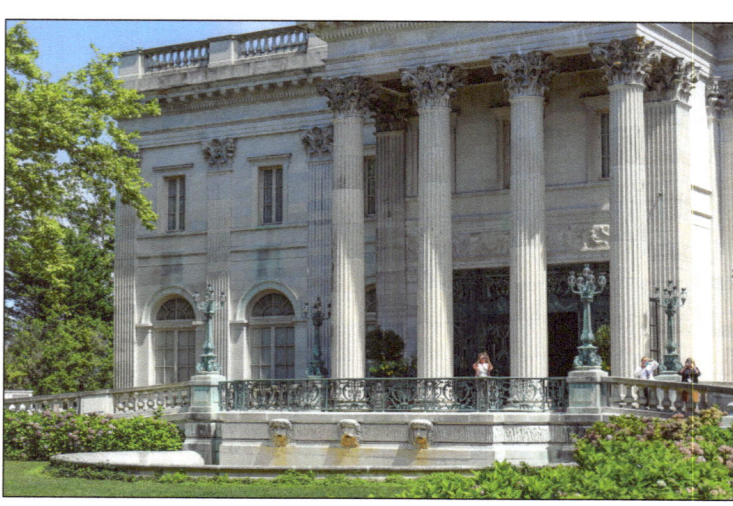
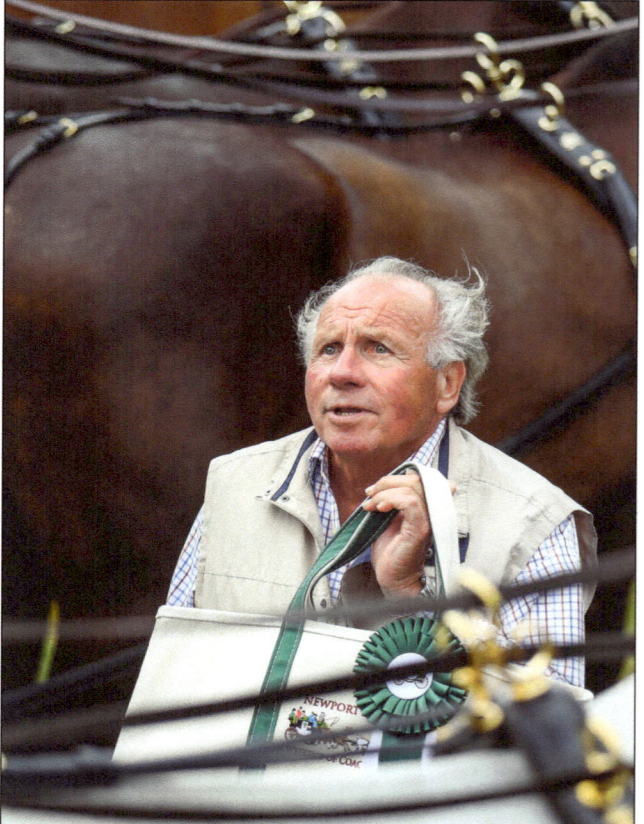

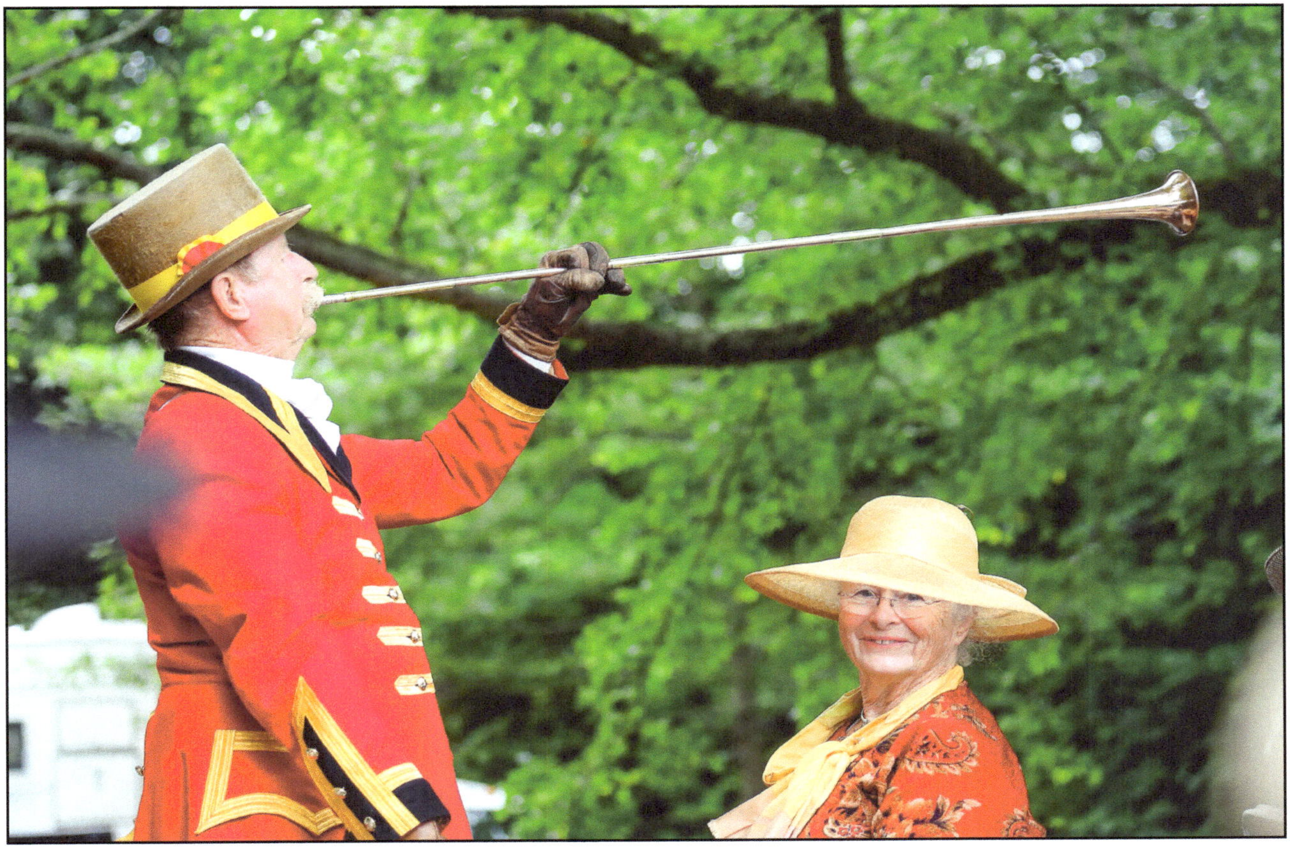

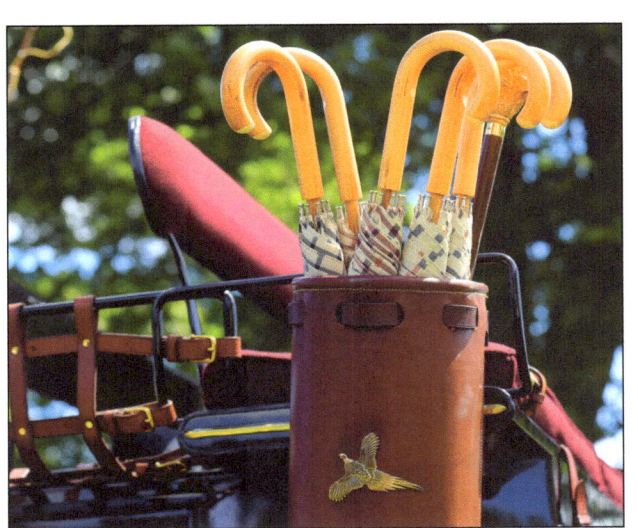
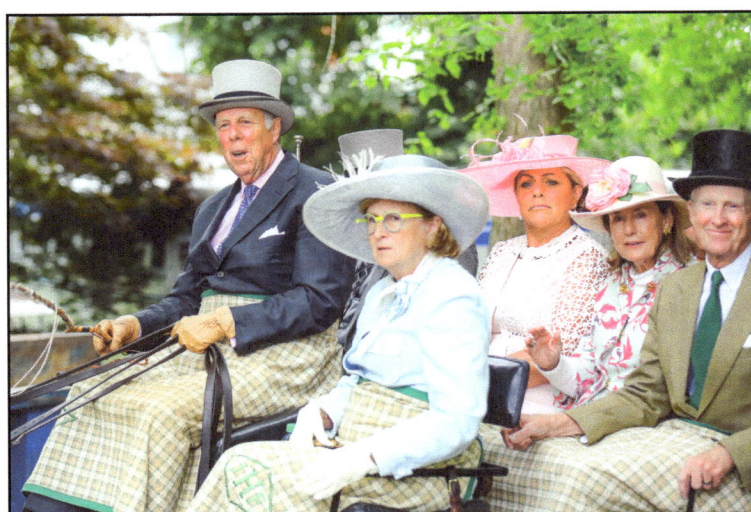

Newport Coaching Weekend

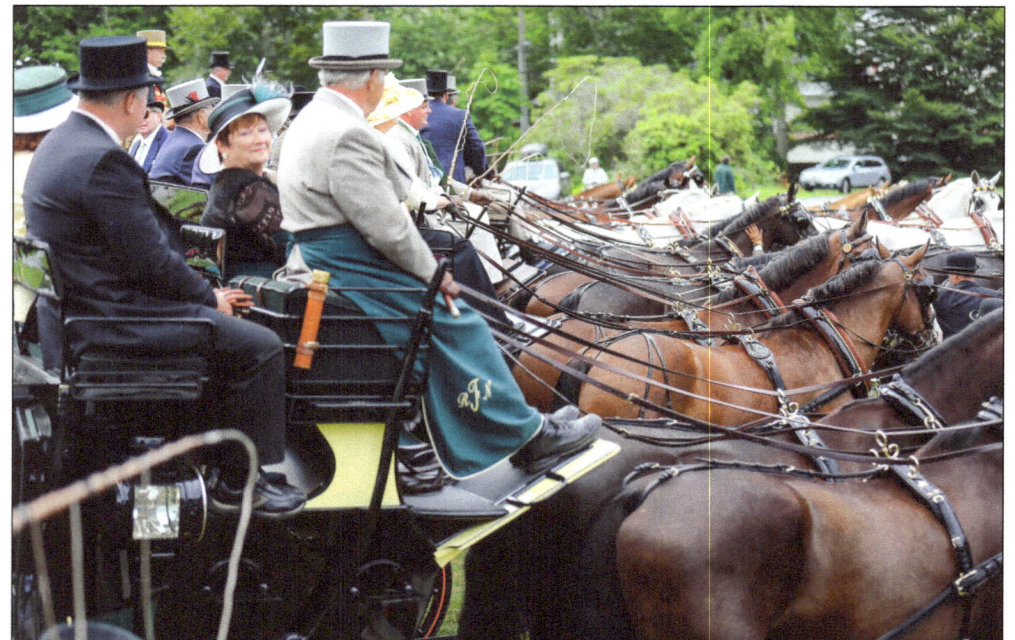
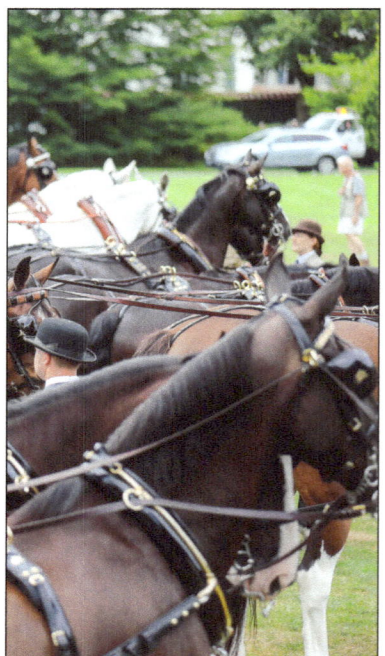
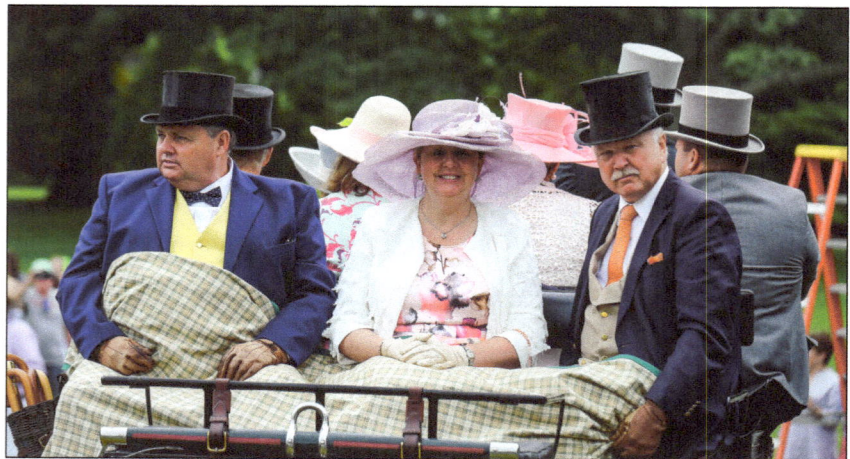
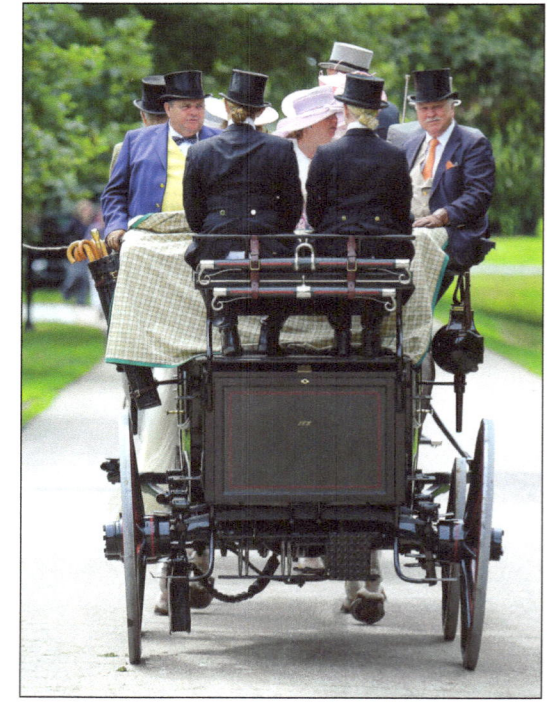

It is impressive to have a view from the top

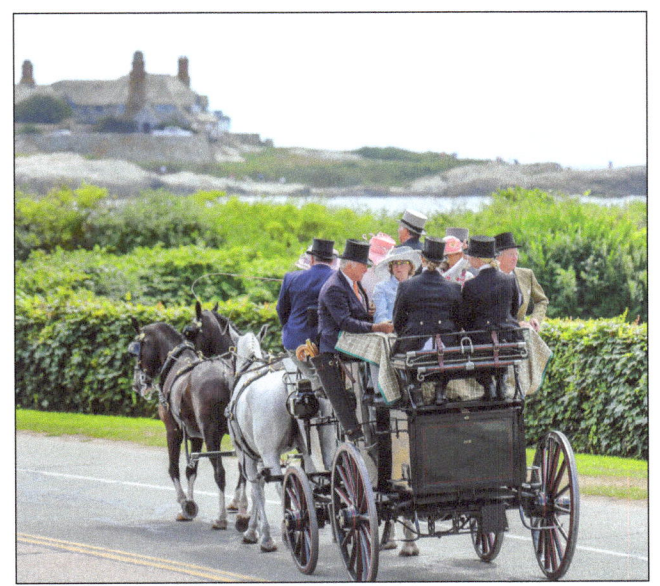
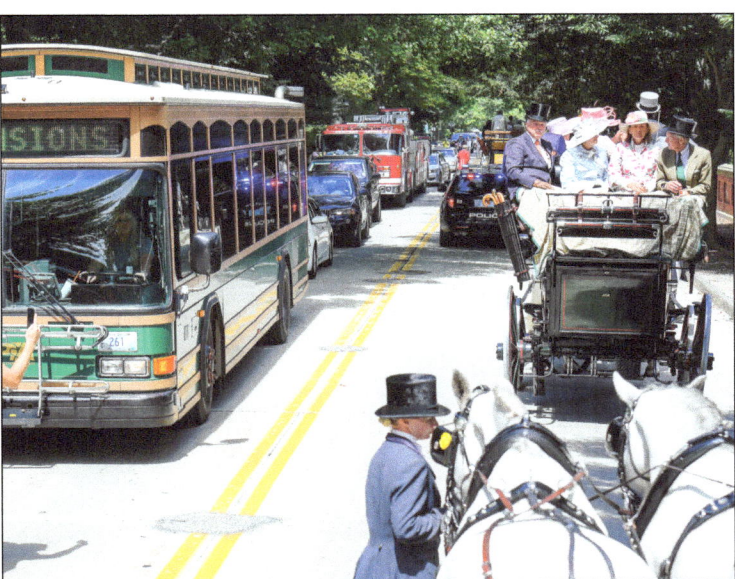

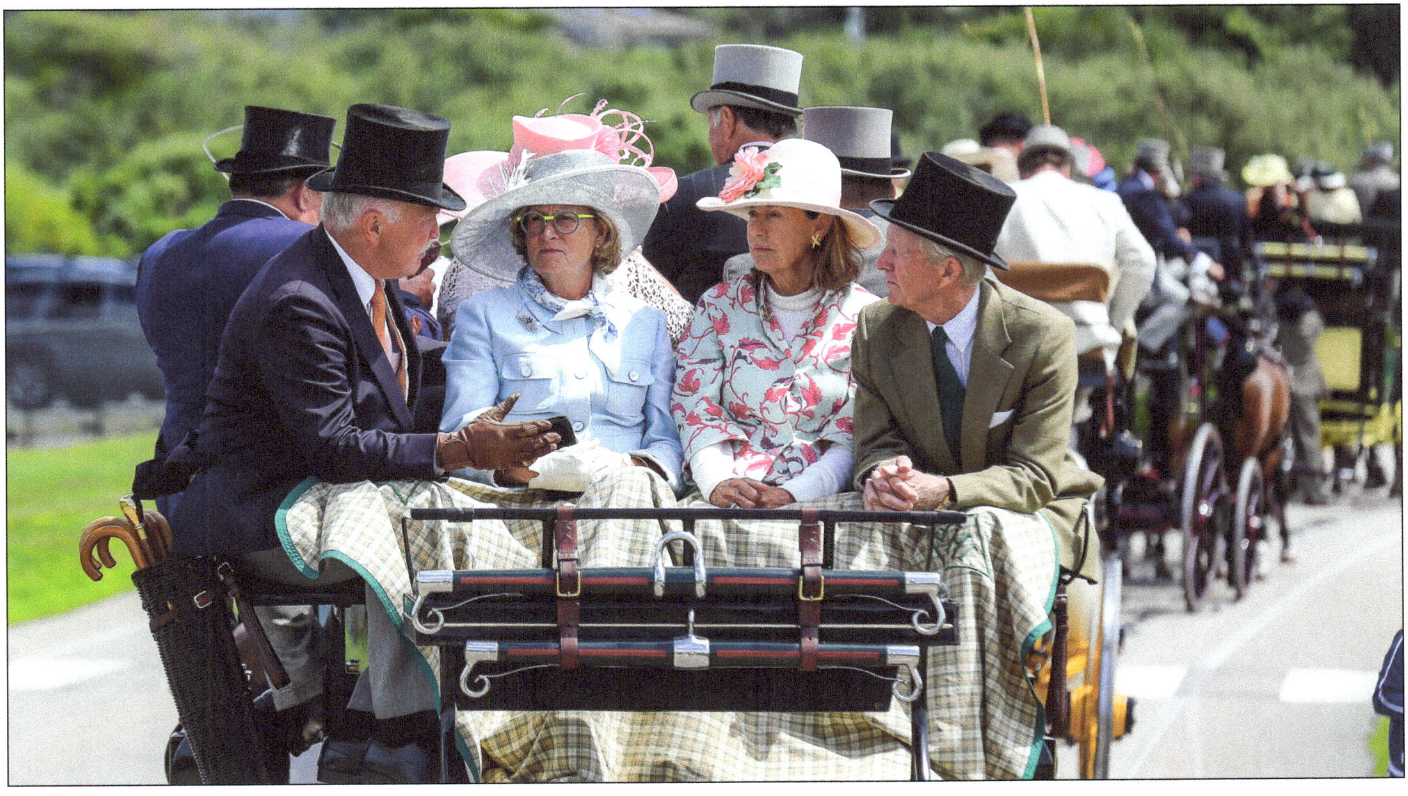

Newport Coaching Weekend

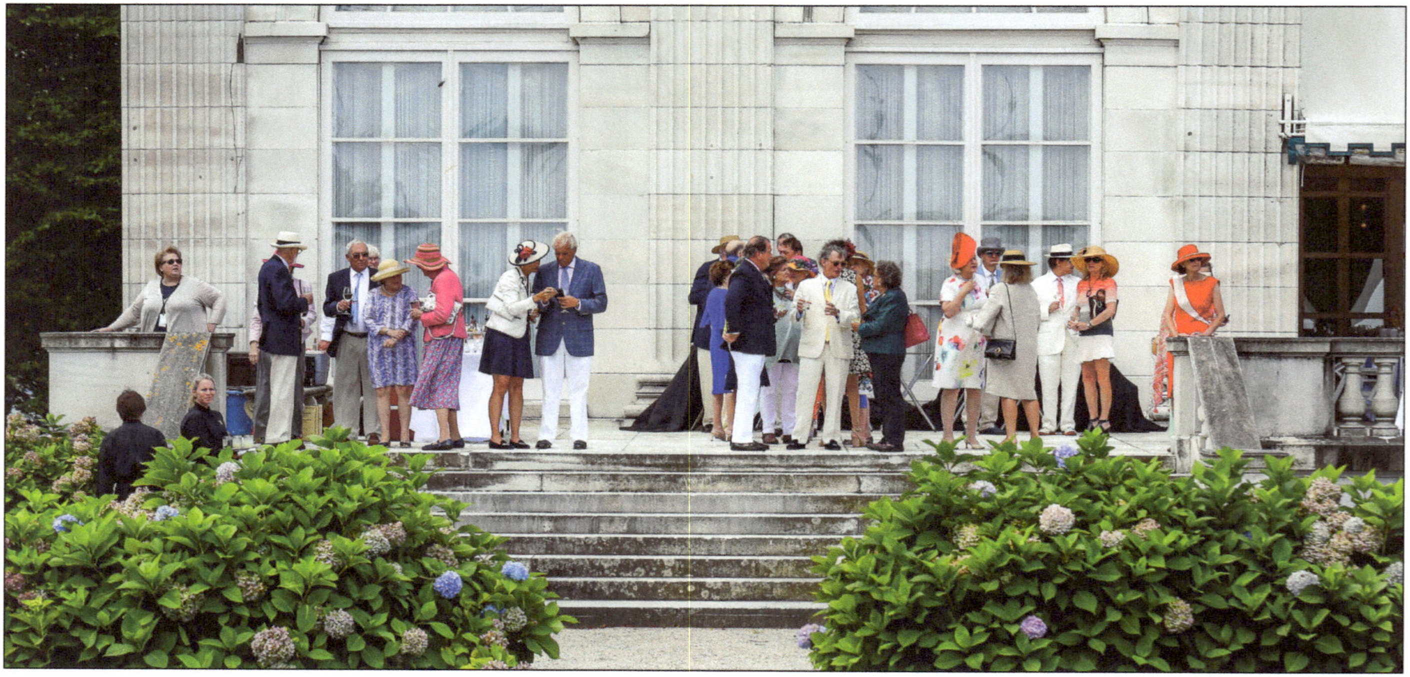

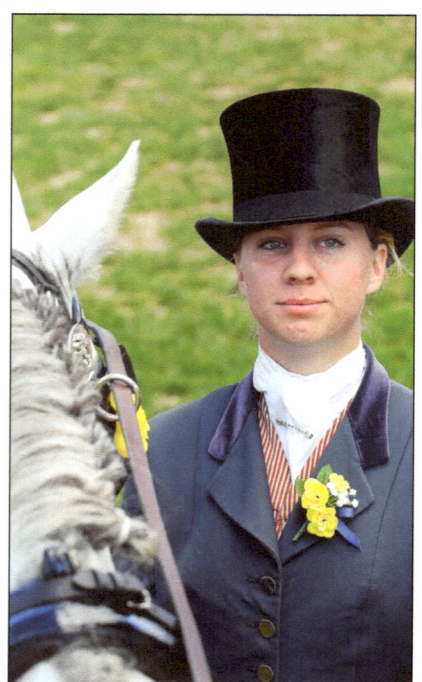
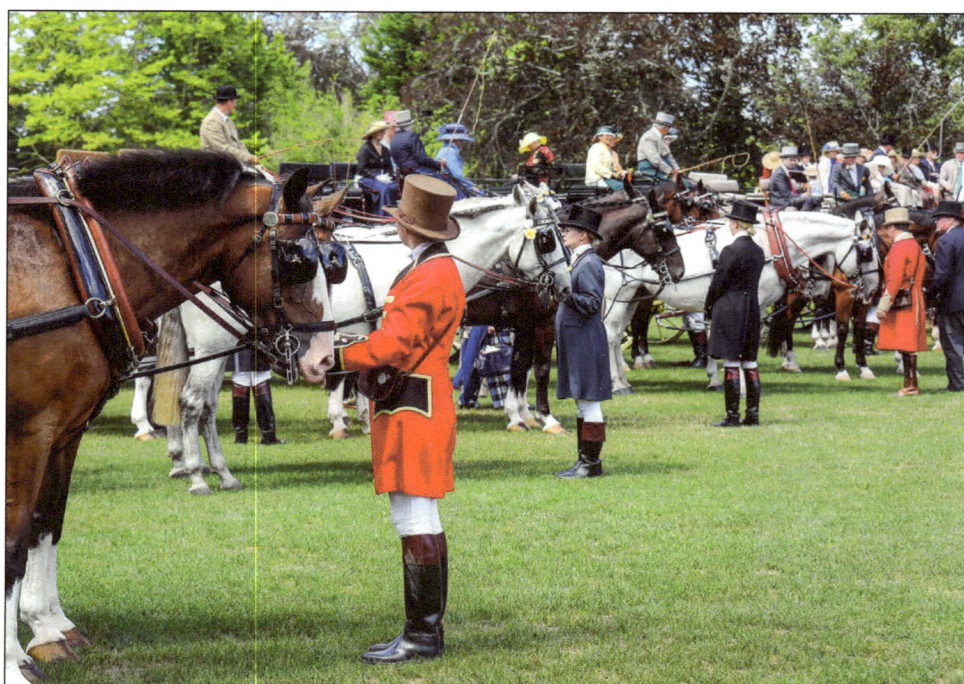

Newport Coaching Weekend

The guard on a Road Coach wears a brightly colored uniform and was originally meant to guard the Royal Mail of the kings and queens of England.

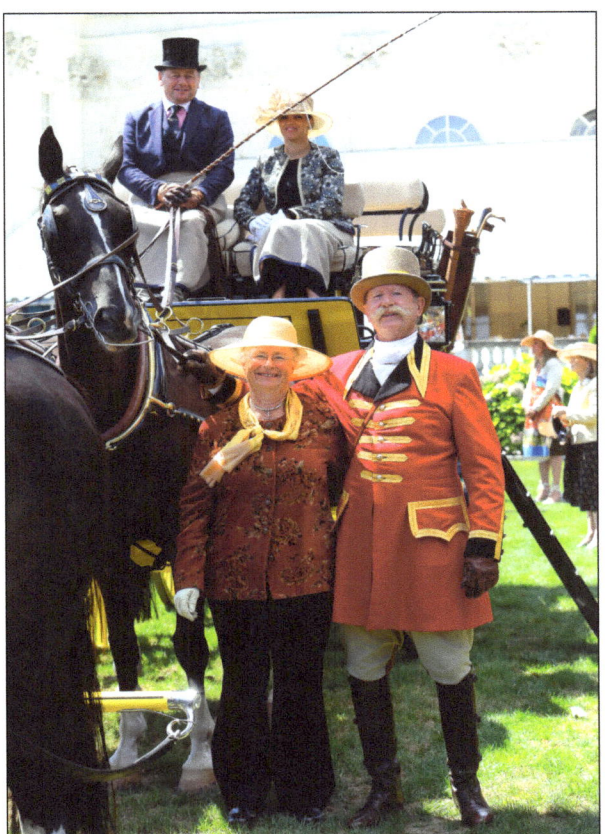

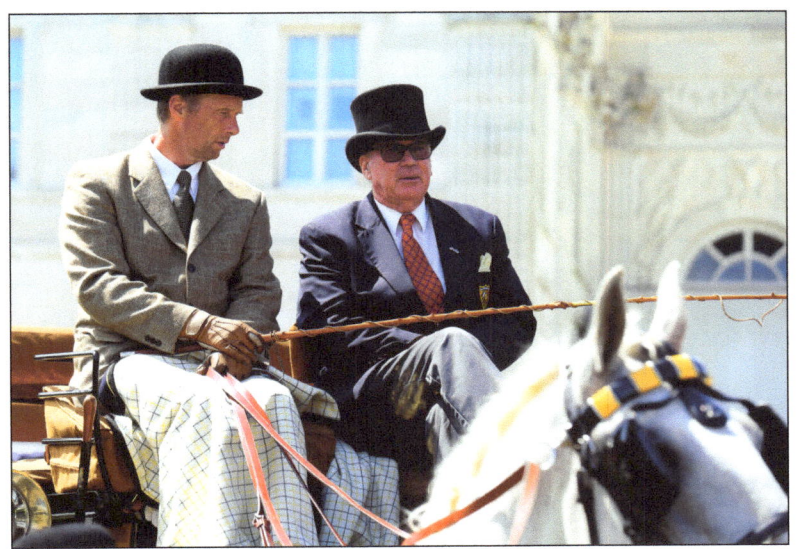

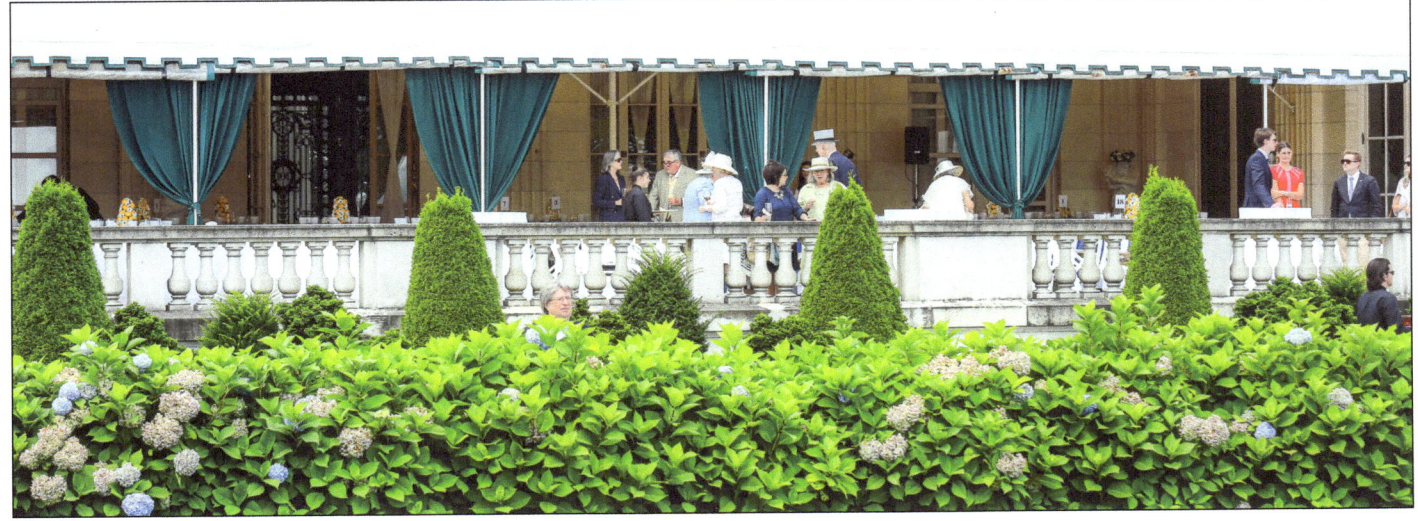

Newport Coaching Weekend · 201

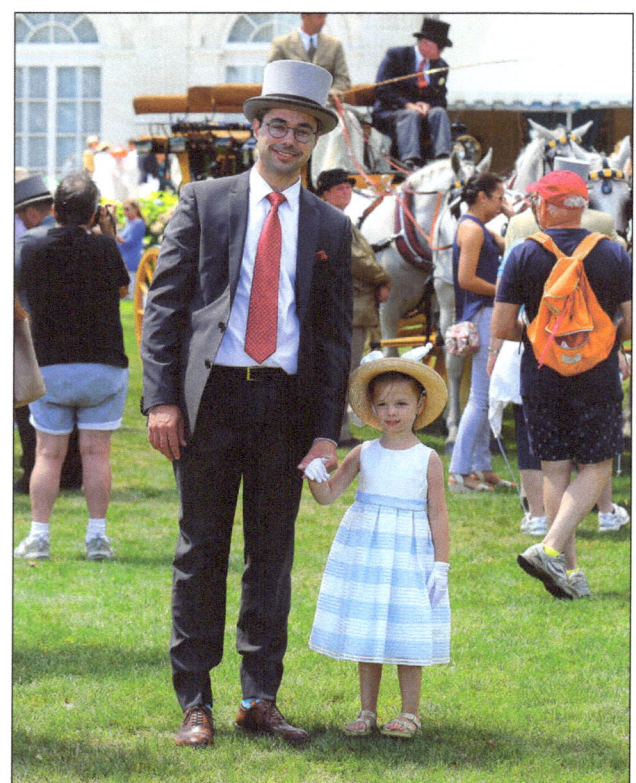

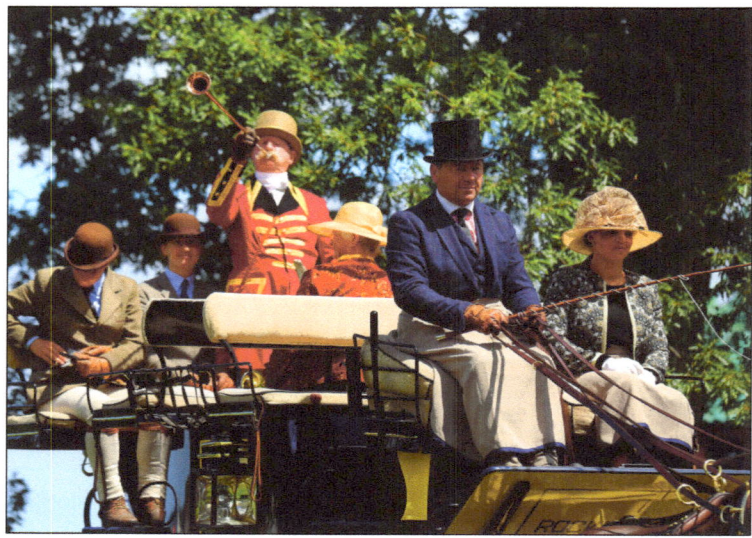

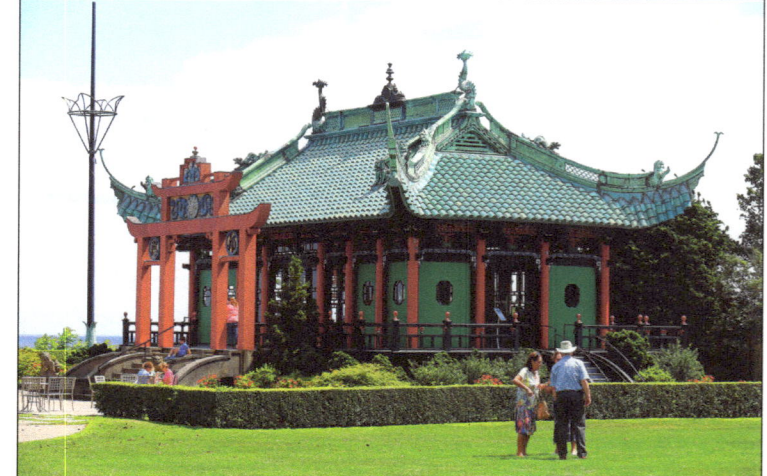

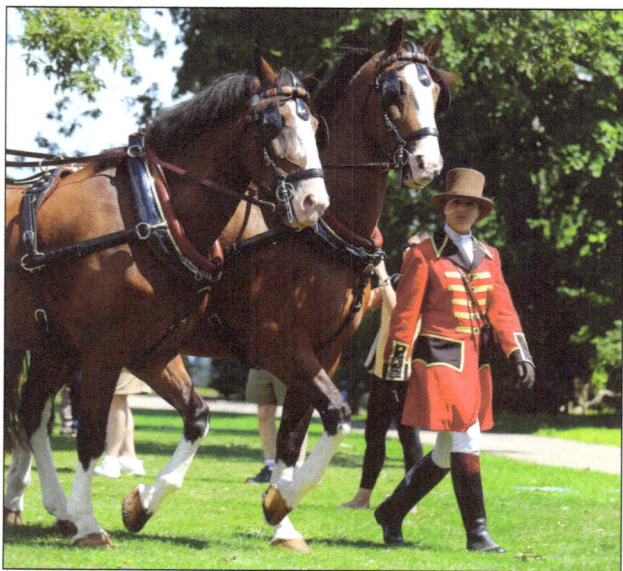

Alva Vanderbilt Belmont built the Chinese Tea House and held rallies for women's right to vote there. The building was modeled after a 12th century Song Dynasty temple.

Newport Coaching Weekend

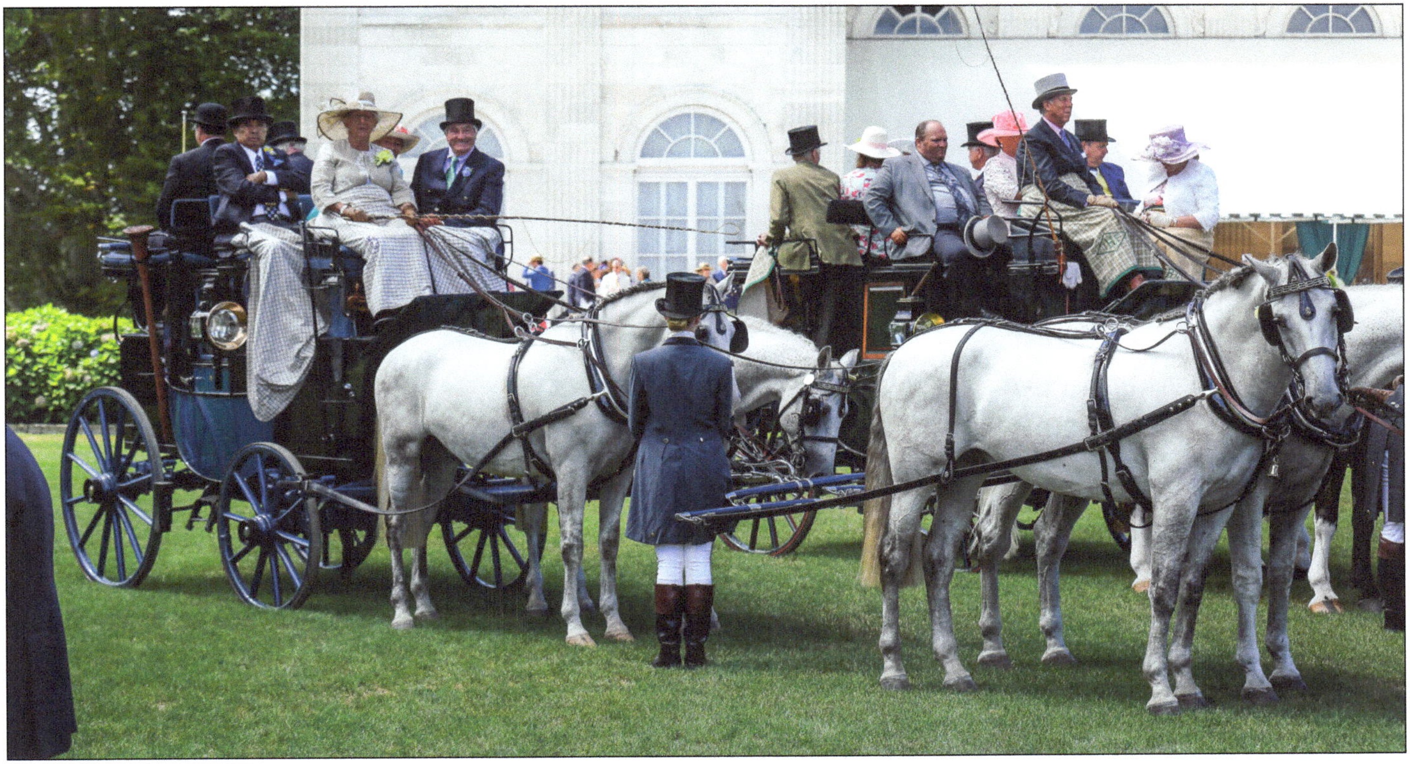

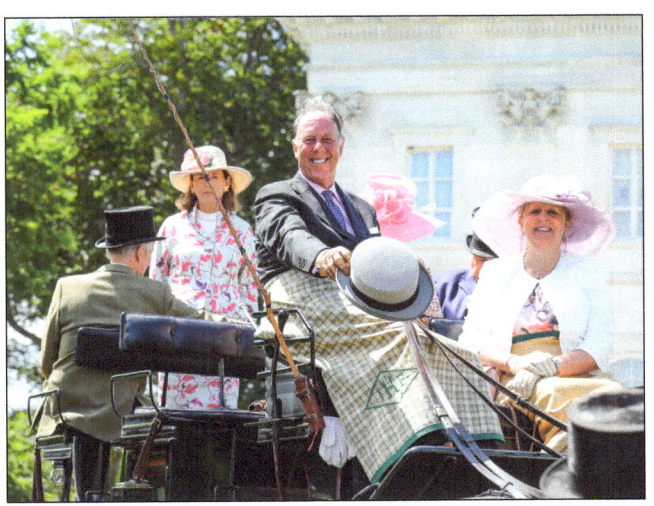
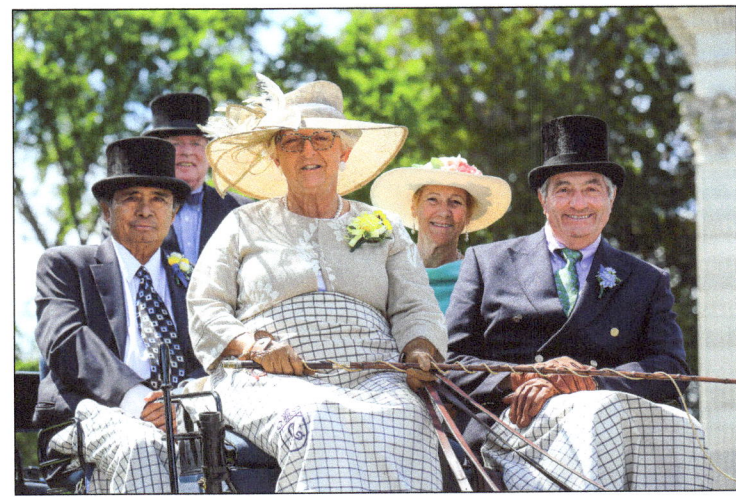

Newport Coaching Weekend

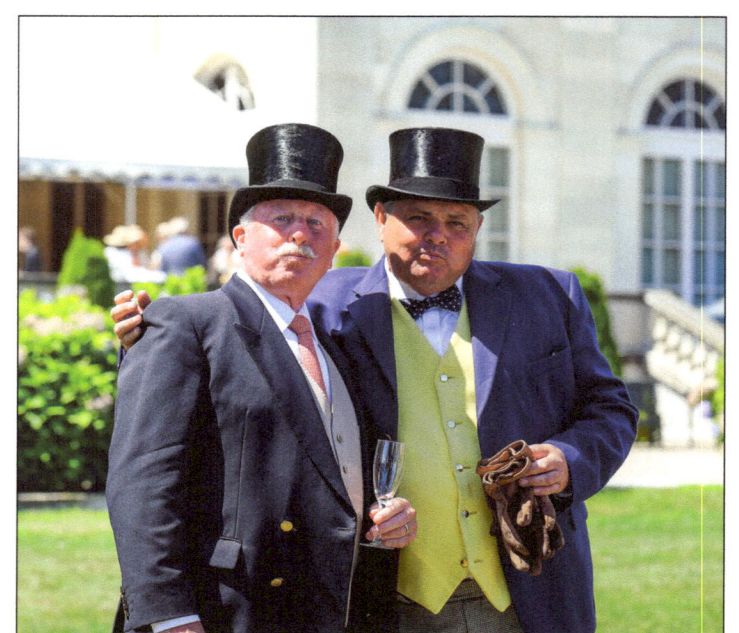
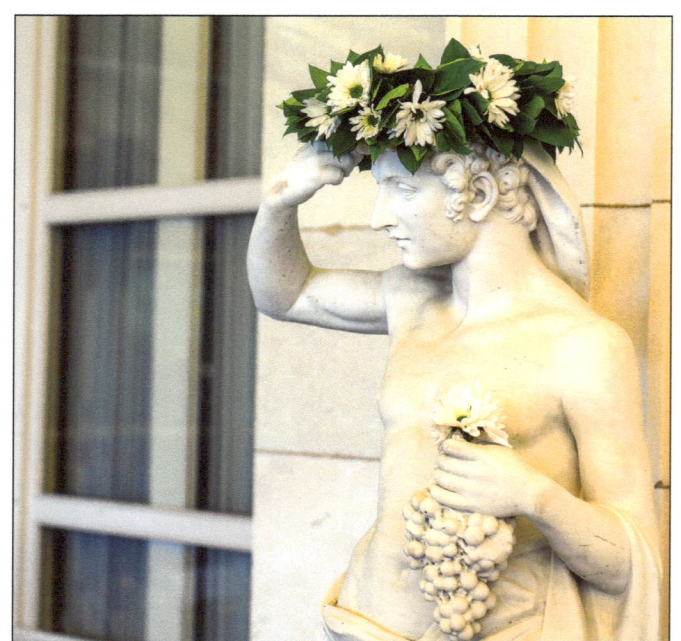
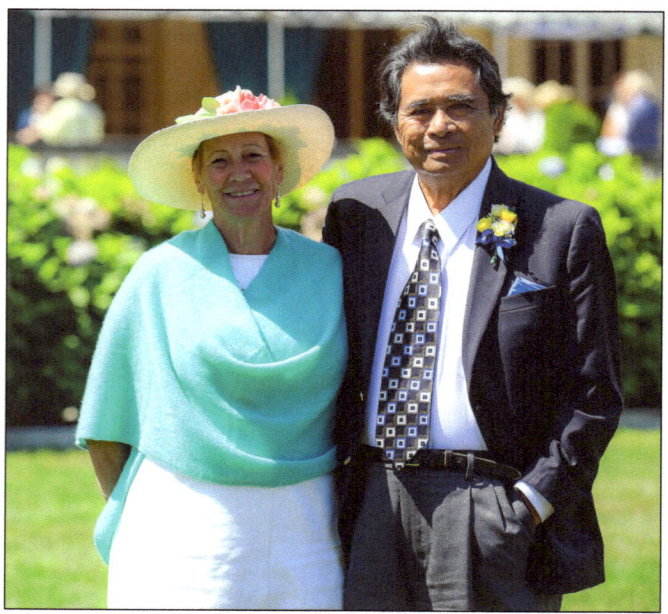
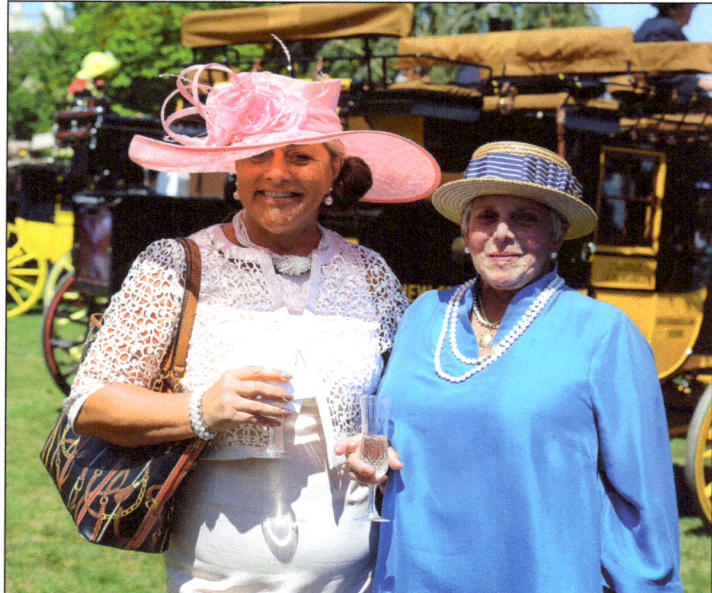

Newport Coaching Weekend

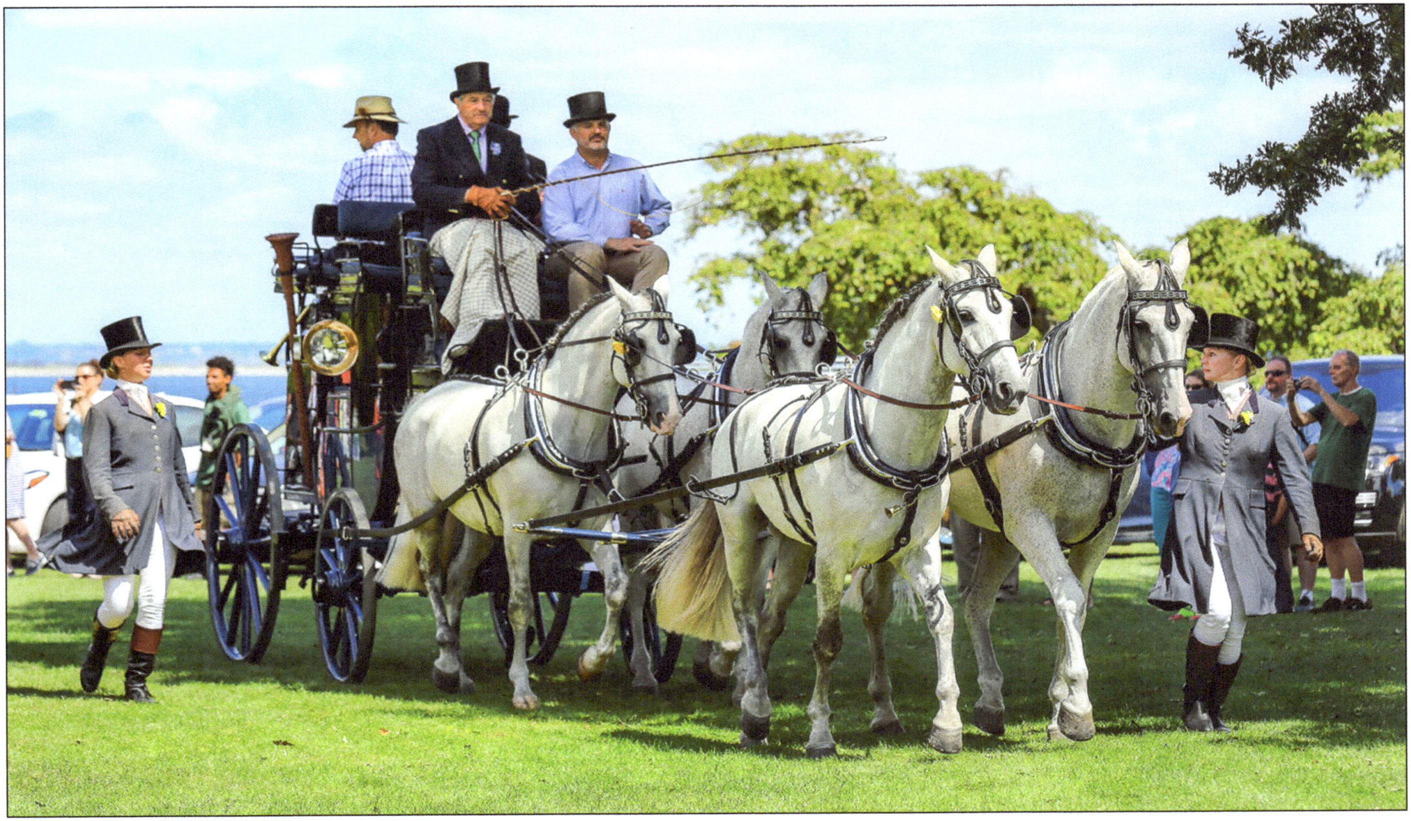

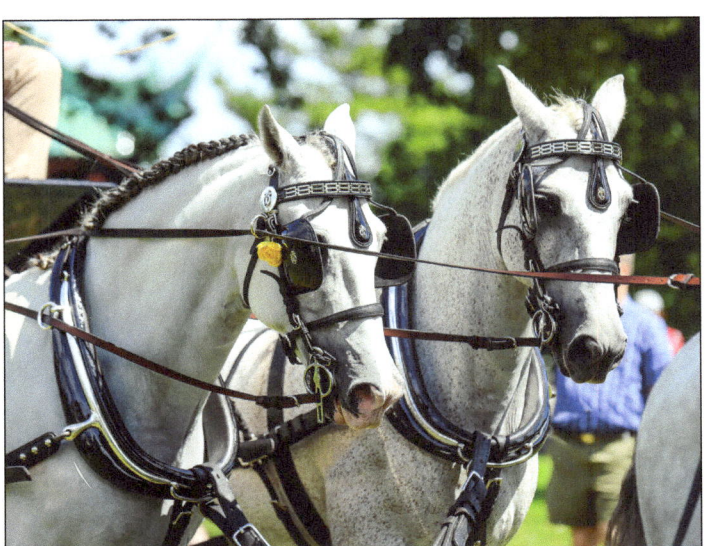
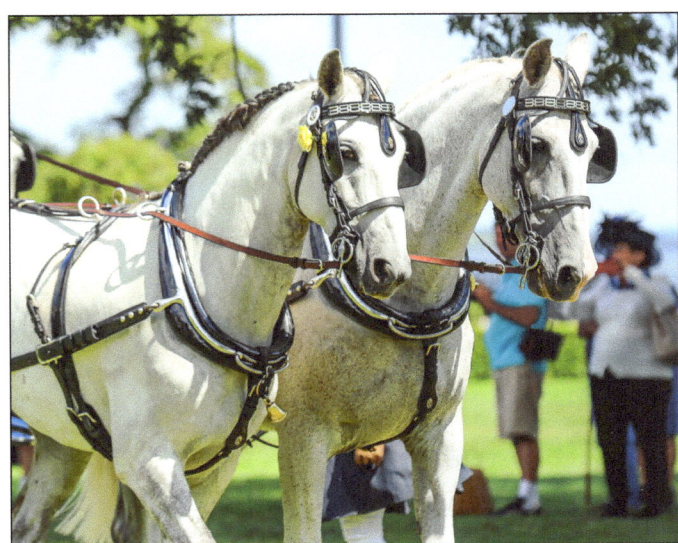

Newport Coaching Weekend

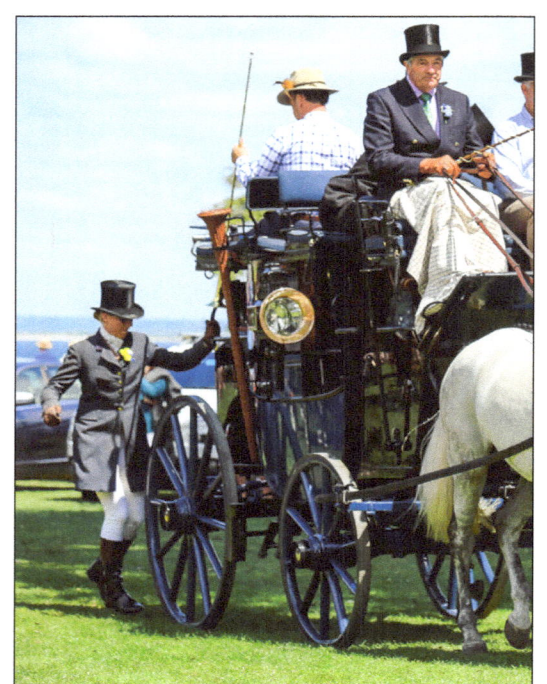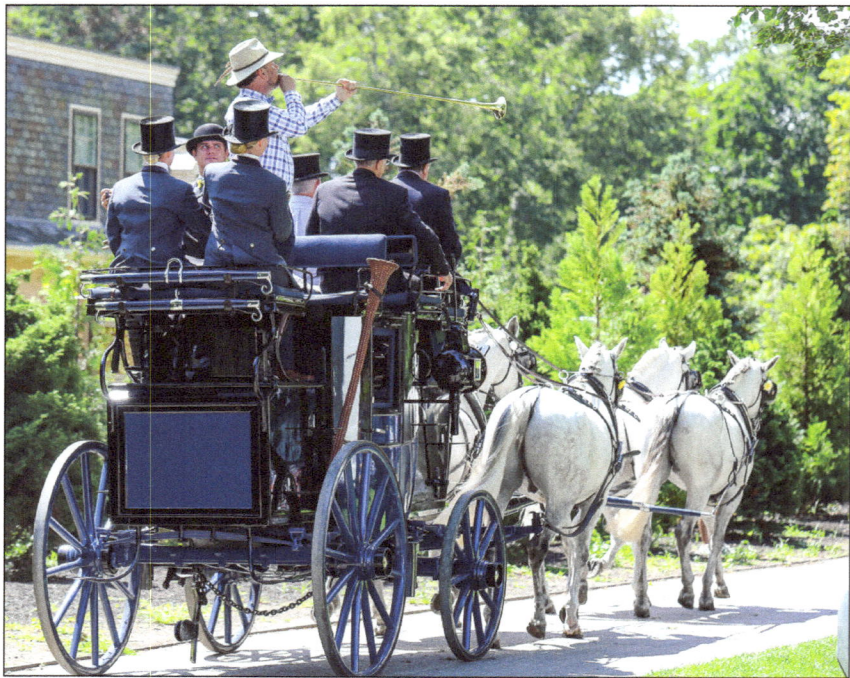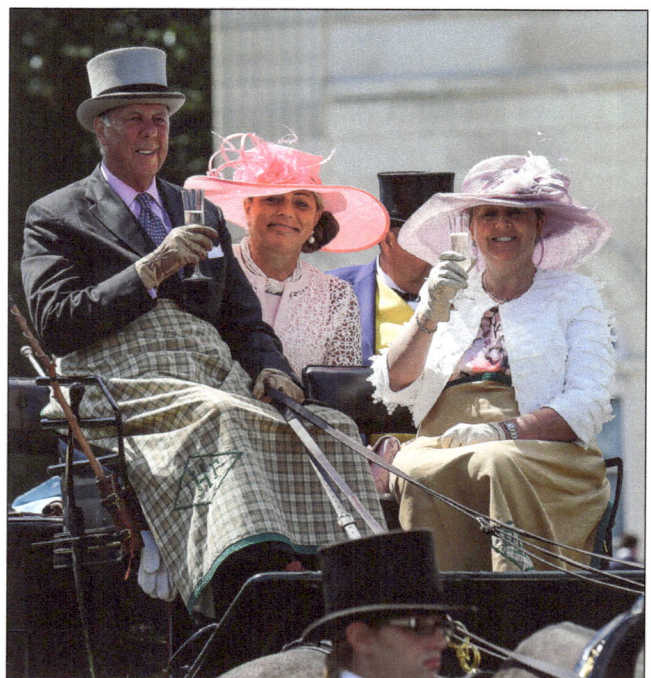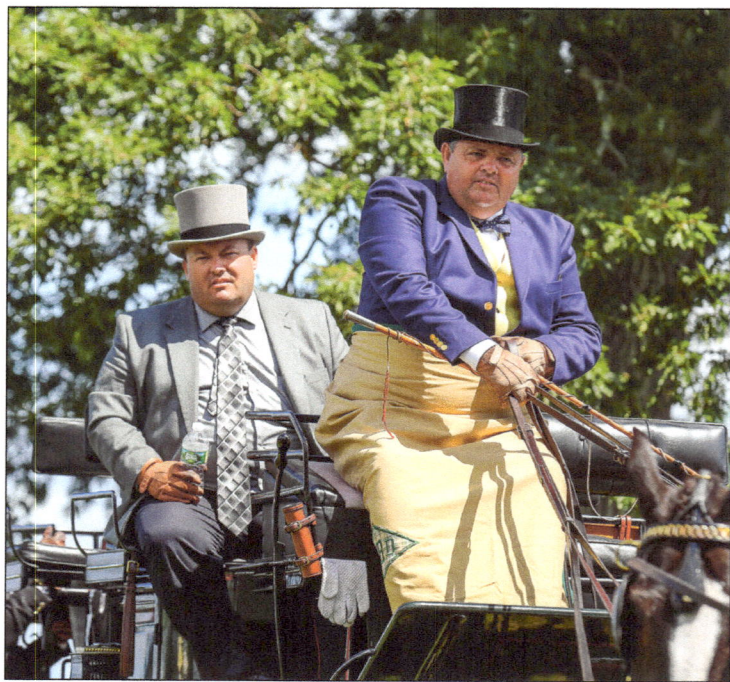

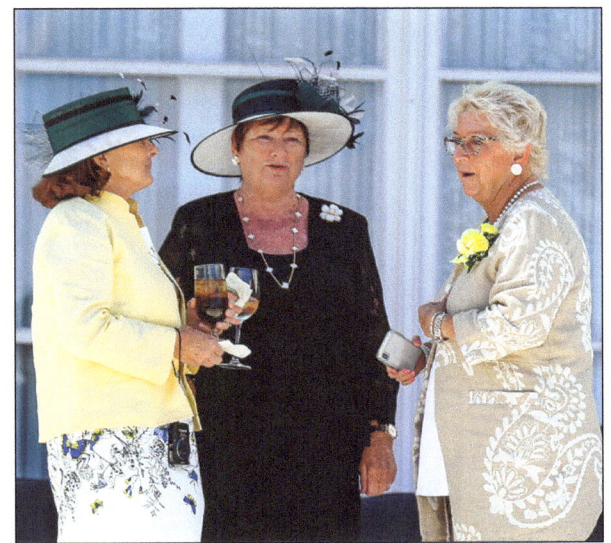
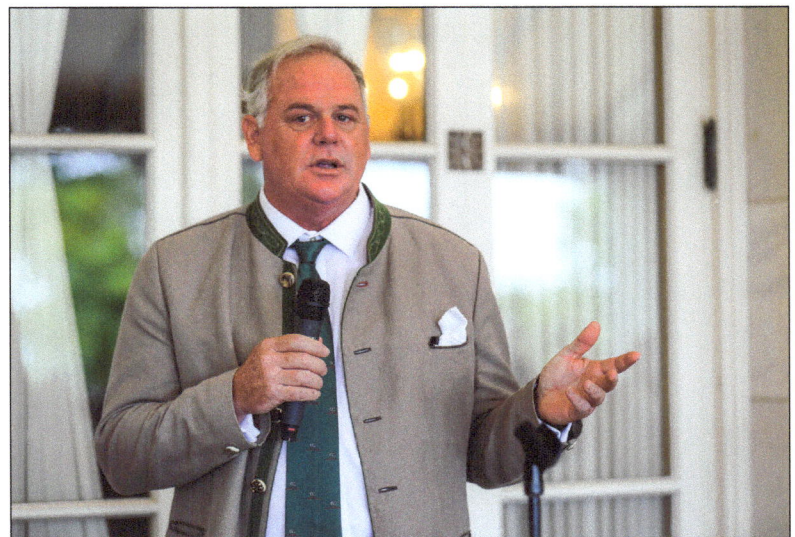
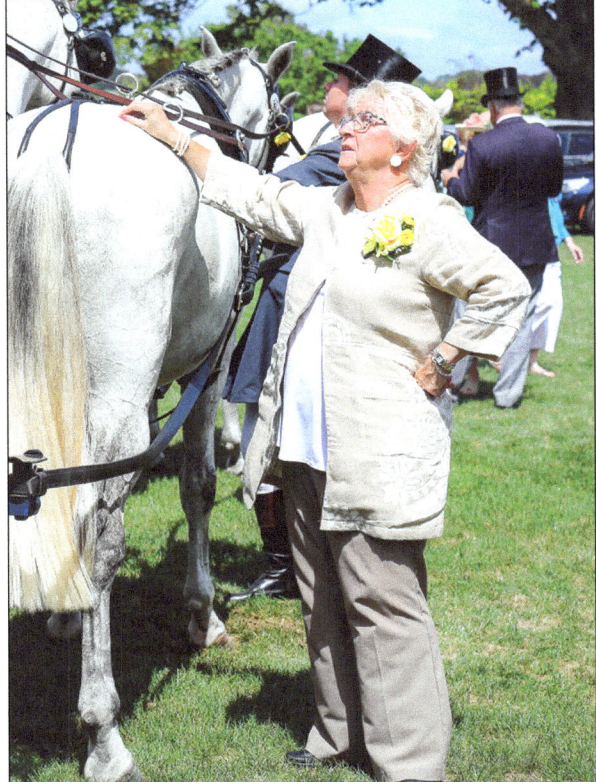
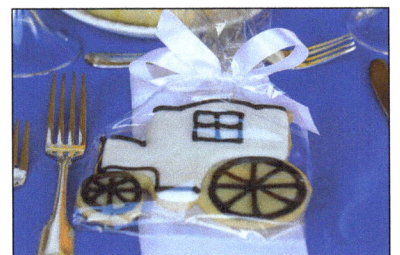
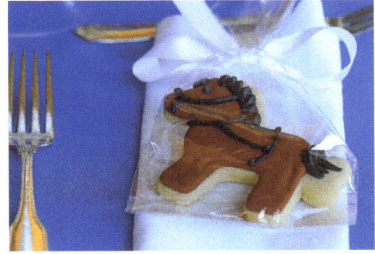
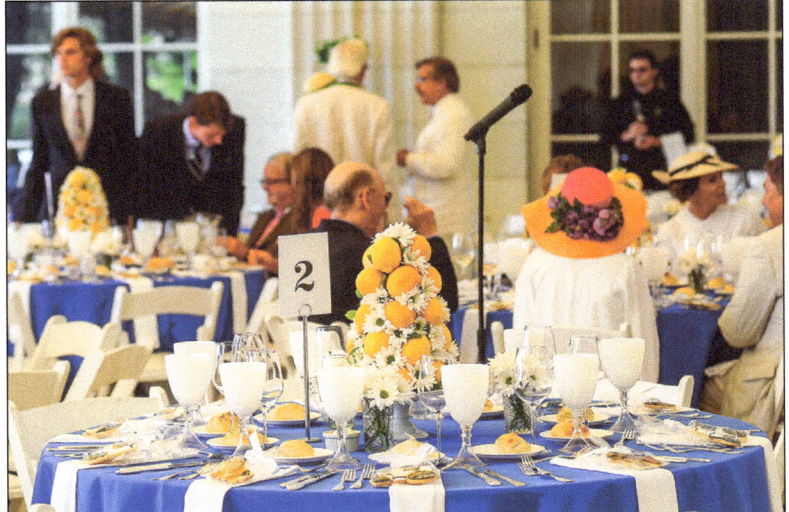

Newport Coaching Weekend

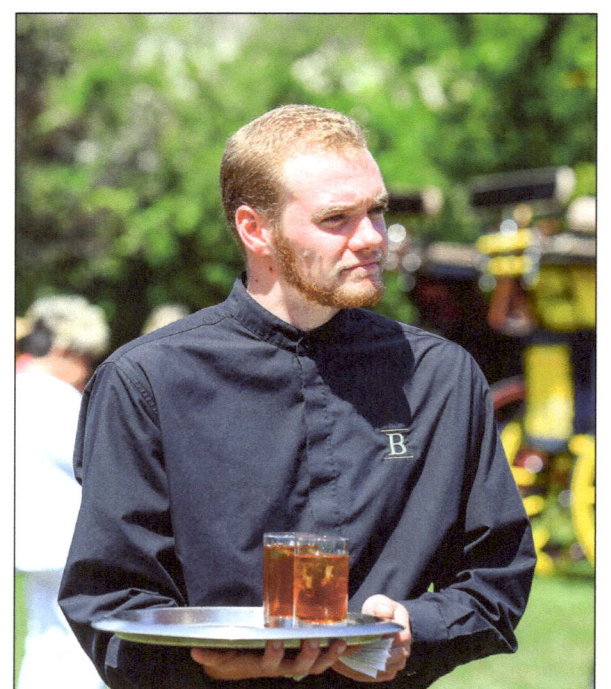
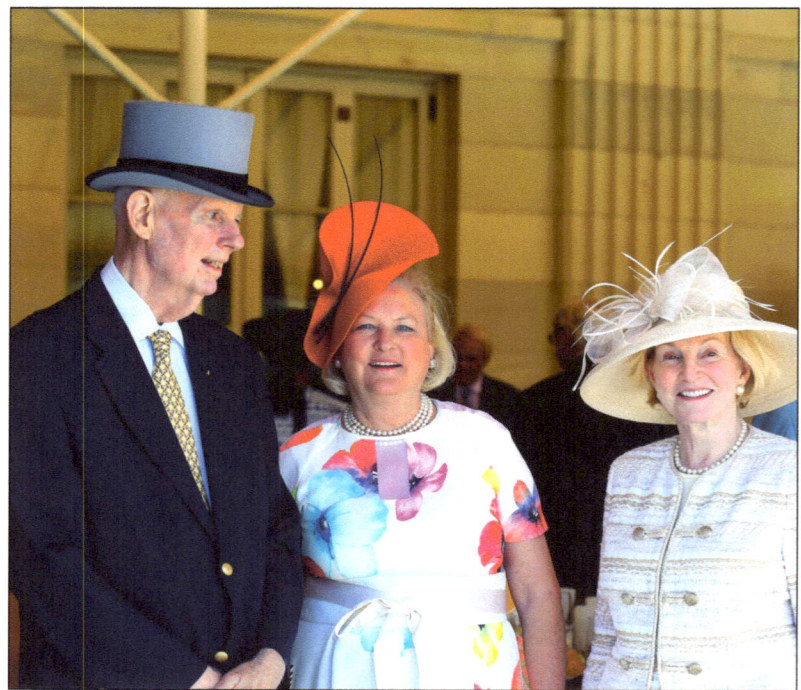
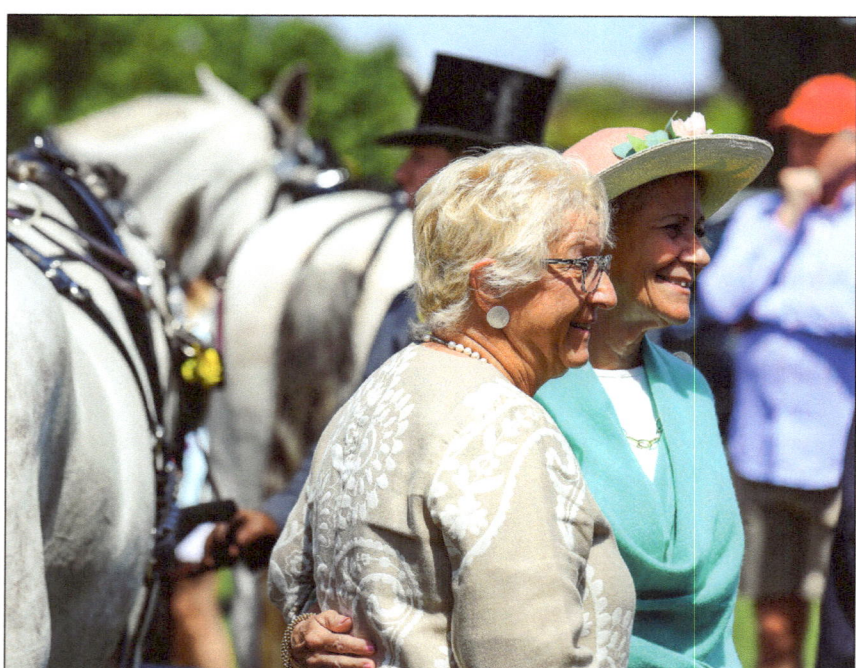
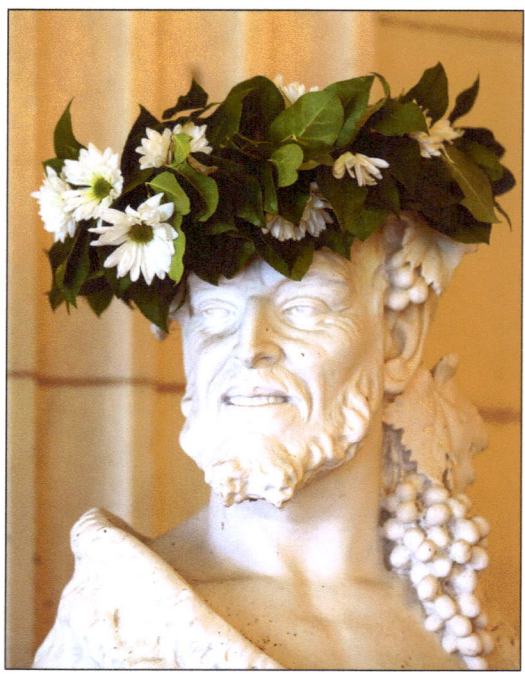

Newport Coaching Weekend

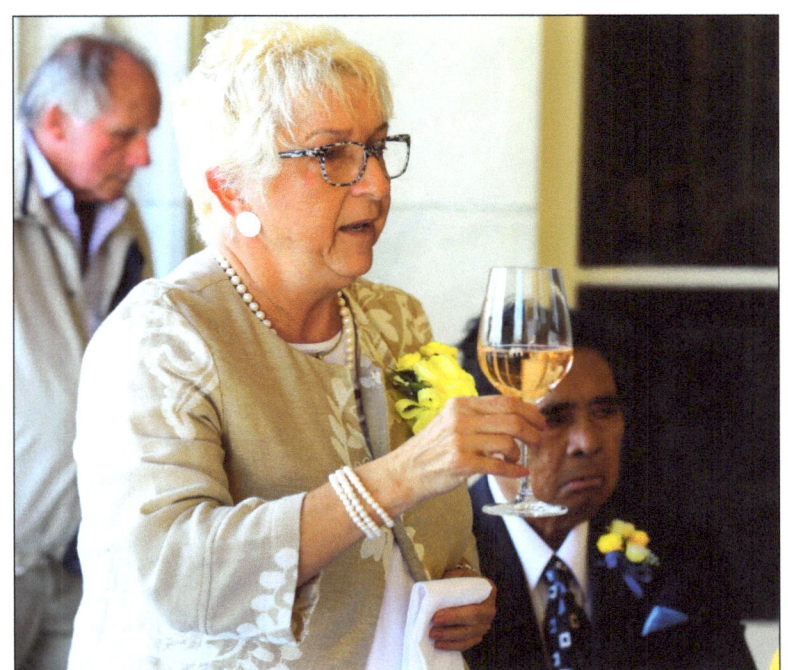
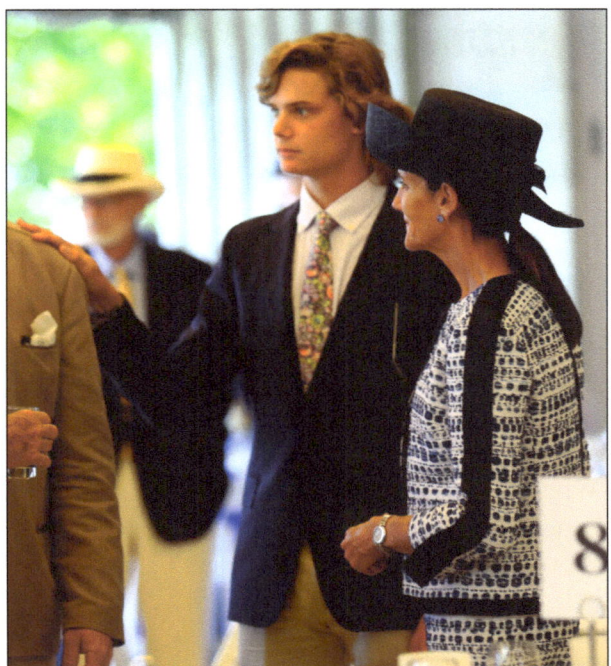
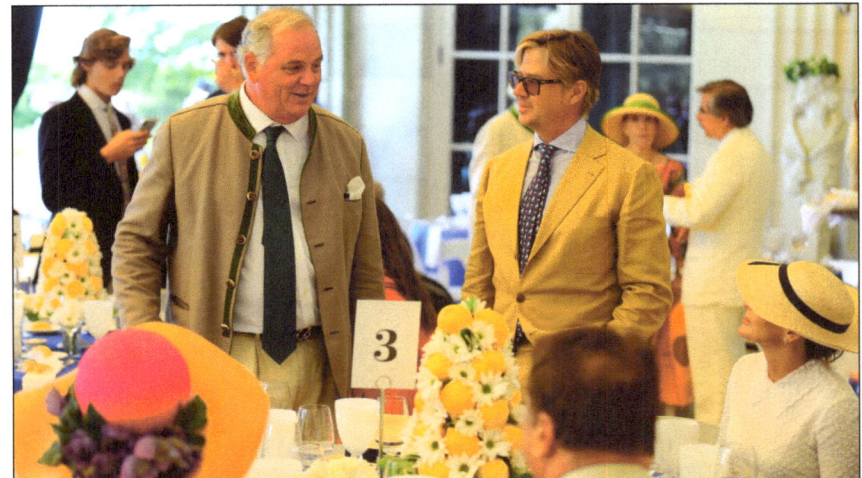
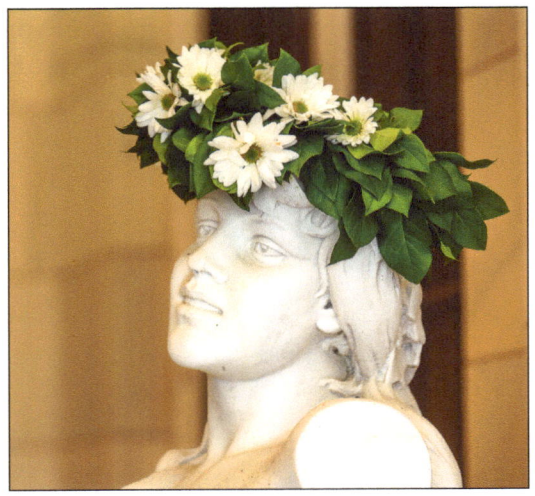

As the weekend came to an end, a toast was offered, "To the Road."
- until we meet again. -Gloria Austin

Newport Coaching Weekend

Newport Locations

MARBLE HOUSE

Marble House is a Gilded Age mansion in Newport, Rhode Island. Designed as a summer cottage for Alva and William Kissam Vanderbilt by the society architect Richard Morris Hunt, it was unparalleled in opulence for an American house when it was completed in 1892. Its temple-front portico, which also serves as a porte-cochère, resembles that of the White House. Located at 596 Bellevue Avenue, it is now open to the public as a museum run by the Preservation Society of Newport County. (cited. https://en.wikipedia.org/wiki/Marble_House)

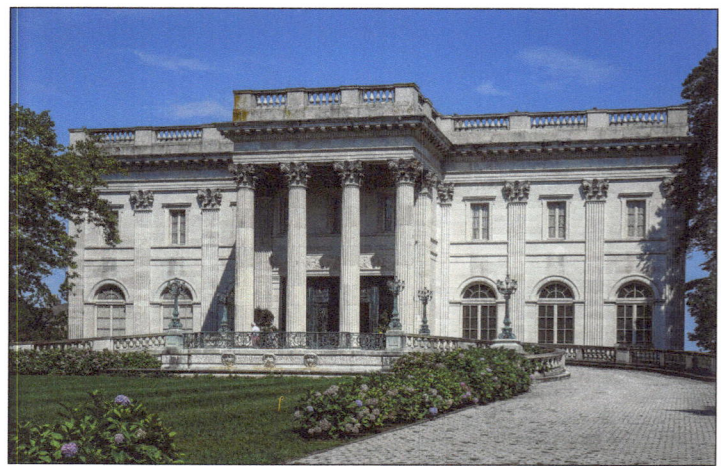

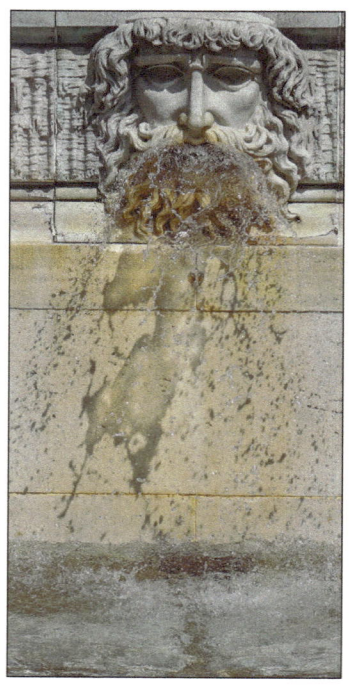

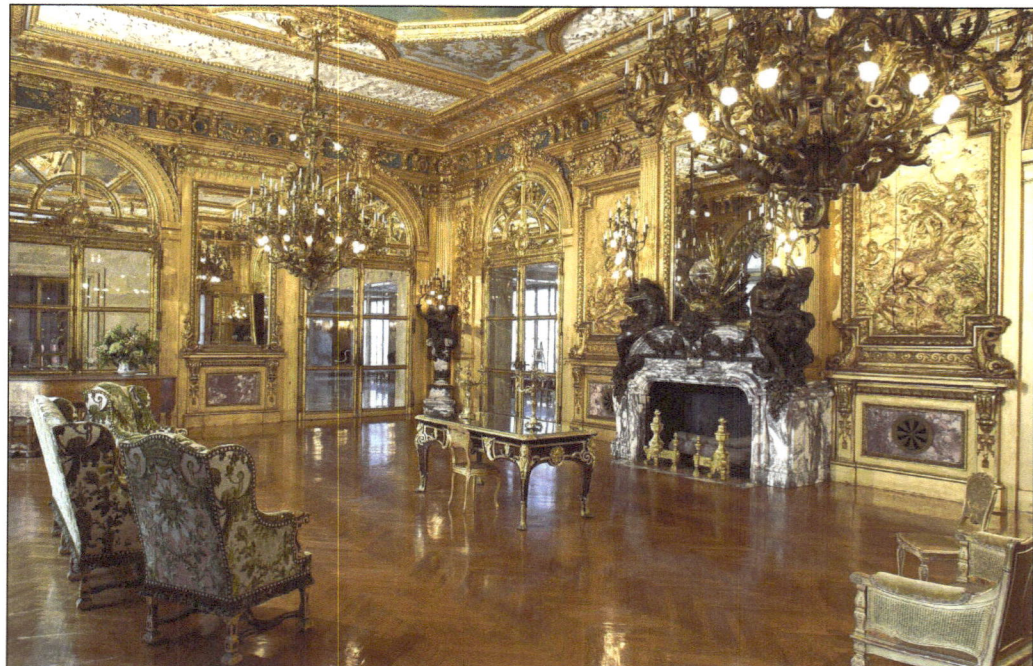

MIRAMAR

Miramar is a 30,000-square-foot (2,800 m2) French neoclassical-style mansion on 7.8 acres (32,000 m2) bordering Bellevue Avenue on Aquidneck Island at Newport, Rhode Island. Overlooking Rhode Island Sound, it was intended as a summer home for the George D. Widener family of Philadelphia. It was designed by Horace Trumbauer, who had earlier designed the nearby Edward Julius Berwind property, The Elms. The gardens were created by Jacques Gréber.

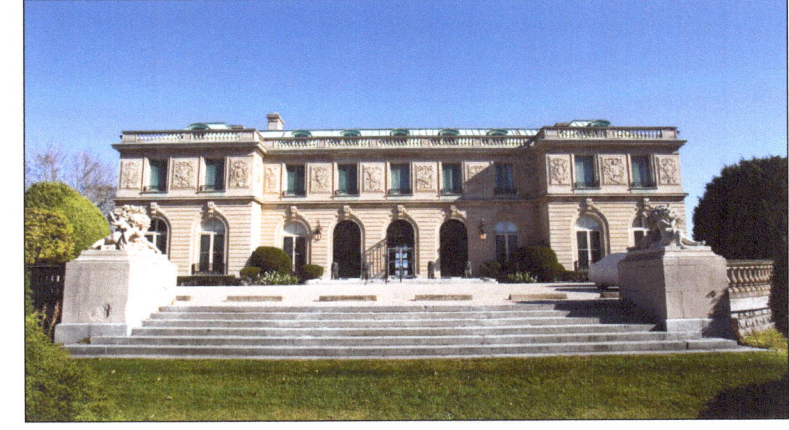

The building and landscaping were still in the design stage when George Widener and his son Harry died aboard the RMS Titanic. His widow, Eleanor Elkins Widener, who was rescued in a lifeboat from the Titanic, completed the project, and construction was undertaken during 1913 and 1914 and opened to friends with a large reception on August 20, 1915. (cited. https://en.wikipedia.org/wiki/Miramar_(mansion)

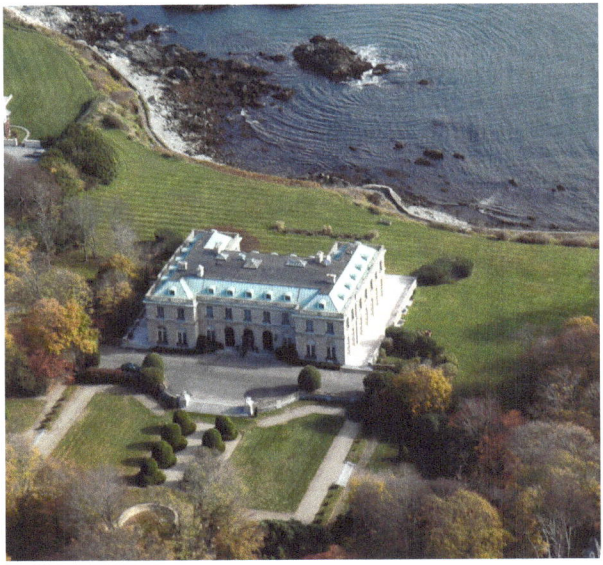

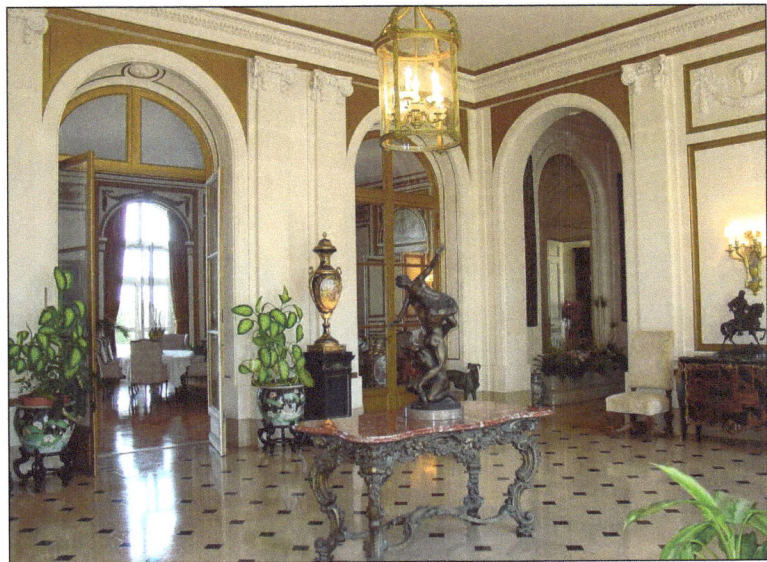

CHATEAU-SUR-MER

Chateau-sur-Mer is a landmark of High Victorian architecture, furniture, wallpapers, ceramics and stenciling. It was the most palatial residence in Newport from its completion in 1852 until the appearance of the Vanderbilt houses in the 1890s.

Chateau-sur-Mer was completed in 1852 as an Italianate villa for William Shepard Wetmore, a merchant in the Old China Trade who was born on January 26, 1801 in St. Albans, Vermont. The architect and builder was Seth C. Bradford, and the structure is a landmark of Victorian architecture, furniture, wallpapers, ceramics, and stenciling, constructed of Fall River Granite. (cited. https://www.discovernewport.org/listing/chateau-sur-mer/251/)

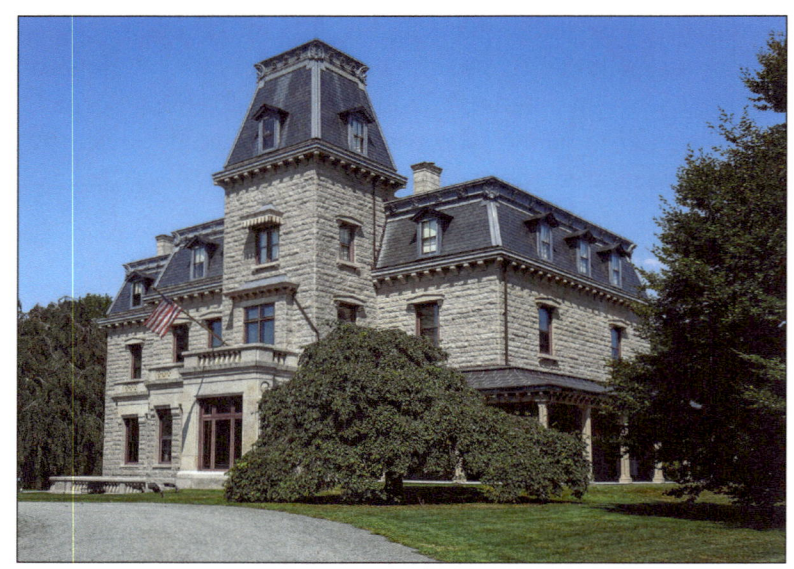

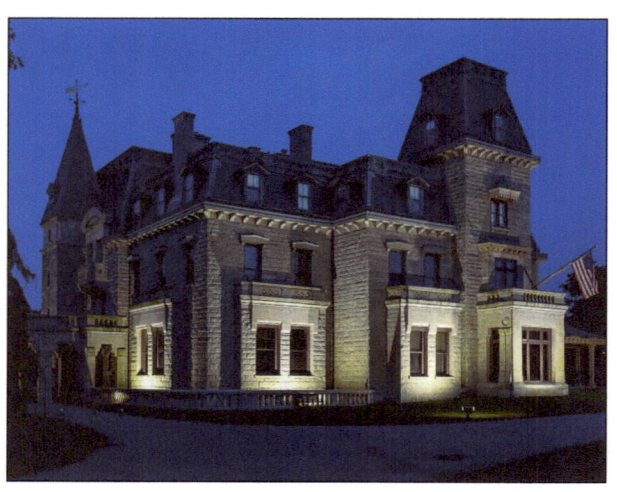

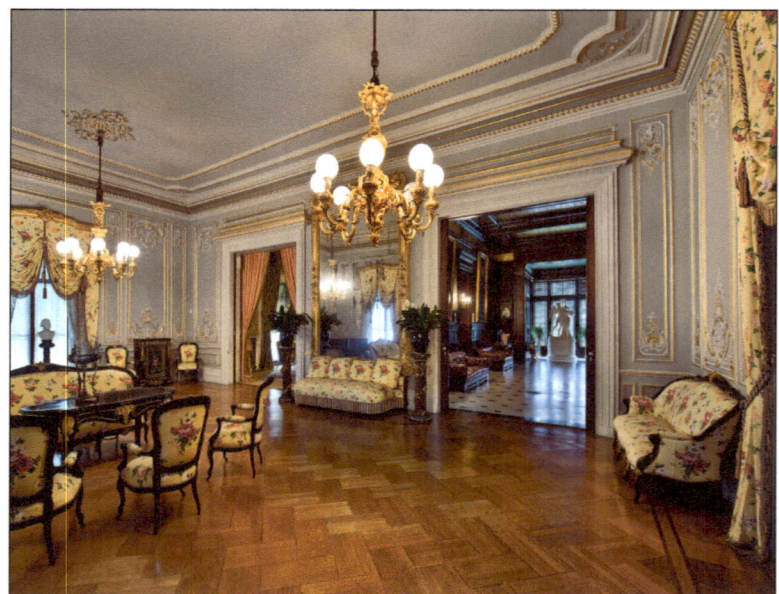

THE LEDGES

Decades before the Gilded Age "cottages" arrived on Bellevue Avenue and the Ocean Drive, The Ledges was commissioned by Robert Maynard Cushing, on a spectacular setting overlooking the Atlantic on the rocky shoreline from Bailey's beach to Gooseberry beach, all of which was farmland at the time, used for grazing sheep. Built-in 1867, The Ledges was artfully designed by John Hubbard Sturgis, a Boston-based architect. He was well regarded for having designed other Newport houses, including Land's End for the fellow Bostonian Samuel Gary Ward, built-in 1864-65, and Frederick William Rhinelander's house on Redwood Street, built-in 1863-64, and now part of the Redwood Library. (cited. https://rentals.liladelman.com/the-ledges-newport)

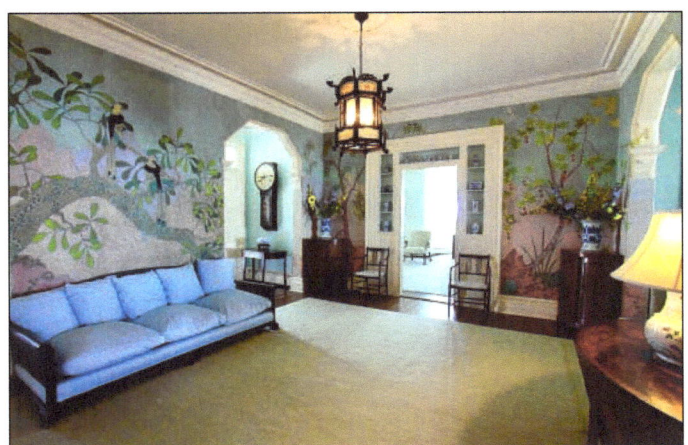

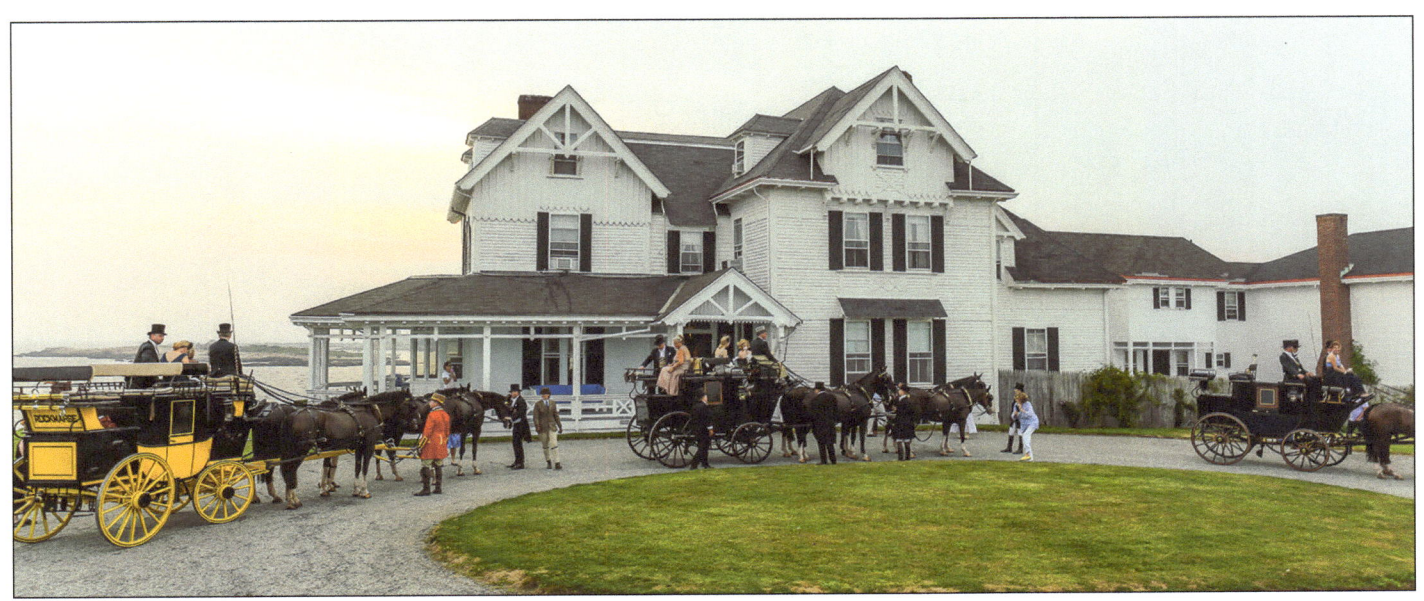

HAMMERSMITH FARM

Hammersmith Farm is a Victorian mansion and estate. It was the childhood home of First Lady Jacqueline Bouvier Kennedy, and the site of the reception for her 1953 wedding to U.S. Senator John F. Kennedy. During his presidency, it was referred to as the "Summer White House". Hammersmith Farm's 28-room main house was built in 1887 for John W. Auchincloss, the great-grandfather of Hugh D. Auchincloss (1897–1976), Jacqueline Kennedy's stepfather. It was erected on what had been originally known as "Hammersmith Island," possibly named after the English hometown of William Brenton, the 17th-century governor of Rhode Island who established the first farm on the site in 1640. It's front lawn overlooks Newport Harbor which is part of Narragansett Bay. This area of Rhode Island is known as the First Horse Capital of the United States. Bred in the late 1600s, The Narragansett Pacer was the first American breed developed in the United States. (cited. https://en.wikipedia.org/wiki/Hammersmith_Farm)

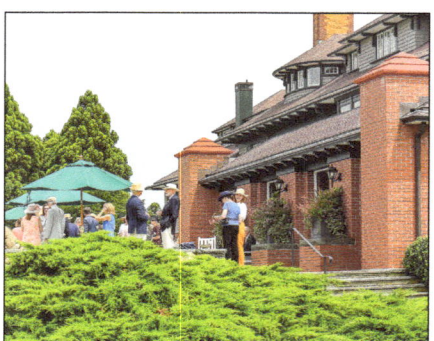
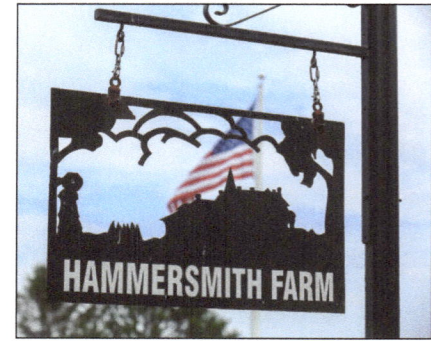

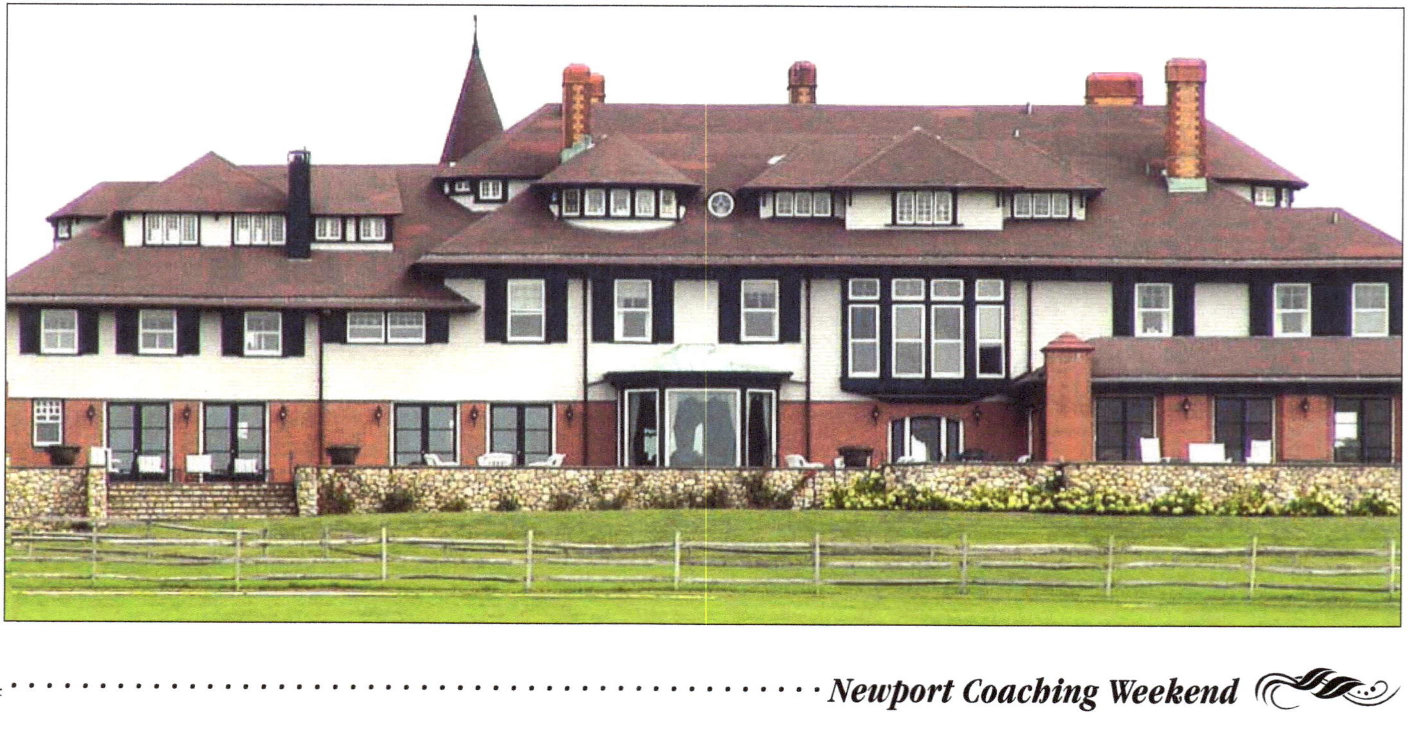

THE BREAKERS

The Breakers is a 70-room Vanderbilt mansion located on Ochre Point Avenue, Newport, Rhode Island, United States. The building became a National Historic Landmark in 1994 and is a contributing property to the Bellevue Avenue Historic District. It is owned and operated by the Preservation Society of Newport County and is open for visits all year.

The mansion was built as the Newport summer home of Cornelius Vanderbilt II, a member of the wealthy United States Vanderbilt family, in an architectural style based on the Italian Renaissance. (cited. https://en.wikipedia.org/wiki/The_Breakers)

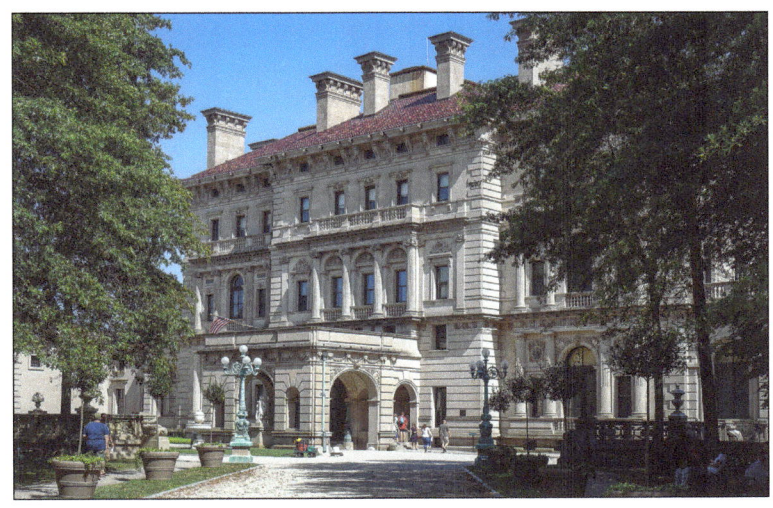

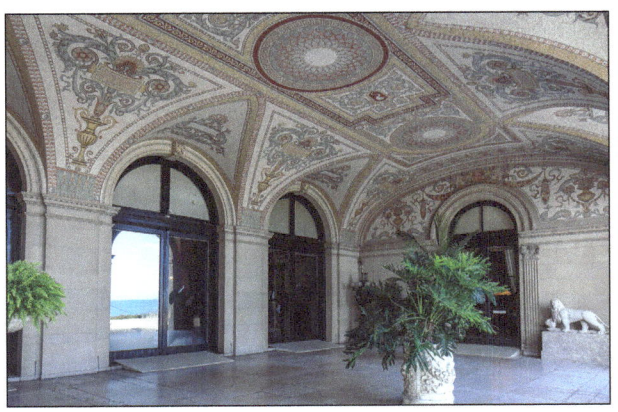

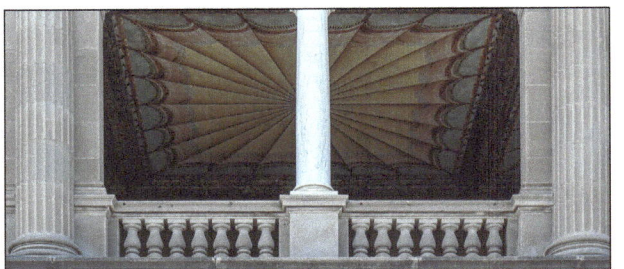

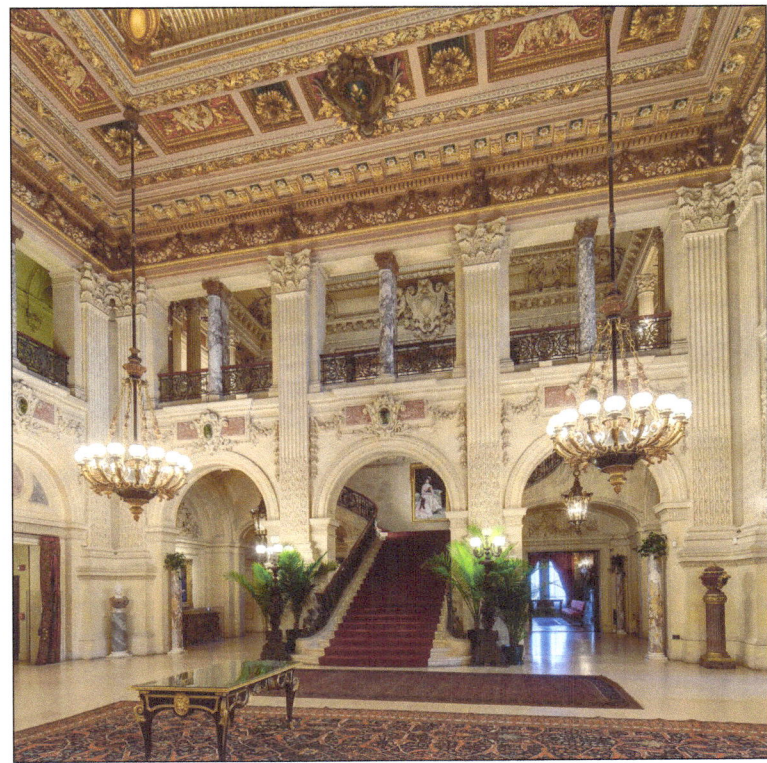

Newport Coaching Weekend · · · · · · · · · · · · · · 215

THE ELMS

The Elms is a large mansion located at 367 Bellevue Avenue, Newport, Rhode Island, completed in 1901. The architect Horace Trumbauer (1868–1938) designed it for the coal baron Edward Julius Berwind (1848–1936), taking inspiration from the 18th century Château d'Asnières in Asnières-sur-Seine, France. C. H. Miller and E. W. Bowditch, working closely with Trumbauer, designed the gardens and landscape. The Preservation Society of Newport County purchased The Elms in 1962, and opened the house to the public. The Elms was added to the National Register of Historic Places in 1971, and designated a National Historic Landmark in 1996. (cited. https://en.wikipedia.org/wiki/The_Elms_(Newport,_Rhode_Island))

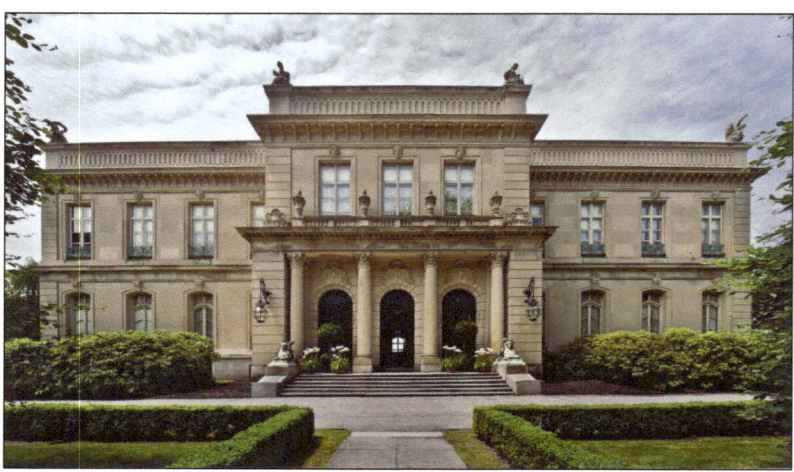

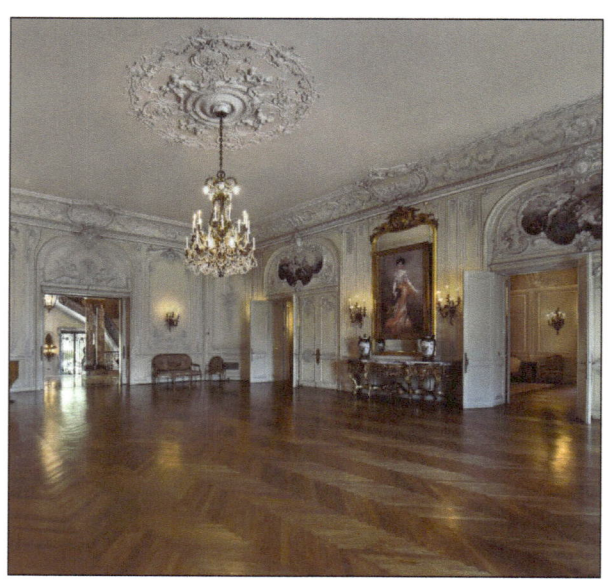

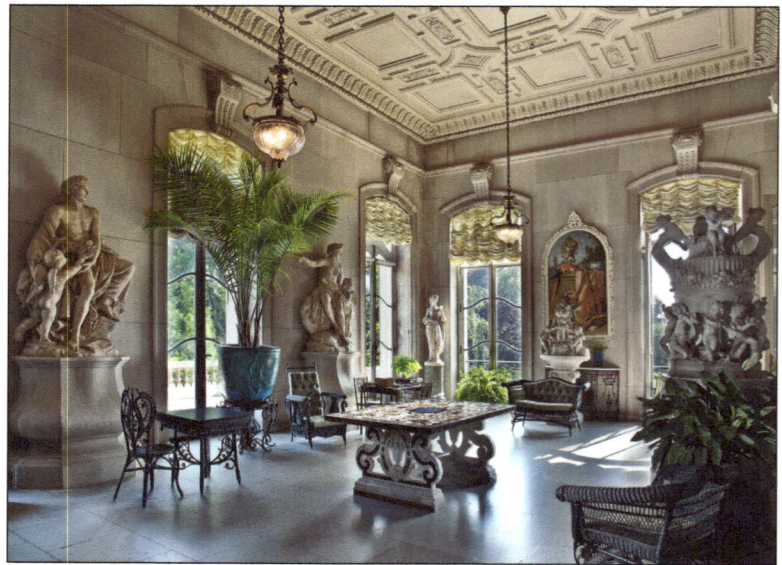

ROSECLIFF

Rosecliff, built 1898–1902, by Theresa Fair Oelrichs, a silver heiress from Nevada, whose father James Graham Fair was one of the four partners in the Comstock Lode. She was the wife of Hermann Oelrichs, an American agent for the Norddeutscher Lloyd steamship line. She and her husband, together with her sister, Virginia Fair, bought the land in 1891 from the estate of George Bancroft. They then commissioned the architectural firm of McKim, Mead, and White to design a summer home suitable for entertaining on a grand scale.

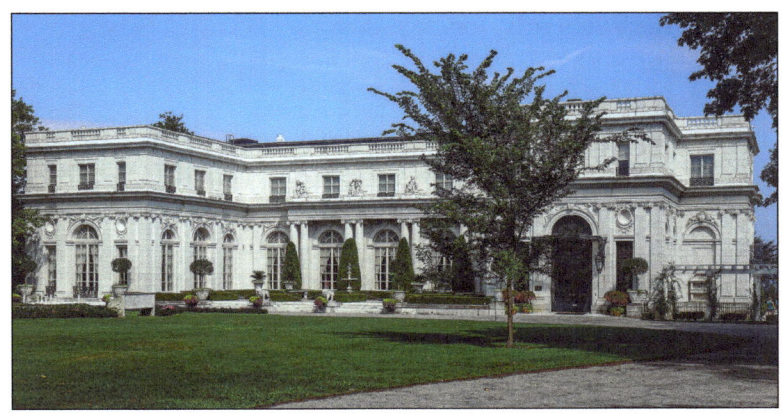

With little opportunity to channel her considerable energy elsewhere, she "threw herself into the social scene with tremendous gusto. She, along with Mrs. Stuyvesant Fish and Mrs. O.H.P. Belmont (of nearby Belcourt), one of the three great hostesses of Newport." (cited. https://en.wikipedia.org/wiki/Rosecliff)

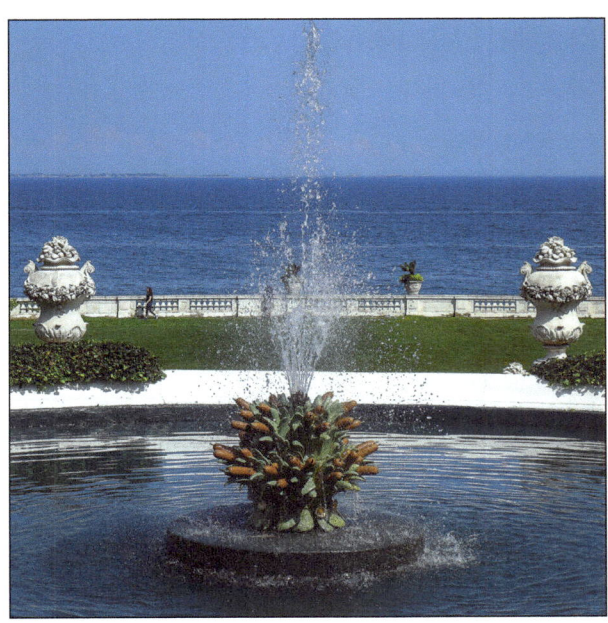
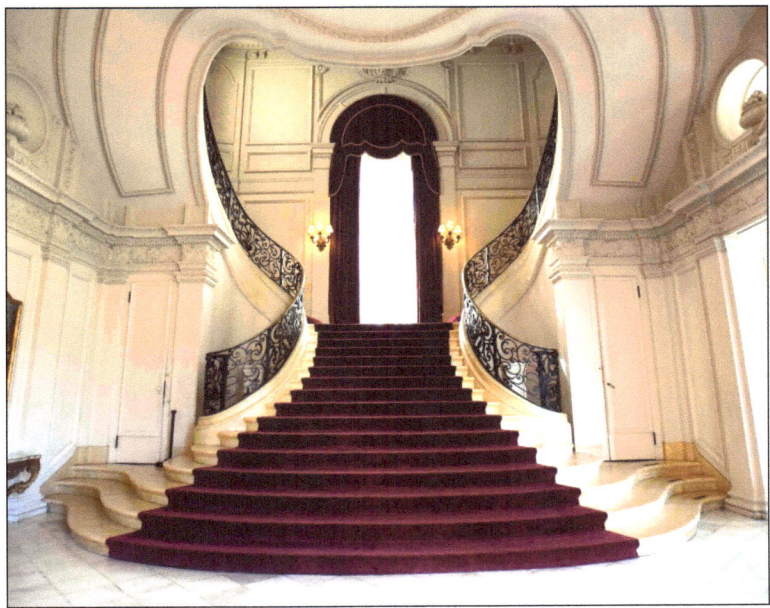

GREENVALE VINEYARDS

Greenvale Vineyards, located along the beautiful Sakonnet River, has been dedicated to quality wine growing since 1982. Owned by the same family since 1863, the vineyard's 100% Estate Grown fruit and award-winning wines are nurtured by an idyllic setting, rich history and commitment to the preservation of open space. Located 6 miles from downtown Newport. It is listed on the National and State Registers of Historic Places. (cited. http://coastalwinetrail.com/greenvale-vineyards/)

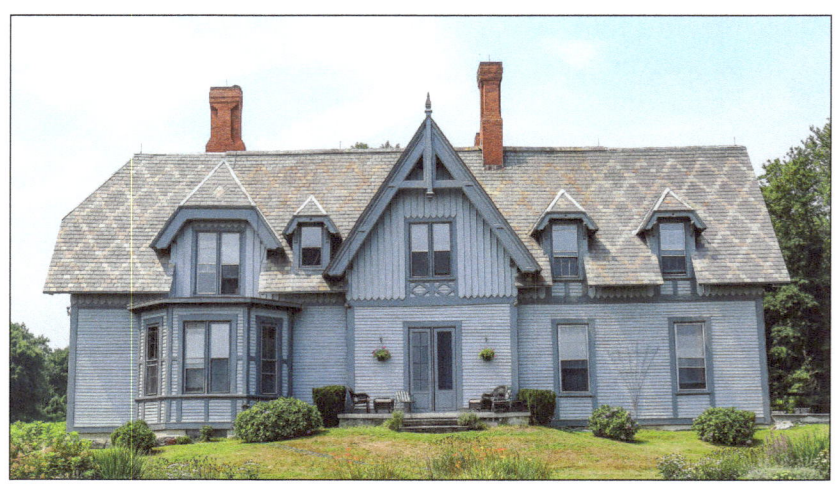

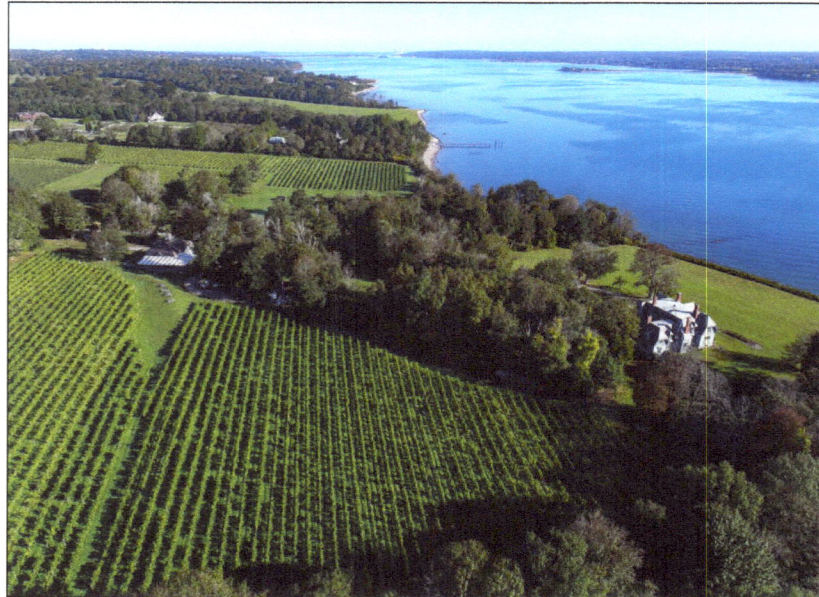

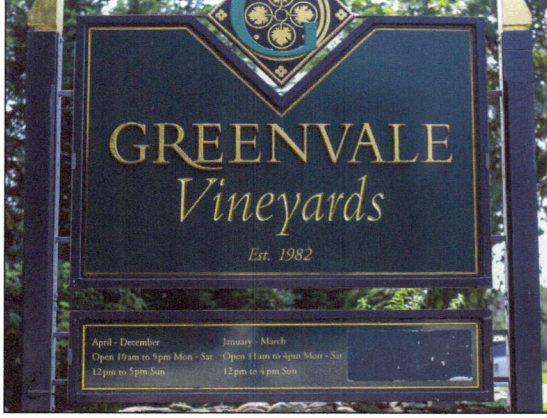

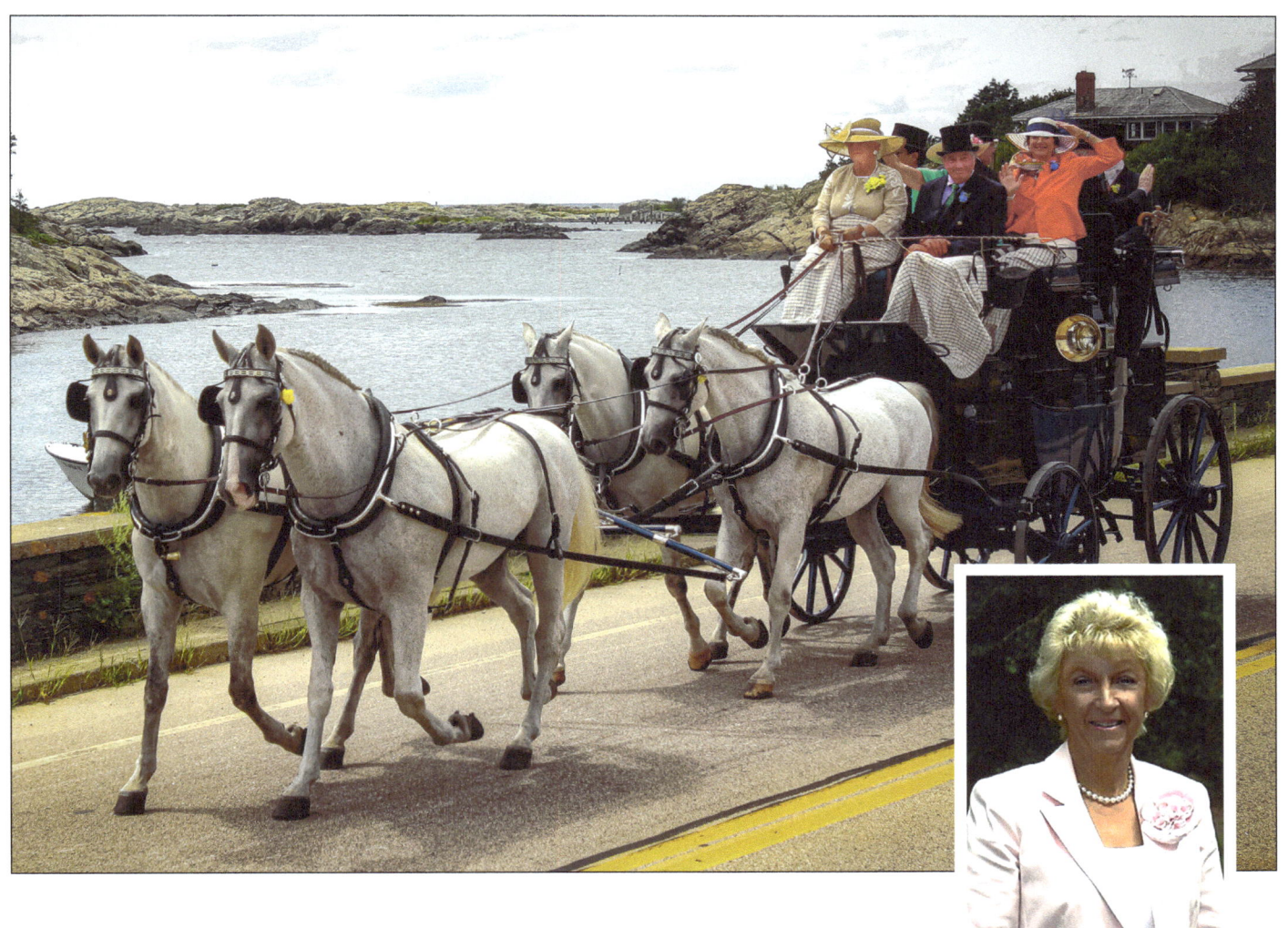

"From Roman roads to the highways of Great Britain, to our modern expressways of this day, let the pathways of life take you where they will. Do not be afraid and keep your friends close as you venture forth on your journey. Thank you for joining me on my travels to the Newport Coaching Weekend. It is one of the most pleasurable experiences one can enjoy in our coaching world."

www.ingramcontent.com/pod-product-compliance
Lightning Source LLC
Chambersburg PA
CBHW041459220426
43661CB00016B/1199

Foreword

Culinary Quickies is a recipe book with a difference written by African Australian chef and entrepreneur Mel Alafaci.

Known as the Queen of Culinary Bling, this sassy, smiley, happy chef will have you creating culinary masterpieces out of everyday ingredients in no time. Chef Mel shares ALL of her culinary secrets and shortcuts, offering practical advice to get you feeling confident and to find your mojo in the kitchen again. Best of all, she will make you extremely efficient and save you time, stress and heartache in the kitchen.

This book is perfect for beginners, intermediate and advanced foodies. The advice, hints and tips given are simple, hilarious and effective. Chef Mel asks all the questions that will challenge you to reconsider how you cook to simplify and streamline the cooking process.

You'll become the foodie you've always wanted to be and start your culinary journey of living happily ever after in your kitchen.

Before we begin..

1

Introduction

2

Reasons you hate cooking.. and how to fix that!

5

How to Shop

Introduction

We all feel like we need a makeover from time to time, especially with our frantic schedules. Makeovers make us feel shiny new and worthwhile again. I always say that recipes should be like your little black dress, or your favourite suit…new earrings + new handbag = new outfit. It's the same for me with cooking. I rehash my favourite old-faithful recipes again and again…new spices + new accompaniments = new recipe.

I'm sure, like me, you often feel that your cooking needs a makeover too. Easily done. In this book, I will not only help you completely makeover your kitchen attitude, but also train you on all the kitchen skills that I think you need to be fabulous in the kitchen. Once you have mastered these skills, you will have the confidence to tackle more and more dishes and in doing so, find your freedom in the kitchen. I really do want you to soar to new culinary heights.

No one should feel stressed and despondent in the kitchen, I do believe that food is a wonderful way of expressing your mood, sharing food with friends and family and letting them know how much you care about them. Cooking also brings friends and family together like nothing else can. If you've said in the last few days, weeks or months that you hate cooking, then this is the book for you.

I also feel that food has a language all of its own; it can break down barriers and bring cultures together. I love to travel; it helps me to find wonderful new ideas on how to interpret and refresh basic ingredients.

Yes, this IS a cookbook with all of my favourite recipes BUT my recipes are written in a very different style than most recipes. Often if you try and cook from a recipe, so many integral parts of the recipe are left out, leaving you frustrated and failing. I will ALWAYS mention the important bits so that you can almost have me right by your side, guiding you all the way. My recipes will train you to be able to handle other recipes more confidently and successfully.

Together, we will be unstoppable in the kitchen!

Reasons you hate cooking.. and how to fix that!

I hear it so often. 'I hate cooking'...

And I can sympathise and understand how we can often feel like that.
The truth is that we all have to cook, I think that's why it can get some people down and make it feel like a tedious chore.
Especially when no one appreciates it when you do cook, or it's all left up to you.
But it can be fun, it can be a fantastic opportunity to bring the family together.
To me, cooking is a therapy, a tonic, my passion. I REALLY do enjoy cooking, I think it feeds my soul and I can enhance my mood by cooking something fabulous and then gobbling it all up!
Perhaps it's because I know ALL of the shortcuts? I always say in my classes if you hate cooking, I can tell you why.

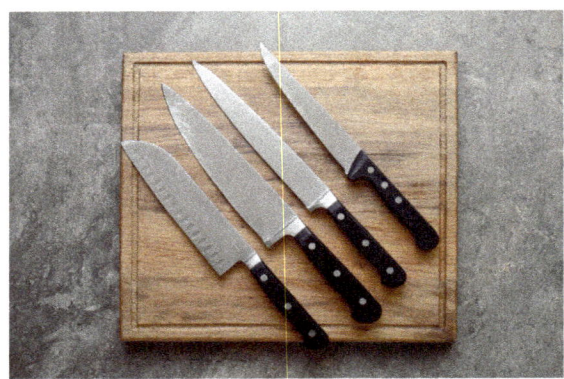

1. YOUR KNIVES ARE BLUNT

If your knives are blunt, you will not enjoy cooking. It is impossible and you know it.
It is pointless having an uber-sexy and expensive knife if the poor thing is so blunt you can barely get it through an Iceberg lettuce. Get them sharpened. Get a professional edge back on that knife by either chatting up your local butcher or getting your knives to a professional sharpener. It isn't expensive to get a professional in; it will make you feel so 'cheffy'. I also have a FREE knife skills course for you to do online, so head to my Instagram, click the link in my bio, scroll down to free knife skills, sign up and do the course online in the comfort of your kitchen.
Then, you can use your kitchen steel to keep it sharp as you go, and you really will find your confidence soar after doing the course.
Once your knife is sharp, you will live happily ever after in the kitchen.
You will dazzle and amaze even yourself with your new culinary prowess! It will practically feel like you have been on a magnificent holiday. You will feel so refreshed. Don't believe me? You know I'm right.

I have a professional knife sharpening service visit the cooking school as necessary, and I also get my knives done at home. It really will change your life and make you excited about chopping down your next ingredients.

2. MENU FATIGUE

If you buy the same dreary ingredients week in and week out OF COURSE you will lose your mojo in the kitchen. I usually have a list of the household basics, but I shop for FRESH produce. And I'm always looking for something I haven't ever tried before. I buy with my eyes and it all depends on what LOOKS fresh and delicious and what is on sale! I would much rather buy seasonal fresh produce than something old, overpriced and on my list.

So buy with your eyes. See what's on special. Try something new. If you have never tried fennel or beef cheeks or fresh turmeric BUY IT and TRY IT. There will be heaps of recipes for anything you may find so be adventurous. The minute you add a new ingredient to a dish it becomes a new dish so remember that. You don't have to learn a repertoire of new recipes; you can simply add a bit of bling to your old ones! Add finely shaved fennel to your next coleslaw…BANG! Sexy fancy 'cheffy' coleslaw. Amazing.

Add veal, chicken or pork mince instead of beef to any of your old favourites…BANG! Glamorous mince. Amazing. Add my favourite spice Ras el Hanout, as a CULINARY SPRAY TAN to your next leg of lamb, roast chicken, mince or even vegetables…BANG! Expensive sounding roast. Amazing! The minute you try a new combination of the same recipe it's a new recipe! I do it all the time!

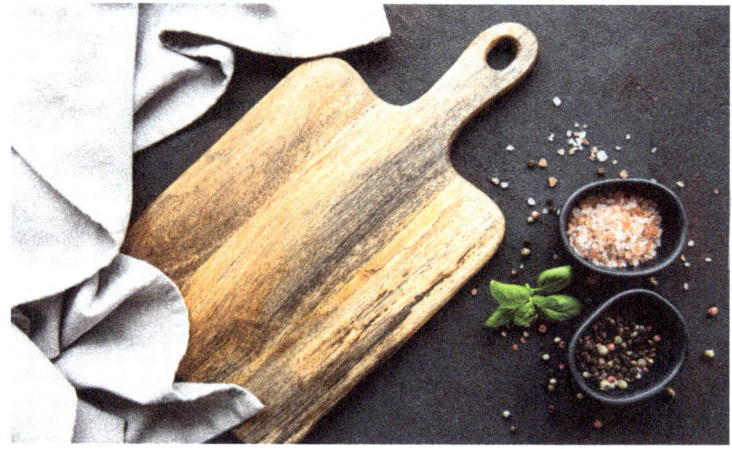

3. YOUR CHOPPING BOARD MOVES AROUND WHEN YOU CHOP

You have no idea how much this upsets me. I've watched many battle it out on a chopping board with the silly thing moving and flapping about OF COURSE you're going to hate chopping. TAKE CONTROL! Put a wet cloth or a plastic mat under the board, and you will be in chopping heaven. It's also MUCH safer, so please try this, and you'll be surprised how such a simple idea can transform your chopping woes. Once your board doesn't move around the counter you will enjoy chopping more!

4. YOU DON'T KNOW THE BASICS

Now, this is quite a broad and loose statement.
What I mean is if you know the basics of cooking, you will have the confidence to try something new.
You need to master basic skills so that you can then feel confident in the kitchen.

Use the right knife for the job; you can't use a paring knife to chop a bunch of parsley finely.
You will need to use a chef's knife or a vegetable cleaver, so make sure to battle it out with the right equipment.
If your mince or your bacon is leaking grey liquid all over the pan when you're cooking, or if your stir-fries are limp and watery and grey, then you need to adjust your cooking method.
Generally, if meat is added to a cold pan and then stirred, it will stew, seep and cook grey every single time.
The more you stir, the more it will stew! You know I'm right! Get the pan nice and hot. Do not use extra virgin olive oil for high-temperature frying; it just can't handle the heat and will smoke and burn before the pan is even hot. Use rice bran, coconut and vegetable oil; these cheap and cheerful oils can handle the heat in the kitchen. Extra virgin olive oil is like a princess: it doesn't like to get hot or sweaty or do any work, but it's really glamorous and is the perfect candidate to bling up and adorn a salad or be drizzled over cooked meat or vegetables - but it's useless at frying at high temperatures!

Remember to manage the heat in your pan.
If you add 650g cold meat drenched in a liquid marinade and, then add it to a small cold pan and then stir, you ARE DEFINITELY going to get a grey, soggy stew and not a stir-fry! Here's the solution, I don't mind repeating it:

- Get the pan swear word hot
- Add a little cheap and cheerful oil (rice bran, canola, etc). Extra virgin olive oil is excellent for dunking bread into, but it's like a princess in the kitchen…it does NOT like to get hot and sweaty and will set off the fire alarm repeatedly.
- Only add the meat to the pan if it SIZZLES!
- Don't stir until the first layer that has hit the pan is browned and sealed; if you are cooking mince, you can attack the lumps with two forks or a whisk. I always add my onion second; that way, I don't have to add extra oil to cook the onions. It makes sense, doesn't it?
- Only stir when the pan has regained its heat; you can lower the temperature in the pan once you are happy it's all sealed and now just needs to cook through.

You will seriously live happily ever after once you know these tricks!

5. YOU DON'T FEEL APPRECIATED

If you've spent an hour or two or more in the kitchen and you don't get a round of applause of course you will feel hard done by!
I always make sure I bling up my meal so when they finally see it, it looks so stunning that they at least murmur wow or oooh or similar! It's incredible what a new dish will do for your reputation!
Learn some quick and easy presentation skills and styles, and you can literally make mac cheese the star of the show!

How to Shop

The biggest problem, as I mentioned, with menu fatigue is having nothing to cook. This is the most obvious reason that you aren't enjoying cooking anymore and can take you to the heights of despair. I have a basic list of ingredients I have in stock all the time so that on those days when I haven't really planned for a real meal, I can still whip something respectable together.

Nothing is better than hitting the markets or supermarkets and taking them up on their specials.
BUT… I don't buy it if it's just too expensive or if it looks old and past its prime.
I rather buy food that is practically busting with happiness and good looks. You know what I mean when it practically jumps out and begs you to take it home! Hasn't happened to you?
It probably has, and then you had second thoughts on how you would cook it or what you would do with it and reverted to your comfort zone. That's okay. I'm here for you now!
Here's an easy breakdown of things I would love you to have in your pantry so that you can mix and match meals.

HERBS & SPICES	TINNED	SALT & PEPPER	NUTS	OTHER	VEG	DAIRY	PROTEIN
Garlic	Butter Beans	Black Salt	Pistachio	Fried Shallot	Onion	Cream	Fish
Ginger	Cannellini Beans	Pink Peppercorns	Macadamia Nuts	Laksa Paste	Cauliflower	Milk	Chicken
Turmeric	ChickPeas	Sichuan Peppercorns	Peanuts	Canola Spray	Frozen Broc	Parmesan	Beef
Ras El Hanout	Chopped Tomato	Flake Salt	Pine nuts	Peanut Oil	Fresh Greens/ Pak Choy/ Baby Spinach etc	Pecorino	Pork
Curry Powder	Tomato Passata	Table and cooking salt	Your choice	Extra Virgin Olive oil	Frozen Peas	Cheddar	Seafood
Chinese 5 Spice	Coconut Cream			Honey or Maple	Asian Kaffir Lime Leave		Tofu
Oregano	Coconut Milk			Mustards			
Marjoram				Rices and Pasta			
Sage							
Paprika							

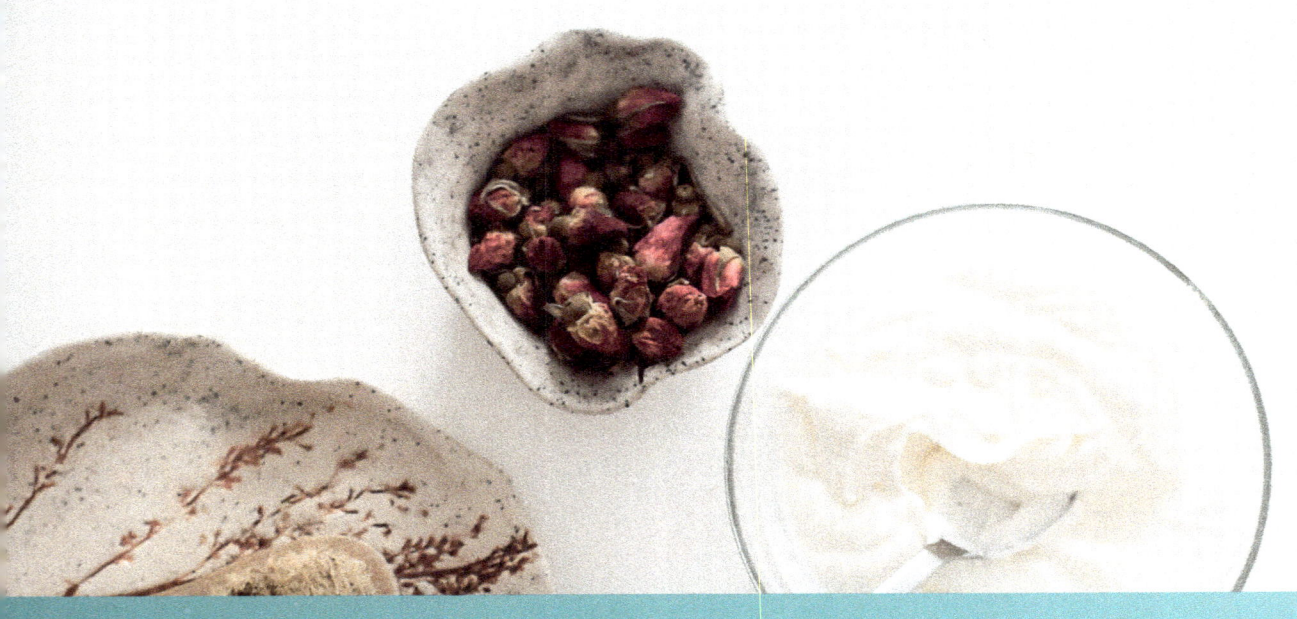

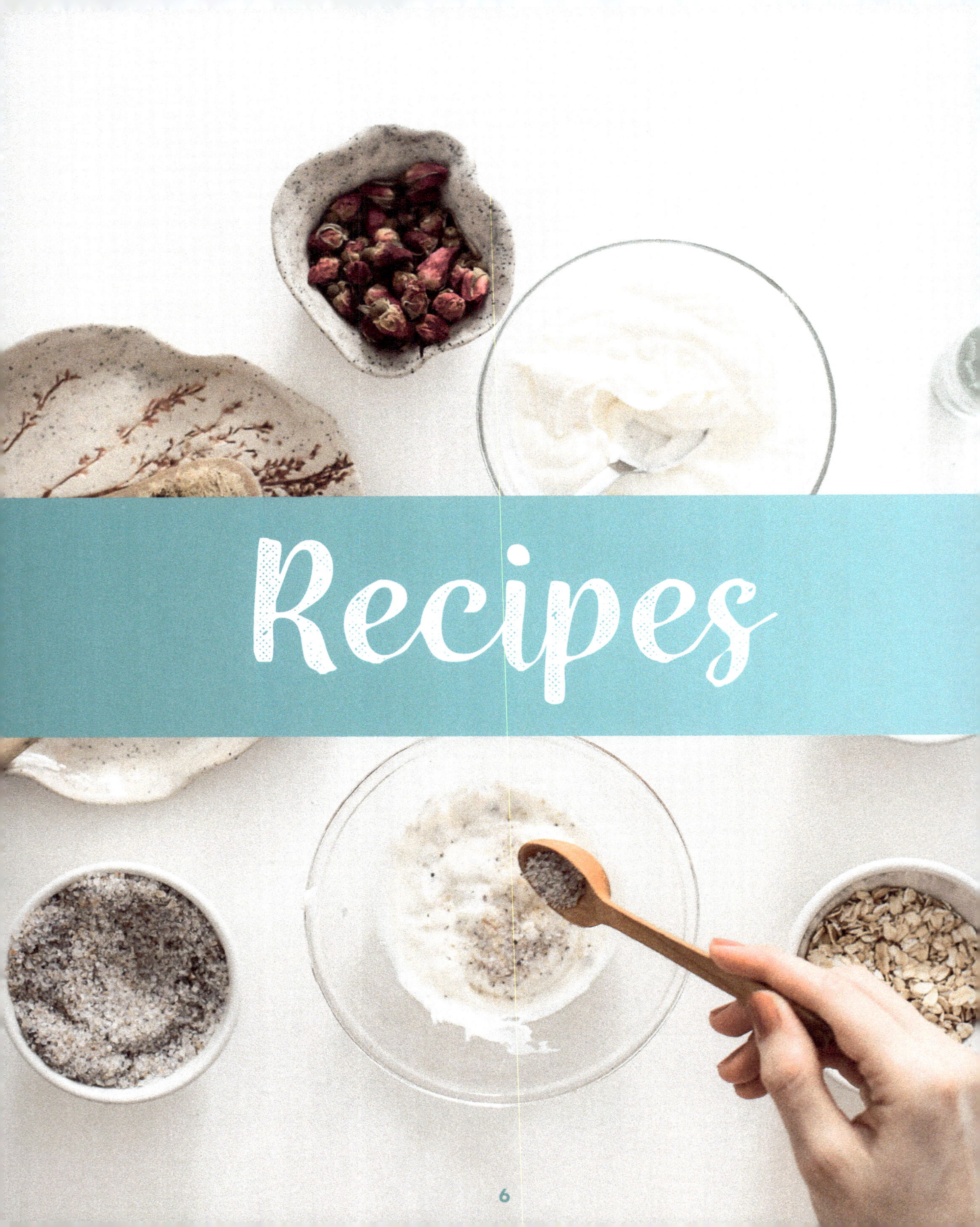

Recipes

Starters

12	Saffron, Lime & Chili infused Butternut Broth with Creamy Chive & Feta Dollop
13	Mushroom Cappuccino with Garlic, Chive & Cheese Croutons
15	The Ultimate Broccoli Salad
16	Pear & Parma Carpaccio
17	Prawn & Strawberry Skewers with Avocado & Lime Salsa
19	Culinary Bark AKA Fragrant Water Biscuits
20	Happy Yellow Butterbean Purée
21	Prosciutto High Heels for Glamorous Platters
23	Around the world with a Baked Brie Fondue

Quickies that you simply must know on the side!

25	Tempura Batter
25	Cream Cheese Pastry

Spice Mixes & Marinades

27	Ras El Hanout
27	Chermoula
27	Nam Jim Sauce
28	Whipped Butters

Quickie Meals

30	Magical Moroccan Mince Stack with Pistachio & Date Gravel
32	Rosti Cottage Pie
33	Cauliflower Paella
34	How to Cook the Perfect Steak
35	Porcini & Sage Cream with Dirty Black Fillet
37	Steak served with Baked Camembert & Fragrant Garlic
39	Beef Tenderloin with Burnt Basil & Black Pepper Butter on Vegetables
41	Steak served with Wasabi Mayonnaise

Recipes

Quickie & Perfectly Sexy Stir Fries

43	Sexy Stir Fry Ingredients
45	Peanut, Chilli, Herb Bling with Petals for Crunch
46	Sweet & Sour Marinade

Quickie Fish Dishes

49	Seared Crispy Skin Fish with Pancetta Bark & Rustic Pea Mash
50	Rustic Pea Purée

Quickie Poultry Dishes

53	One Pan Suntanned Chicken
54	Sticky Chicken with Toasted Sesame Seeds, Chickpeas & Rocket
55	How to Roast Sesame Seeds
57	Plump Sweet Potato, Sage, Bacon Stuffed Roast Chicken
58	Chilli & Pumpkin Stuffing
60	Tremendously Moist Terrific Turkey

Quickie Lamb Dishes

63	Fragrant Lamb Shoulder with Sticky Figs, Pistachio & Lemon Gravel
65	Suntanned Pan-Lamb with Dates, Mint & Pistachio Bling

Recipes

Quickie Pork Dishes

67	Pork Belly with perfect Crackling on Butterbean Purée
69	Perfect Crackling Every Time
70	Beautiful Suntanned Beer-Braised Pork Belly, Caramelised apples & Onions
71	Twice-Cooked Sticky Plum & Ginger Pork Rashers

Quickie Sides & Accompaniments

73	Chiang Mai Curry Paste
74	Famous Roasted Red Capsicum Purée
75	Gourmet Mash

Quickie Desserts & Cakes

77	Easy Panna Cotta
79	Lightest & Fluffiest Butter Cake
81	Vanilla Apple Lattice Pie
83	Carrot Cake
84	Health Muffins
86	Versatile Cheesecake
87	Mel's Family Recipe Telephone Pudding
88	White Chocolate Mousse with Vanilla & Berry Cream
89	Chef Mel's Ultimate Hot Chocolate Sauce
90	Cape Brandy Pudding: The Ultimate Winter Warmer
91	Basic Scones
94	Pumpkin, Parsley & Parmesan Scones
95	Death by Chocolate Brownie Platter
96	Chocolate Tiles
97	Complexion-Busting Chocolate Salami

THE LITTLE BLACK BOOK OF Culinary Bling

Contents

103	Culinary Lingo: It's all about the description
104	Culinary Weapons: The tools of the trade
105	Culinary Bling: Adding interest to your plate
109	Culinary Trinkets: Adding charm and accessories to your food
112	Culinary Spray Tans & Salts: Adding colour and flavour
113	Culinary Flavour Dusts: Adding personality to your meal
114	Culinary High Heels: Adding height to your meal

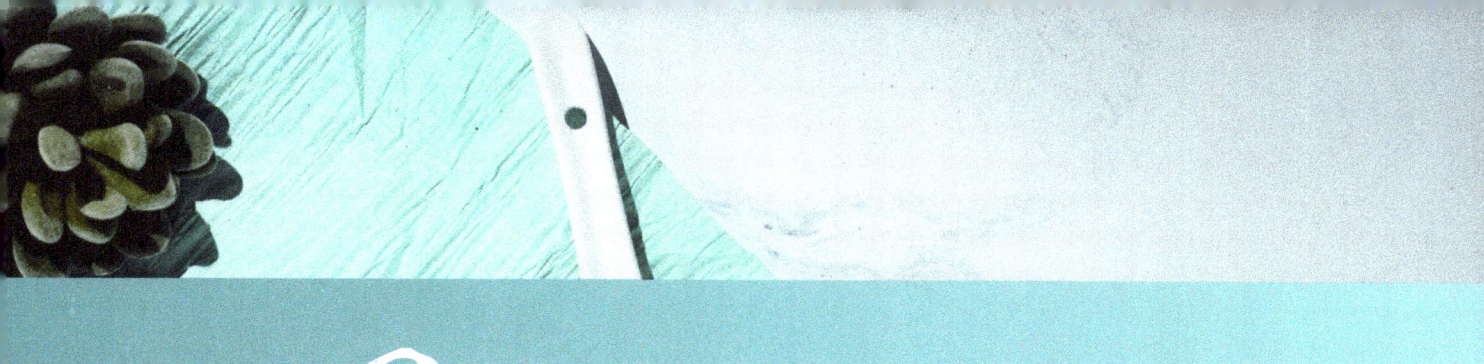

Starters

SEXY SOUPS | SALADS & OTHER QUICKIE STARTERS

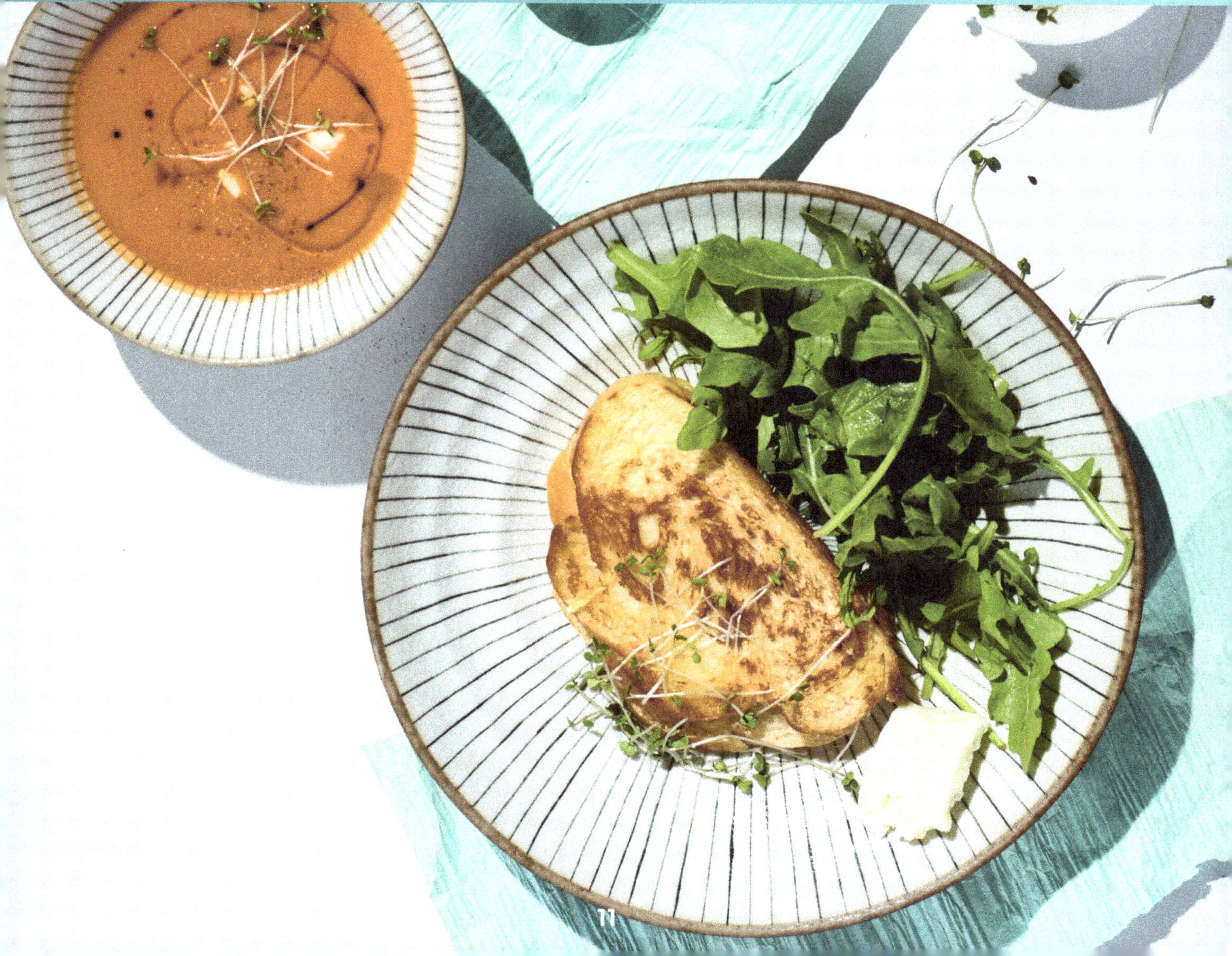

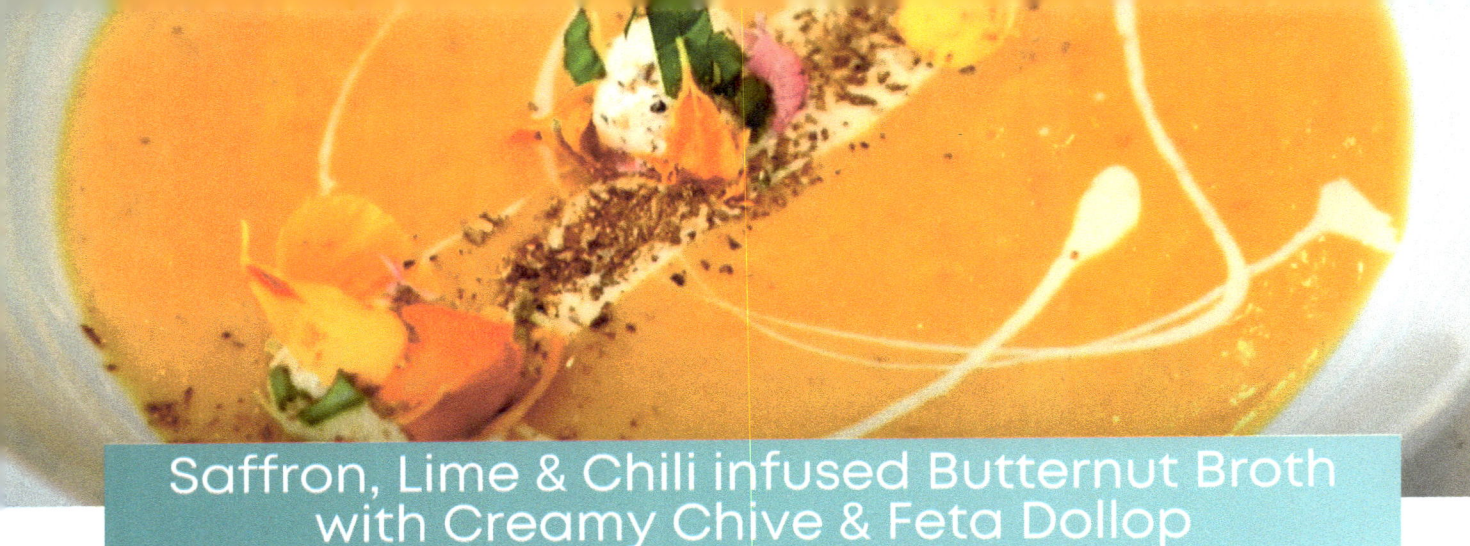

Saffron, Lime & Chili infused Butternut Broth with Creamy Chive & Feta Dollop

SERVINGS: 6-8

INGREDIENTS

2 teaspoons butter or olive oil
2 medium onions chopped
2 cloves garlic, crushed
2 good pinches of saffron
or use 1 teaspoon of turmeric powder instead
600g -1 kg butternut, sweet potato or pumpkin
cubed into 1 or 2 cm cubes (perfect way to use leftovers)
2 litres of good chicken or vegetable stock
Salt and pepper to season
Zest of one lime

1 small chilli crushed (or use more if you like!)
2 tablespoons Parmesan cheese or use mature cheddar (optional)
80 – 100 ml fresh cream
100 g Danish-style feta mixed into a paste with
1 bunch of chives or spring onions, finely chopped
Alternatively, use Greek feta blended with a few tablespoons of cream until smooth!

METHOD

Nothing is more satisfying than a healthy and nutritious bowl of fabulous pumpkin or butternut soup to warm the cockles of your heart. Here's a really easy and very sexy soup for you to try. It's all about adding a delicious dollop of creamy chive and feta for some texture, flavour and culinary bling. Not everyone can get their hands on saffron so do not fear, I have accounted for that in the recipe. Read on fabulous foodie.

Fry the onions in the oil or butter with the garlic until just soft. Now add the saffron or turmeric and finely cubed butternut and the stock. Allow to come to a boil and cook for about 15 -25 minutes until the butternut is soft. Now add the zest, chilli and cheese (optional) as well as the **fresh cream**.
Remove from heat and blend with a stick blender, and blend until ridiculously velvety and smooth. If this is too thick for your liking add some more stock and thin it down.
When you serve simply garnish with dollops of feta and chives, and even some fried shallots for crunch!

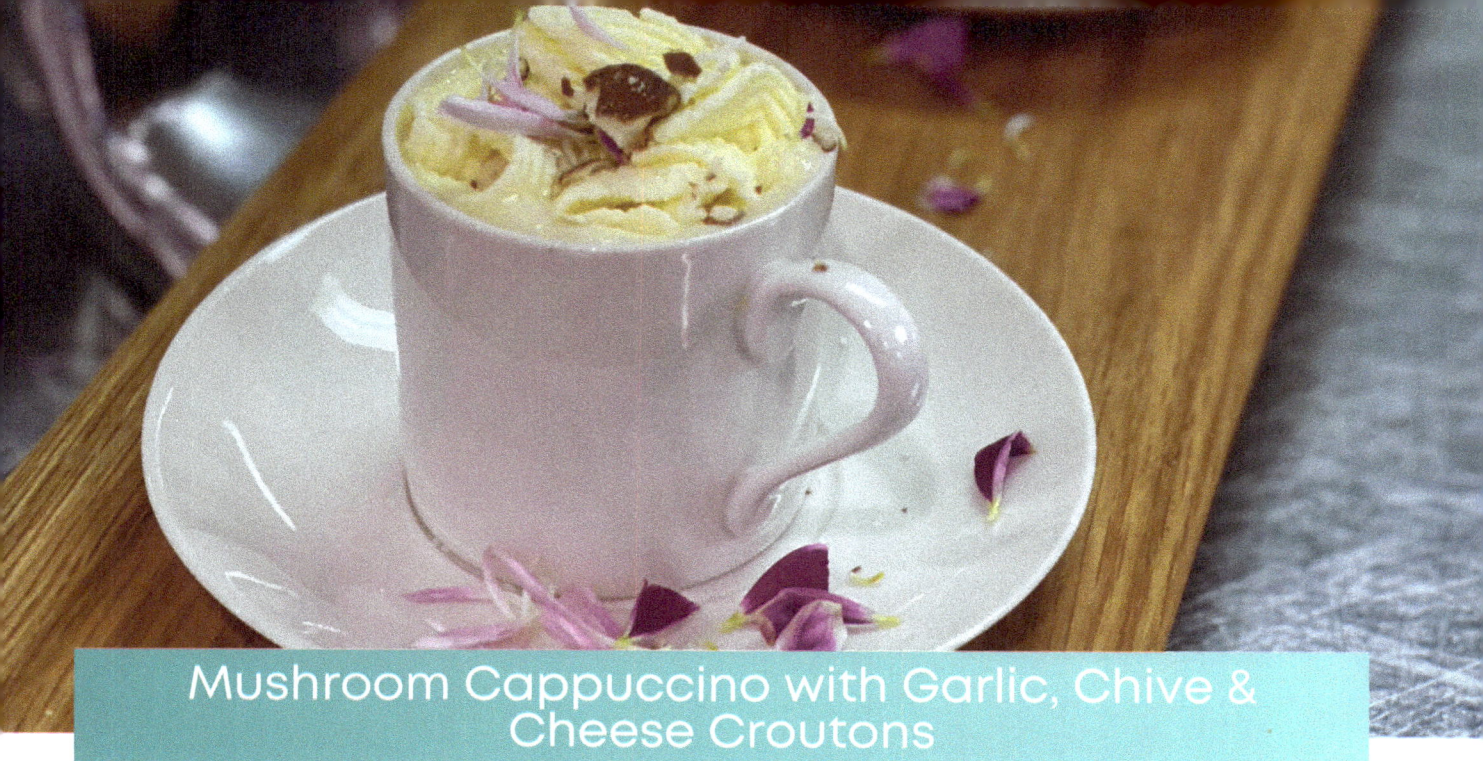

Mushroom Cappuccino with Garlic, Chive & Cheese Croutons

SERVINGS: 4-6

INGREDIENTS

1 small onion, finely chopped
1 clove garlic, crushed
500 g mushrooms
500 ml stock, mushroom or vegetable
10 ml corn flour to thicken
100 ml pouring cream
100 ml cream, whipped
Season with salt and pepper
4 slices baguette slices, toasted, then topped with Parmesan, chives and garlic

METHOD

Fry the onion in oil or butter until soft and fragrant, then add the garlic and sliced mushrooms. Sauté until soft, then add the stock and corn flour and allow to cook through.
Season with salt and pepper, serve in a teacup with a saucer, and then top with whipped cream and serve with the croutons.
Add pouring cream... delicious.

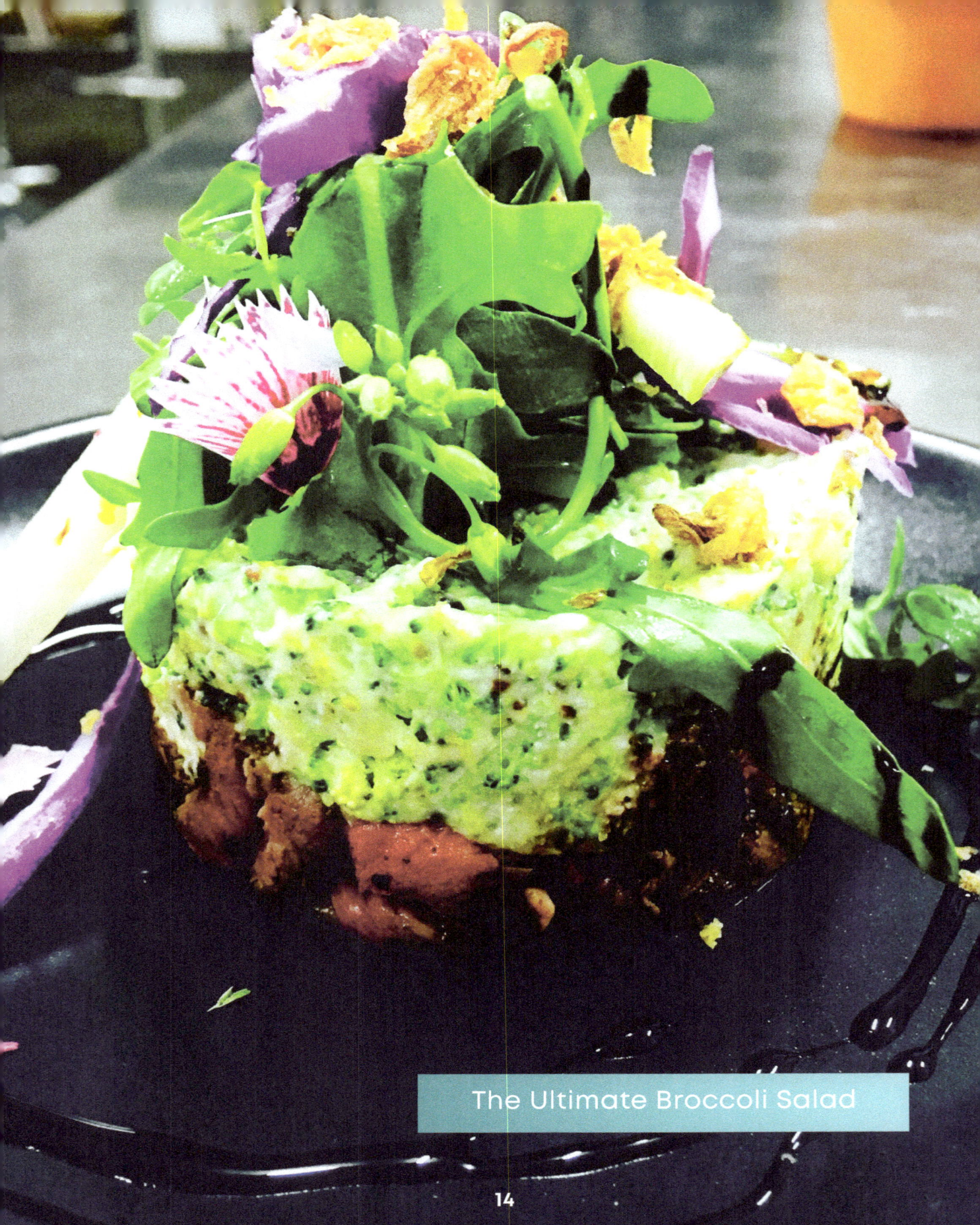
The Ultimate Broccoli Salad

The Ultimate Broccoli Salad

SERVINGS: 4-6

INGREDIENTS

1 small head of broccoli, rinsed and then chopped (about four cups)
1 pink lady apple, sliced
1 baby bulb fennel finely chopped (optional)
1 cup plain fat-free yogurt
1 tablespoon grainy mustard
Salt and freshly ground pepper

METHOD

**Bursting with goodness and taste, this unusual salad takes almost no time to prepare and is not cooked.
Don't worry about eating broccoli raw; it tastes even better this way, I promise!
Another thing is that you can add just about anything else to it, depending on your favourites.
Lean bacon bits, smoked chicken, cheeses...it can be quite glamorous, actually.**

This is your basic salad, which is divine just as it is….
If you start making it often, though, you may want to 'spice' it up and add some protein to make it a main course salad. You can see how I've layered this in the photo on the previous page.

**Add fresh baby spinach leaves and rocket leaves.
Roughly chopped basil.
Sliced smoked chicken breasts
Rare roast beef sliced or shaved.
Cooked lean bacon bits.
Low-fat feta.
Dried Cranberries.**

The possibilities are endless!

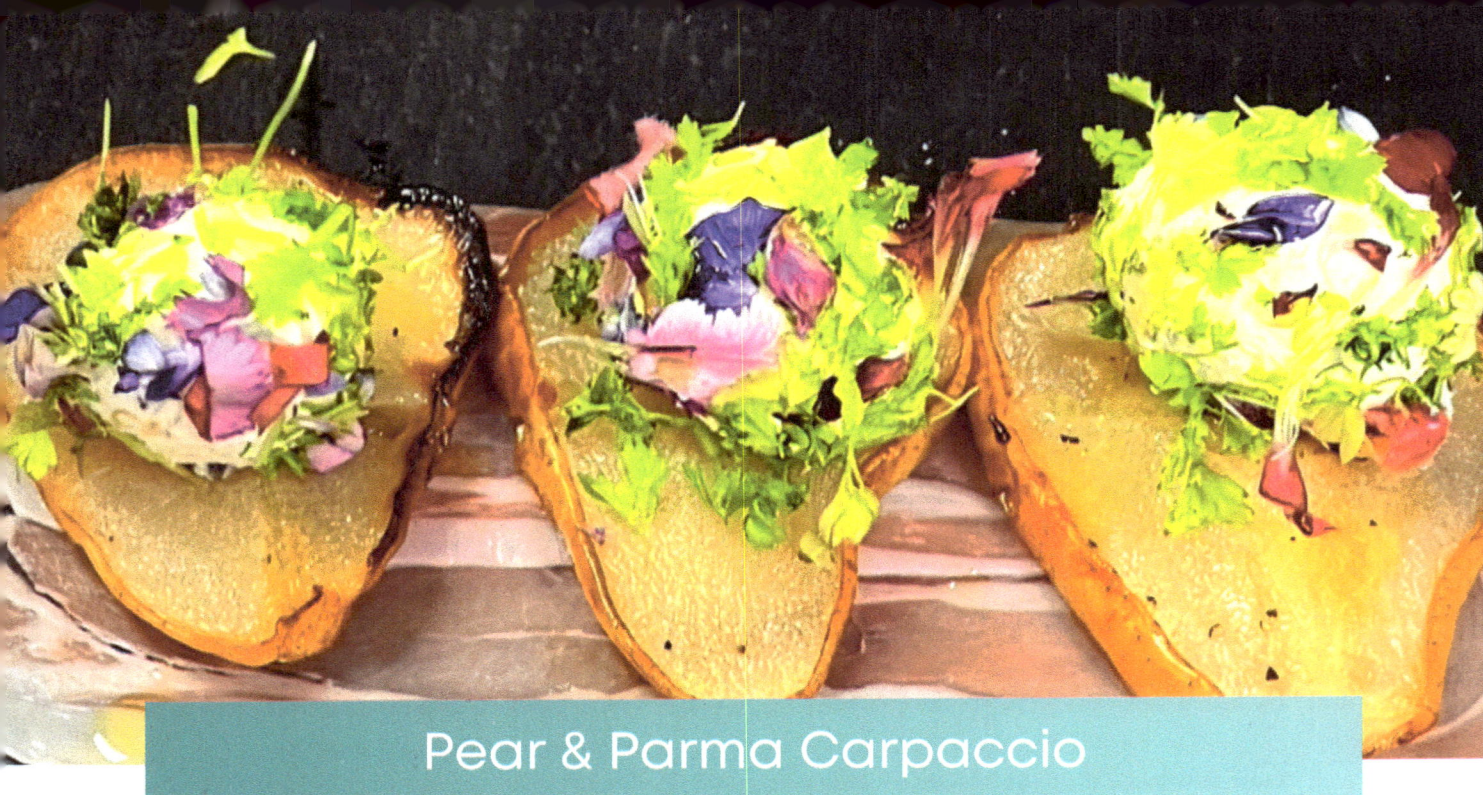

Pear & Parma Carpaccio

SERVINGS: 4-6

INGREDIENTS

2-3 pears/apples/quince sliced thickly and roasted
2-3 sliced prosciutto or parma per person
1 tablespoon goats cheese/cream cheese per person
edible flowers and herb fronds
chives chopped up and placed in a bowl

DRESSING
20ml honey
80ml verjuice
50ml olive oil
(all mixed together)
salt and pepper to taste

METHOD

Place the sliced pears/apples/quince on a greased baking tray and then bake at 225-250°C for about 20-25 minutes until dried and crisp! Place one slice of parma ham/prosciutto onto a plate.
Mix the goat's cheese in a bowl until nice and smooth.
Roll 1 tablespoon of the cheese into a ball and then roll through the chopped-up herbs and petals. And top onto your baked fruit slice.
Serve with micro herbs, rocket, and some of the dressing.

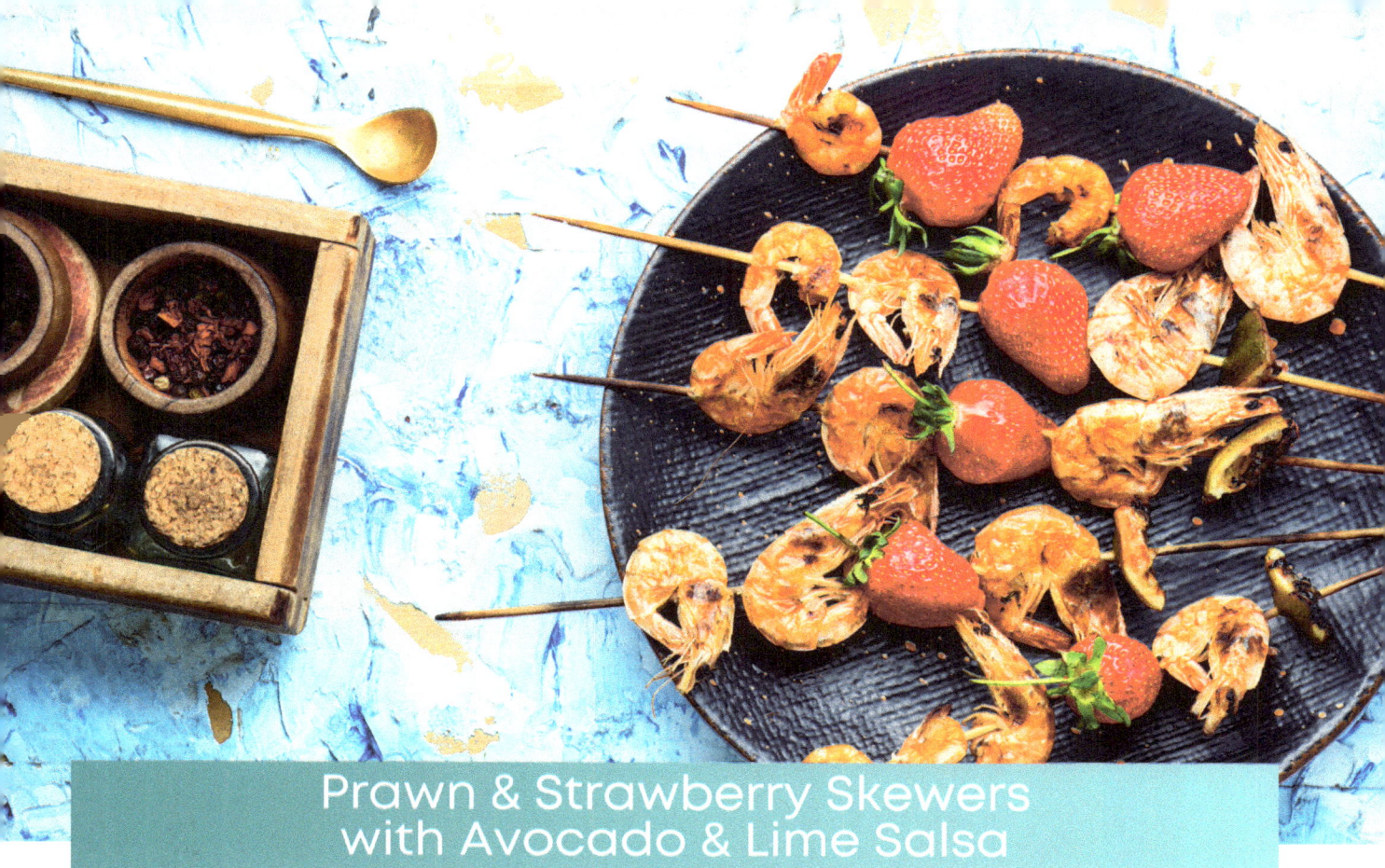

Prawn & Strawberry Skewers with Avocado & Lime Salsa

SERVINGS: 4-6

INGREDIENTS

300g - 500g prawn meat, flash-fried in 1 tablespoon butter
1 punnet strawberries, hulled and halved, *or use mango if in season*
3 ripe avocados, halved and skin removed, cubed
1 small red onion finely chopped *or a bunch of spring onions*
2 red or green chillies, sliced or chopped
2 small ripe tomatoes finely chopped
fresh lime to squeeze
Salt and freshly ground pepper

METHOD

Cook the prawns hot and fast in 1 tablespoon butter until cooked; allow to cool.
Place the cooked prawns, strawberries and chillies on the skewers.

Make the salsa by gently mixing the cubed avo, chopped onions, chillies, tomatoes and lime juice. Season well. Serve drizzled over the skewers..so fresh and delicious with all the flavours working together!

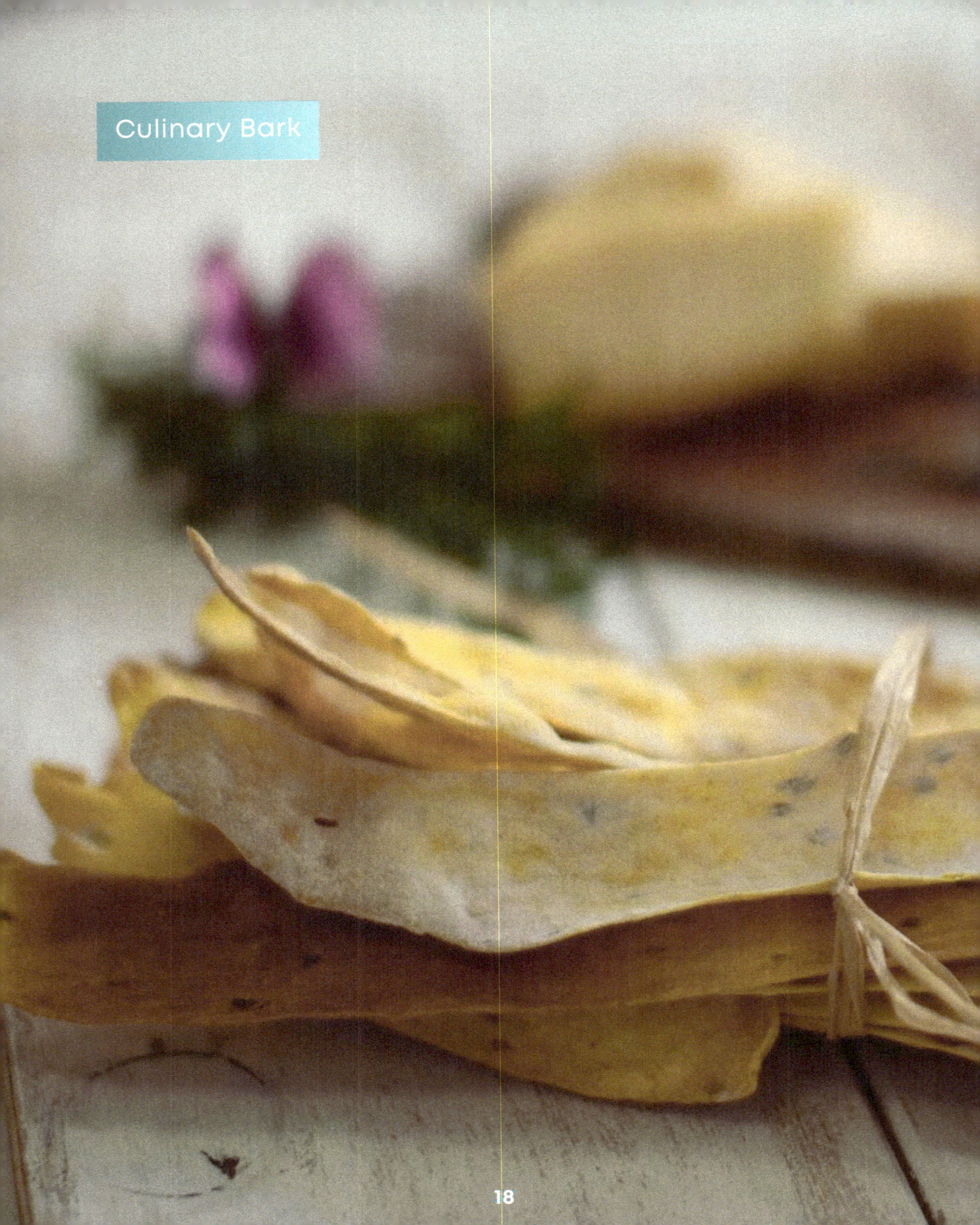

Culinary Bark

Culinary Bark AKA Fragrant Water Biscuits

SERVINGS: 6-8

INGREDIENTS

1 cup plain flour
80ml water and 20ml melted butter/olive oil
(must be 100ml or just a bit more liquid in total to bind)
Seasoning to match your cheese
(nigella seeds, pink pepper, black salt, lavender, rosemary)
BLING - Petals, spices, etc., depending on what you need to match!

METHOD

When was the last time you were given a round of applause when you served your cheese board at a party? If the answer is no, perhaps you must swap from the dreary store-bought water crackers and super-expensive lavish and start making your own designer culinary bark.

Not only will these inexpensive water biscuits or lavosh bling up your next cheeseboard, charcuterie platter or just plain old hummus, but you will save yourself SO much money as these are so easy on the pocket. They don't take long at all; you can make them just before you need them OR bake them a few weeks or months in advance and store them in the fridge or freezer in an airtight container. Head to my YouTube videos to see how these are made if you want, but these are super easy.
You can also then match the water cracker to the cheese or dip or ingredient they will serve as a platform for.
Think lemon zest and cracked black pepper and dill for smoked salmon pate. Think rose petals and Nigella seeds for a Middle Eastern Dip or hummus. Think black salt and rosemary for a deliciously creamy brie or camembert. Have fun and create! About a teaspoon of each bling should be enough to get noticed.
Poppy seeds and pepper would be just as groovy!

Mix flour, water/oil, seasonings and bling until combined. To prevent the dough from being annoying and sticking to your hands, sprinkle it and the counter surface with a dredging of flour. Always do this before handling the dough. Knead for about 3 minutes until the dough is nice and soft and pliable. Take a teaspoonful of dough and roll it out into long, thin biscuits, making sure you use lots of flour underneath or roll in between two pieces of baking paper to make sure they don't stick to the counter. Bake hot and fast on an ungreased baking tray for about 3-8 minutes at 200°C. They should be brittle and not too brown! Store them in an airtight container until you want to use them.

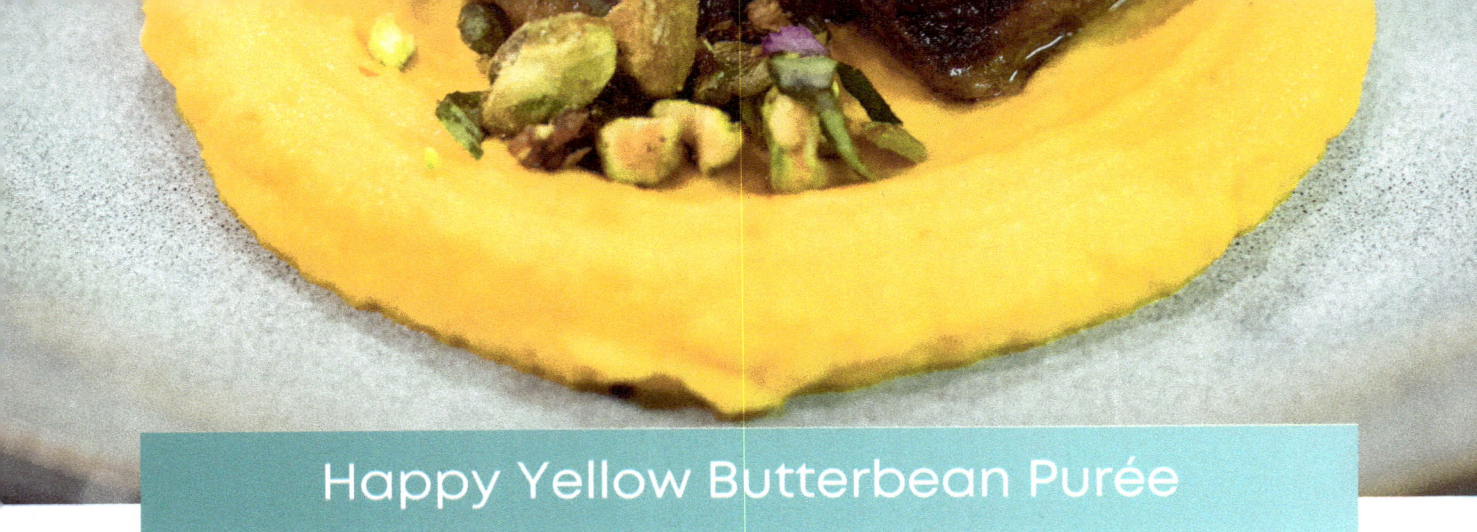

Happy Yellow Butterbean Purée

SERVINGS: 6

INGREDIENTS

2 tins butterbeans, drained
1/4 cup cream or milk *or simply use stock if you want to omit dairy*
1 chicken/mushroom/vegetable stock cube or use a teaspoon of stock powder
1 clove garlic, crushed
¼ teaspoon turmeric
¼ veggie or chicken stock cube to taste

METHOD

Guys this recipe is just too easy. If you have any roast carrots, butternut or sweet potato left over in the fridge, feel free to throw about half a cup of that roasted goodness in here too.

Place all ingredients in a large saucepan and heat over a really low heat, stirring regularly for about 10 minutes until wonderfully hot. Once the beans are heated through, simply mash with the metal head of a stick blender OR place in a food processor once cooled slightly.
Either process completely, or leave slightly chunky for a more rustic mash!
Feel free to add hot water to make this puree thinner if you don't want it as thick.
You can make this as thick or as thin as you like. And if you have leftovers, you can repurpose this as a sexy dip (drizzle with olive oil, crushed pistachios and dukkah).
Serve either serve chunky or as a puree.

NOTE

You can change the flavour of these beans to suit or match your meal. These beans can take on multiple personalities so have fun!
Add a teaspoon of chopped rosemary if you are matching lamb.
Add a teaspoon of grainy mustard or horseradish if you are matching beef or pork.
Add a teaspoon of curry powder if you are serving this with a curry.
Add smoked garlic and smoked paprika to match a Spanish theme.

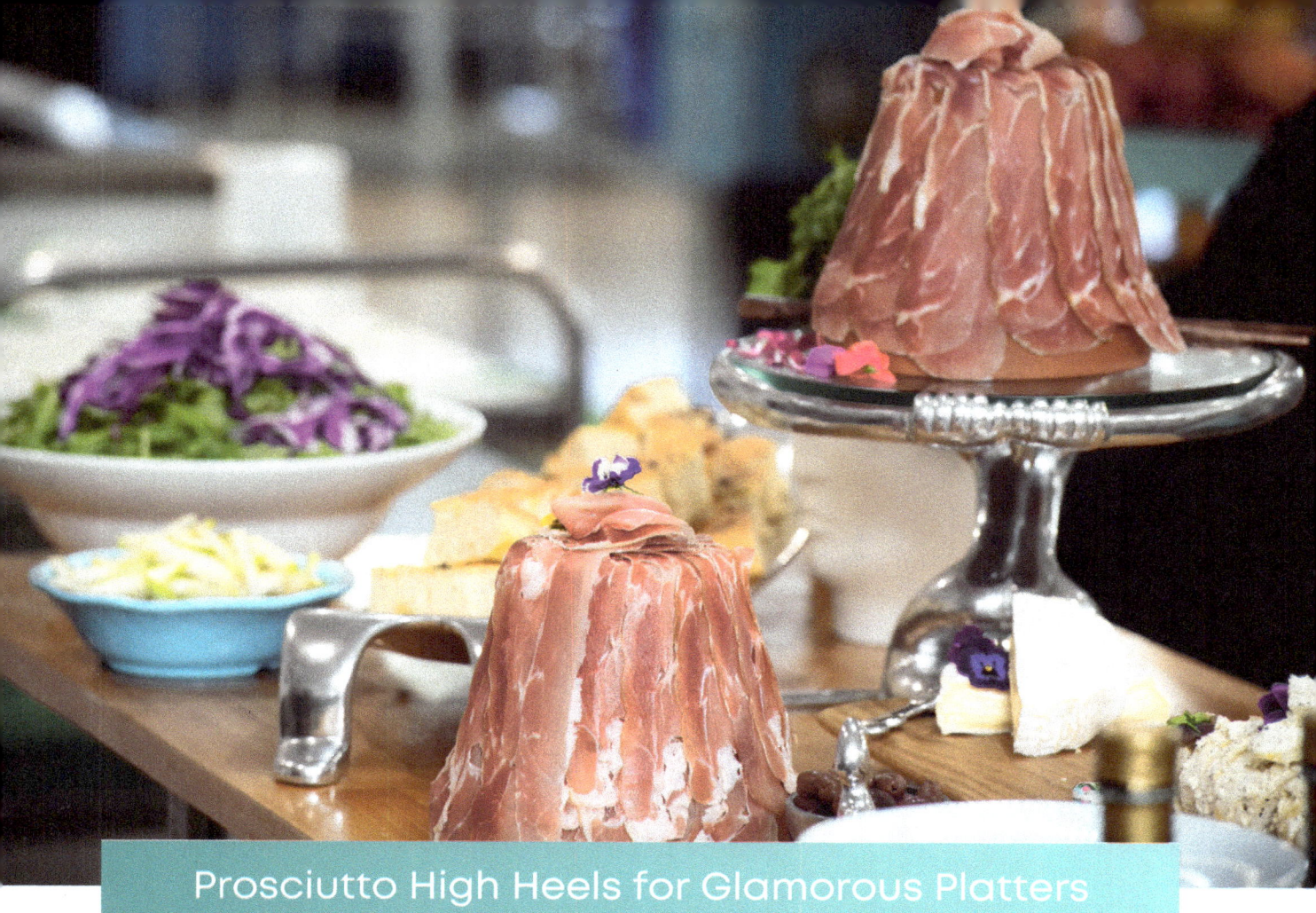

Prosciutto High Heels for Glamorous Platters

SERVINGS: 4-6

INGREDIENTS

16-20 slices of prosciutto/parma ham cut to 1mm thickness at your deli
1 medium terracotta pot or similar vessel
Figs or herbs or edible flowers to garnish

METHOD

Turn the terracotta pot upside down and then start draping the prosciutto or parma ham over the pot with the fat side presenting on the outside.
Continue to drape until you have covered the bowl, I usually allow 2-3 slices per person depending on what this is being served with.
Garnish with cut figs, petals, or sprigs of fresh herbs.
You can do this the day before and then wrap it with cling film or plastic wrap.
It's perfect for cheese boards, and feasting platters and is highly mobile and so very glamorous!

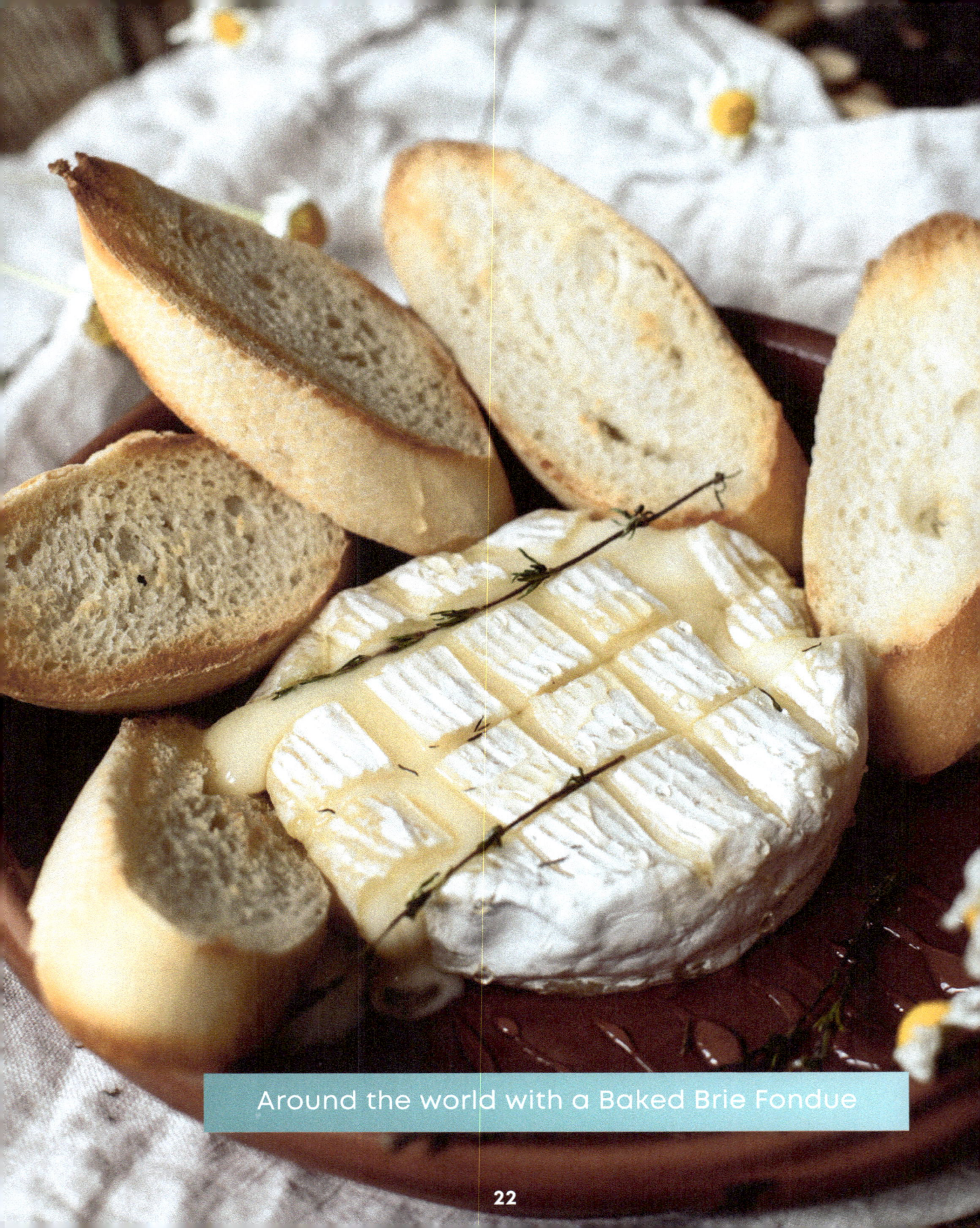

Around the world with a Baked Brie Fondue

Around the world with a Baked Brie Fondue

METHOD

This is a gorgeous and glamorous take on the everyday cheeseboard. Baking Brie or even a delicious Camembert will transform it into the most delicious baked oozy cheesy treat, and the best part is that it's super simple.

We can also transform this fantastic fondue into many global flavours by adding a few glorious ingredients to change the theme. Try these or try your own idea; you'll be doing this dish for many years to come. You'll have travelled the world in no time!

For all the recipes below, start with brie and place it on an ovenproof plate, I use a soup bowl or similar (most of them are ovenproof!)

FRENCH INFLUENCE

Make a paste with 1 clove of minced garlic and 1 teaspoon of chopped tarragon/rosemary/thyme and the rub over the cheese to coat it in this fragrant paste. Bake for 8-12 minutes in a hot oven of 200c until it has puffed up and the cheese is oozy and melting. Garnish with freshly chopped edible petals like roses, borage, pansies, dianthus or carnations.

MIDDLE EASTERN INFLUENCE

Place a tablespoon of creamed or plain honey on the cheese and bake for 8-12 minutes in a hot oven of 200c until it has puffed up and the cheese is oozy and melting and the honey is caramelised and melted. Now add a teaspoon of chopped nuts and a light dusting of cumin powder or ras el hanout spice and serve garnished with the petals I've mentioned above.

AFRICAN INFLUENCE

Bake for 8-12 minutes in a hot oven of 200c until it has puffed up and the cheese is oozy and melting. Garnish with freshly chopped chilli, biltong/jerky chopped up really fine and a little bit of lemon or lime zest...garnish with petals and serve.

SPANISH INFLUENCE

Chop about 80g chorizo sausage up until it looks like mince, fry quickly in a hot pan until just browning, add 2 tablespoons finely sliced onion and a hefty sprinkle of paprika. Add a teaspoon of lemon zest and then place this on the cheese and bake for 8-12 minutes in a hot oven of 200c until it has puffed up and the cheese is oozy and melting. Garnish with strips of fire-roasted capsicum diced finely and a sprinkle of freshly chopped parsley.

STICKY ASIAN

Mix 1 tablespoon of plum jam to a paste with half a teaspoon of fresh ginger and place on top of the cheese. Bake for 8-12 minutes in a hot oven of 200c until it puffed up and the cheese is oozy and melting.

Quickies that you simply must know on the side!

TEMPURA | PASTRY | SPICE MIXES | MARINADES | WHIPPED BUTTERS

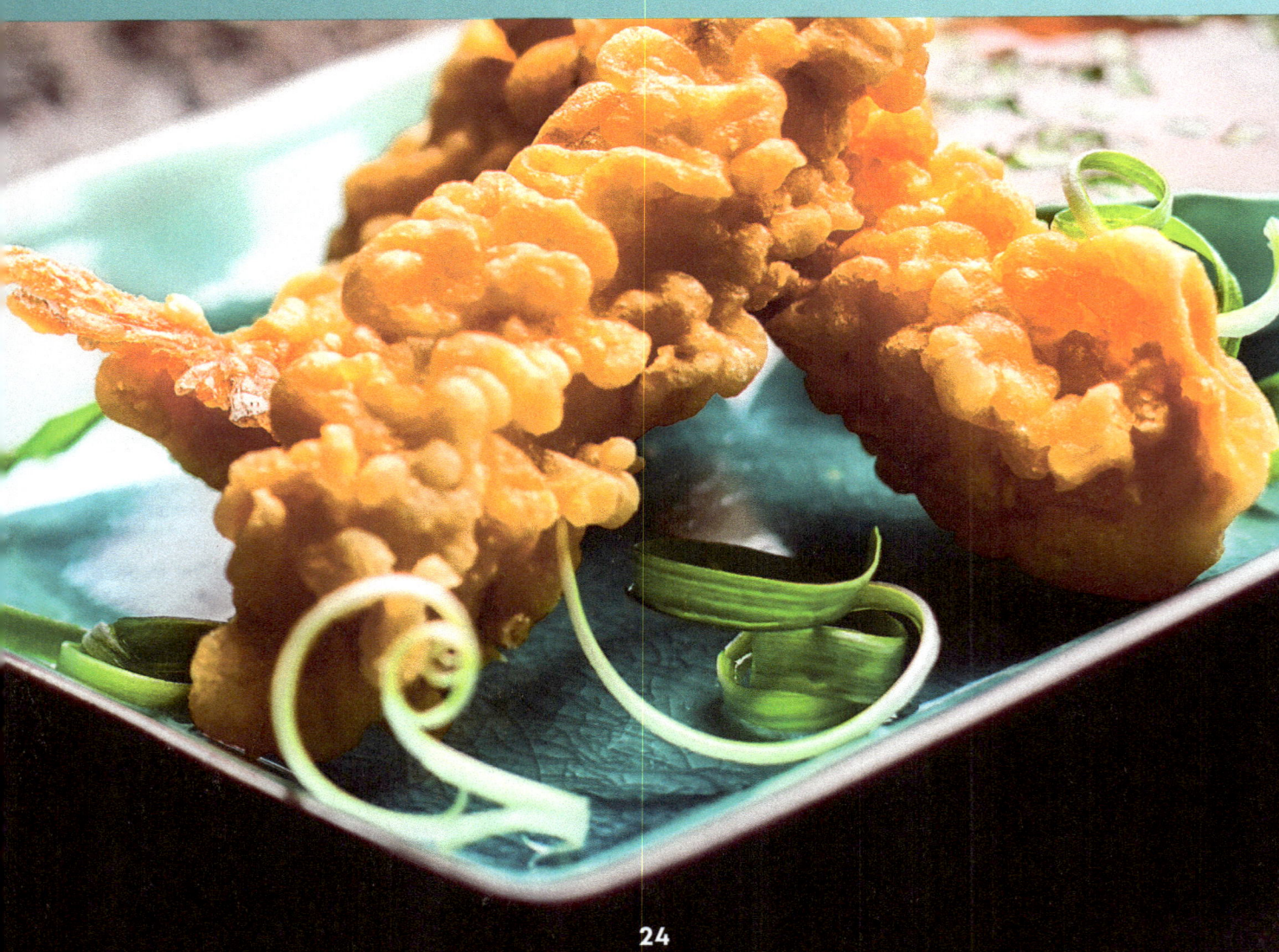

Tempura Batter

SERVINGS: 4-6

INGREDIENTS

½ cup cornflour
½ cup plain flour
1.5 cup soda or water ICE COLD
1 egg beaten

METHOD

The trick to an excellent crunchy batter is using freezing-cold liquid! Place ingredients in a bowl and mix to make a thin runny batter. Dust the item to be coated in a bit of flour, then into the batter and straight into some waiting hot vegetable oil. Cook till golden and then drain and serve!

Cream Cheese Pastry

SERVINGS: 4-8

INGREDIENTS

125g butter
200g flour
Pinch salt
125g cream cheese or crème fraîche

BLING: Add matching bling to really show your guests you care!
Add 1 teaspoon black pepper and 1 teaspoon lemon zest to really get a round of applause for this, you can really mix and match it depending on your filling!

METHOD

Grate the butter into the flour and then pinch in till the flour resembles breadcrumbs, and the butter is evenly distributed. Add the salt, bling, and cream cheese and mix through or use a food processor to combine. Do not overwork the dough! Roll into a dough ball, then cover and chill for about an hour before rolling out and using as desired! Perfect for sweet or savoury dishes.

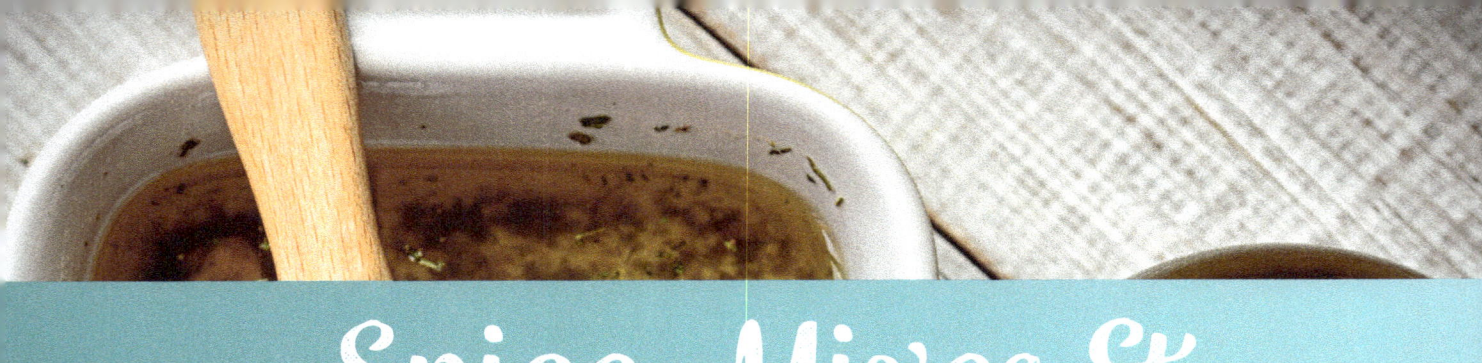

Spice Mixes & Marinades

"SECRETS, ESPECIALLY WITH COOKING, ARE BEST SHARED SO THAT THE CUISINE LIVES ON."
– BO SONGVISAVA

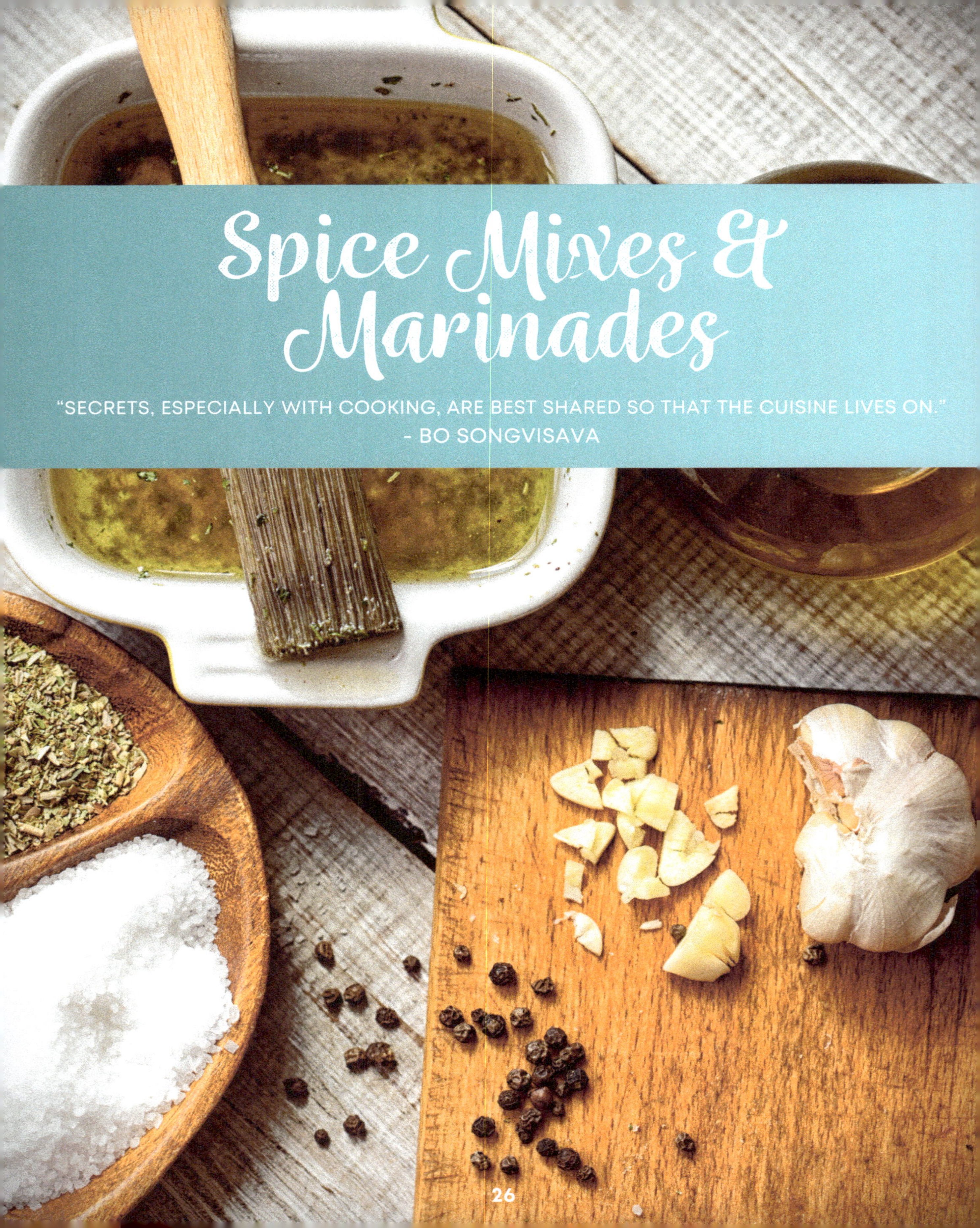

Ras El Hanout

INGREDIENTS

- 2 teaspoons black peppercorns
- 1 teaspoon ground ginger
- 2 teaspoon cumin seeds
- 2 teaspoon coriander seeds
- 1 teaspoon cinnamon
- 1 teaspoon nutmeg
- ½ teaspoon cardamom
- 1 teaspoon paprika
- ¼ teaspoon cloves
- 3 teaspoons turmeric
- 1 teaspoon salt
- 1 teaspoon ground allspice
- 1 teaspoon safflower or rose petals

METHOD

Either pound in a pestle and mortar or blend in a grinder to form a fragrant powder.

Chermoula

INGREDIENTS

- 1 cup oil
- 1 teaspoon ground cumin
- 1 teaspoon chilli powder
- 1 teaspoon salt
- 1 large red onion minced or finely chopped
- 3 cloves garlic
- 1 teaspoon turmeric
- 1 teaspoon black pepper
- 1 teaspoon paprika
- 1 teaspoon ground cinnamon
- 1 cup coriander leaves
- 1 cup parsley leaves

METHOD

Simply whizz together in a food processor. Delicious as a drizzle over almost anything.

Nam Jim Sauce

INGREDIENTS

- Half cup fresh coriander/use roots too!
- 2 teaspoons minced ginger
- 1-3 red and or green chilli (use more if you like!)
- 60ml fresh lime juice
- 30-45 ml fish sauce
  (balance to your preferred taste, I like mine saltier!)
- 1 tablespoon palm or brown sugar
- 1 cup red onion chopped
- 1 tablespoon peanut/avocado or vegetable oil
- 3 tablespoons mint chopped

METHOD

Place all ingredients into a food processor or blender and simply whizz together.

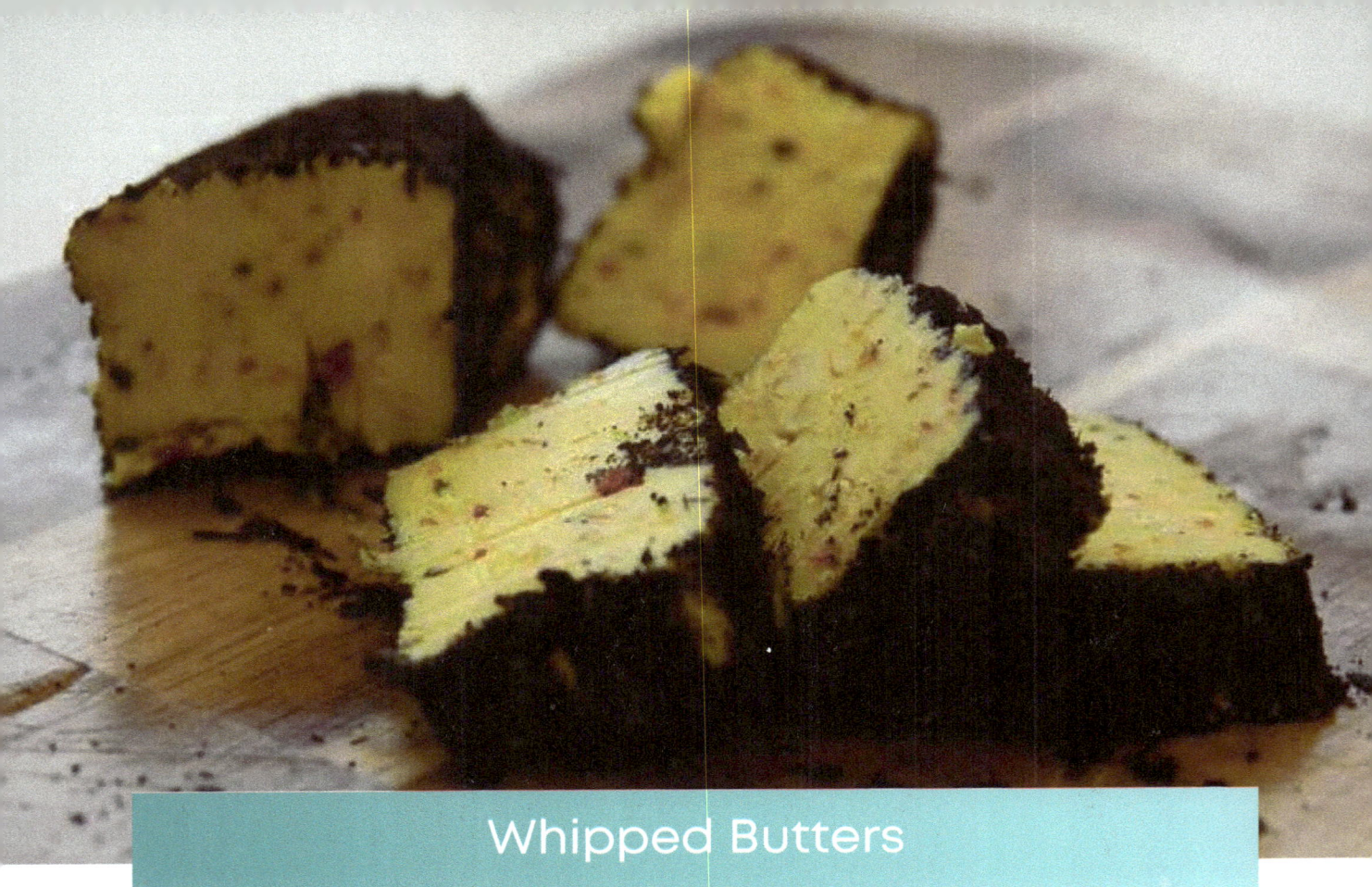

Whipped Butters

Whipped butters are so sexy and so easy.
By whipping butter you get the most amazingly light texture and colour from it.
It's a real transformation!

METHOD

Simply cube salted or unsalted butter and place in your mixer with the whisk attachment.
Allow to beat until pale and fluffy, this will take some time.
At first, it will just look thick and yellow, and then as it heats and whisks it will become lighter and fluffier and practically heavenly. Now you add the bling you need to match the dish you are serving this with.
Whip about 250g at a time because this can be left in the fridge or freezer until needed.
Then, you need at least two tablespoons of your chosen bling to make this shine.

VARIATONS

Think truffle tapenade through your whipped butter.
Think food processed to a powder-dried mushroom whipped butter.
Think turmeric, chilli and Thai lime leaf whipped butter.
Think chive and cracked black pepper whipped butter.
Think garlic, chives and parsley whipped butter.

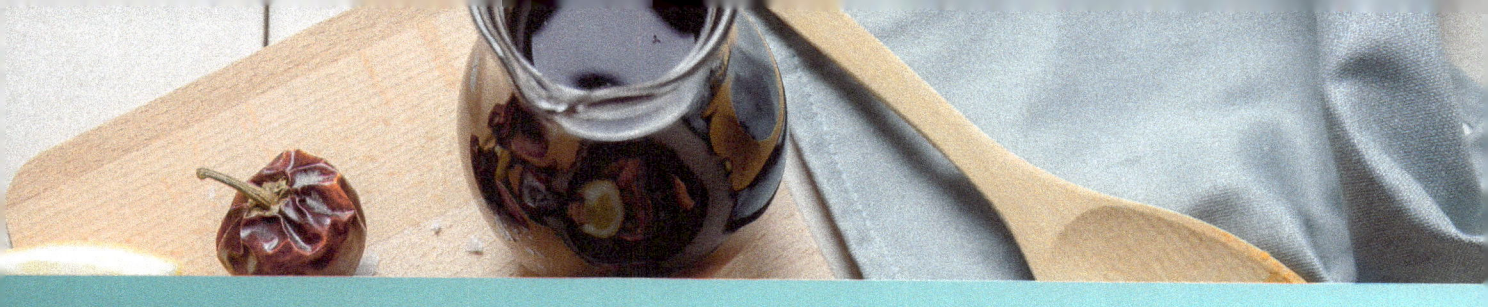

Quickie Meals

MINCE | PIES | PAELLA | STEAKS

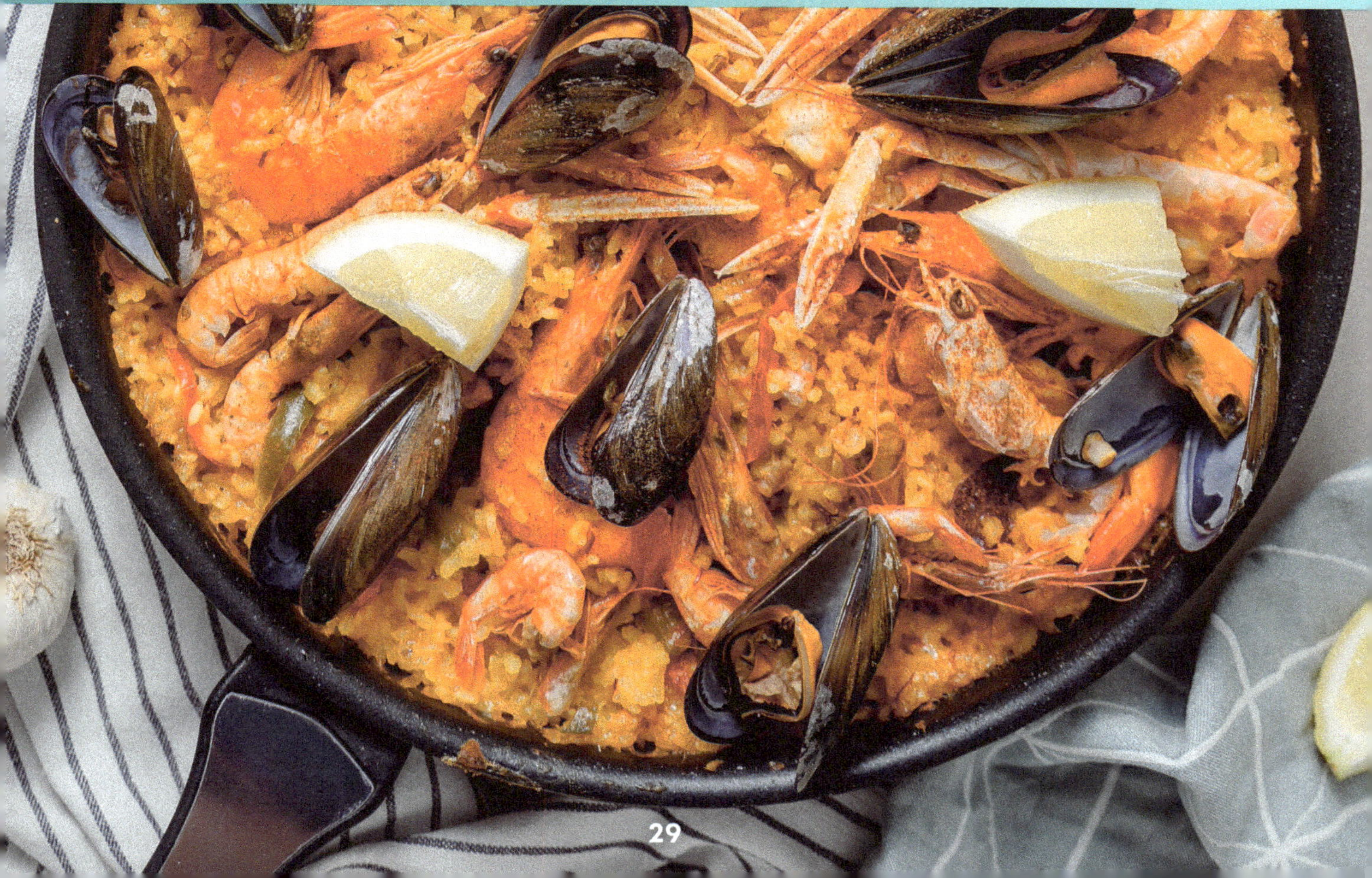

Magical Moroccan Mince Stack with Pistachio & Date Gravel

SERVINGS: 4-6

INGREDIENTS

MOROCCAN MINCE STACK

2 squirts of canola or rice bran cooking spray
800g lean beef mince
(fluff this up with your hands so it's nice, loose, fluffy & and not in 1 big block)
1 large onion, finely diced
1 clove garlic, crushed (optional)
1 tablespoon Ras el Hanout
(you can make your own using 1 teaspoon cumin powder, 1/2 teaspoon cardamom powder and 1/2 teaspoon coriander/cilantro powder)
1 teaspoon turmeric
1/2 cup finely diced fennel
or you could use grated carrot/zucchini
1 tin chickpeas, drained & rinsed
1 cup or tin chopped tomatoes
2 tablespoons tomato paste or passata
1 vegetable or beef stock cube crumbled to a powder
Salt and pepper to season
About 1 teaspoon of lemon zest

PISTACHIO & DATE GRAVEL

1-2 tablespoons pistachios, *bashed or chopped to a nice coarse gravel*
2 tablespoons finely chopped dates
Dried rose petals, but if you don't have that:
grate in some lemon zest (1/2 teaspoon) and 1 tablespoon finely chopped parsley or coriander/cilantro for colour

METHOD

Grease a large pan with the oil spray and heat the pan until it's just about smoking hot. The mince MUST sizzle when it hits the pan.

Now add the mince you have broken up in the packaging or a bowl so it is loose and fluffy already. Put the mince into the pan. IT SHOULD SIZZLE nice and loud and sexy.

DO NOT STIR. I know you are worried about this burning and you are also worried about lumps, but let the mince brown and seal on the first side you put down FIRST and let the pan heat up again and THEN you can stir ever so slightly just to get some more mince onto the base of the pan. My favourite mince 'fluffer' is one of those cheap plastic-coated whisks you get at the supermarket with only about 4 loops. If you don't have one of those use a strong plastic spoon or egg flip to break down the mince.

Once the mince is brown and fragrant and sexy ALL BY ITSELF, then and only then, do you add the finely chopped onion and garlic. There should be a good amount of fat rendered out of the mince during your amazing sizzling at a nice high heat.

You can stir as much as you like now by the way. That mince is SEALED off!

Now add the spices, stock powder and seasoning and stir through. Amazing colour isn't it? Finally, add the chopped tomatoes and passata and the chickpeas and you're practically done. Turn down the heat and let that all cook through and then add the lemon zest and it's ready to serve. This way of cooking will not only save you time, BUT it will add valuable flavour and vibrant personality to your otherwise boring mince. I love to get creative with my mince and change the spices thus changing the flavour. I pack mine into a food stacker and serve it with a yogurt swirl, the pistachio and date gravel, and just a twist of fresh, peppery rocket leaves.

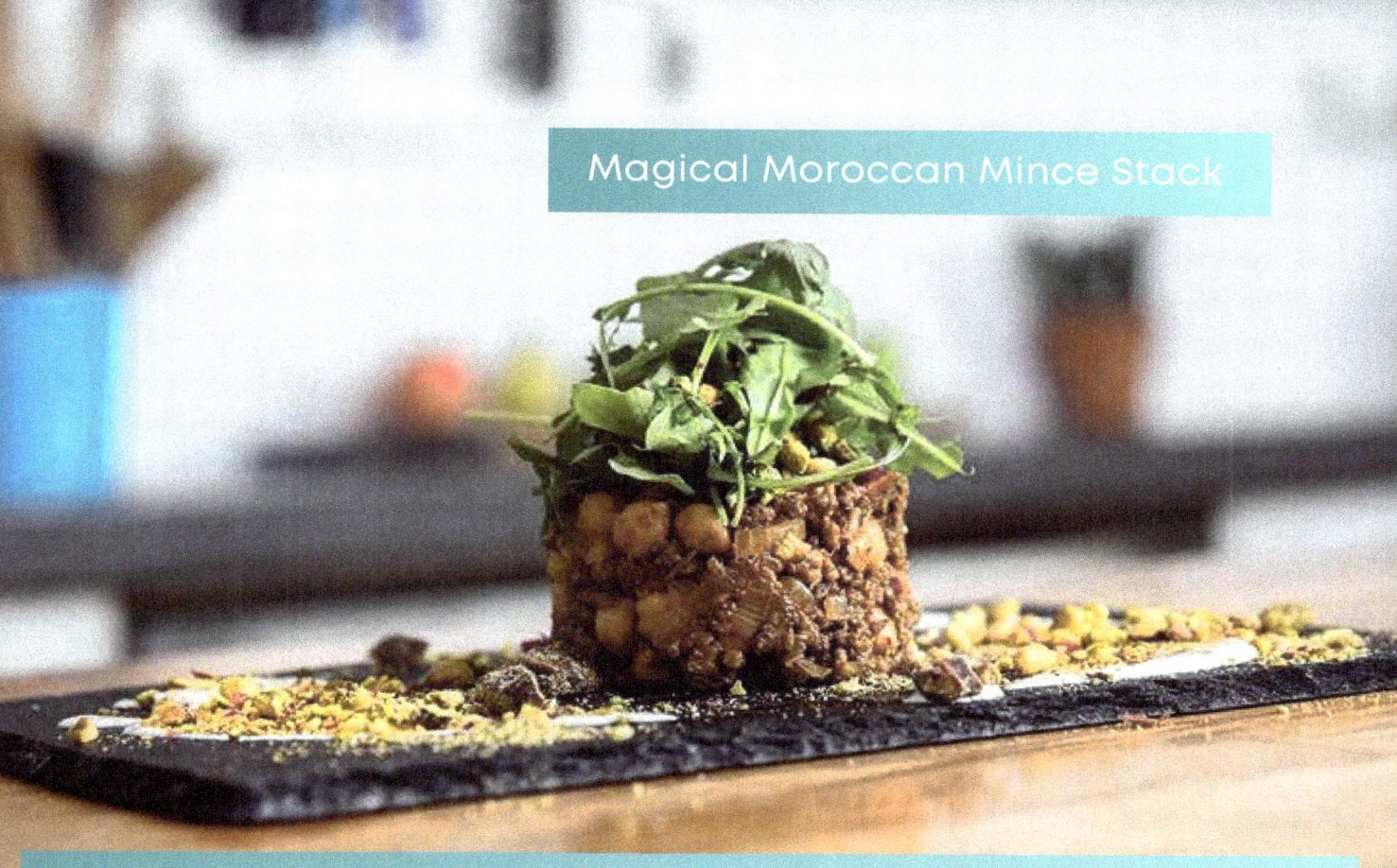

Magical Moroccan Mince Stack

Want to give your Mince a Make-Over?

Now that you can cook mince perfectly, why not change the theme and the style of your mince. I like to take my mince around the world!

Try These Variations
(instead of the ras el hanout but ALWAYS leave the turmeric in)

SPANISH

1 tablespoon smoked paprika for a Spanish Style mince.
You could also add some finely diced or chopped chorizo to this to really make it Spanish.

INDIAN

1 tablespoon curry powder to make an Indian-style mince.
Add chopped chilli and fresh coriander and then serve!

CHINESE

5 spice is another favourite

Rosti Cottage Pie

SERVINGS: 4-6

INGREDIENTS

750 g lean beef mince
2 medium onions chopped finely
2 cloves garlic, crushed
1 pinch ground nutmeg (optional)
250 ml beef or vegetable stock
4 tomatoes finely chopped (1 tin)
2 tablespoons tomato paste
1 tablespoon fresh herbs (thyme, oregano, sage)
4 medium potatoes cooked but still firm (allow to cool before grating)
50 ml butter melted
1 tablespoon chopped parsley or chives to garnish

METHOD

Heat a heavy-based saucepan until swear word hot. Now add the mince into the pan, but do not stir until the first layer you have put down has browned up. Only then must you stir!

Fry the minced meat hot and fast until all the meat has browned off; now add the onions and garlic and allow to cook through. Add the nutmeg and the stock, and the remaining ingredients and allow to cook through. Season to taste and then transfer into a suitable oven-proof baking dish.

Use the grated cooked potato over the top of the meat sauce and then brush with melted butter, and grill for a fantastic finish. Garnish with chopped herbs!

NOTE:
Use this recipe to top your favourite vegetables instead and make a vegetarian culinary delight! Use spinach and feta, roasted vegetables of your choice…anything goes!

Cauliflower Paella

SERVINGS: 4-6

INGREDIENTS

10-30ml oil
450-600g chicken pieces of your choice cut into pieces no larger than your palm
(optional; you can keep this vegetarian and use eggplant or zucchini)
1 tablespoon smoked or sweet Paprika
1 teaspoon ground turmeric
1 cup chicken stock
80g chorizo sausage or bacon, finely diced or minced
1 onion minced or finely chopped
1 head cauliflower food processed or chopped really fine (to make cauliflower rice)
1 teaspoon garlic paste
Juice and zest of one lemon
1 cup peas, snow peas or beans
80g fire-roasted capsicum (from your deli or house-made) or red capsicum sliced fresh

METHOD

**Nothing can beat a traditional Paella, but if time isn't on your side and you still want amazing flavour and a touch of glamour for a weeknight meal, you just have to try my cauliflower paella.
Bursting with flavour and personality, this is one you will use again and again.**

Coat the chicken in the paprika and turmeric. Grease and heat a large Paella pan until sizzling hot. Add vegetable oil, chorizo sausage or bacon to the sizzling hot pan and allow to brown. Add onion and stir through. When the onions are soft, add the chicken. Brown the first side of the chicken to seal in the flavour and moisture. Once browned, turn over and do the second side.
Add the stock and then reduce heat and allow the chicken to cook through for a few minutes and for the stock to reduce. About 5 minutes.
Add the cauliflower 'rice' and stir through; reduce heat and allow to cook gently for about 5-10 minutes until tender. Add the lemon zest and juice and stir through. Add the vegetables and cook for a minute or two (I like mine still crunchy!), and then check the seasoning.
Serve hot!

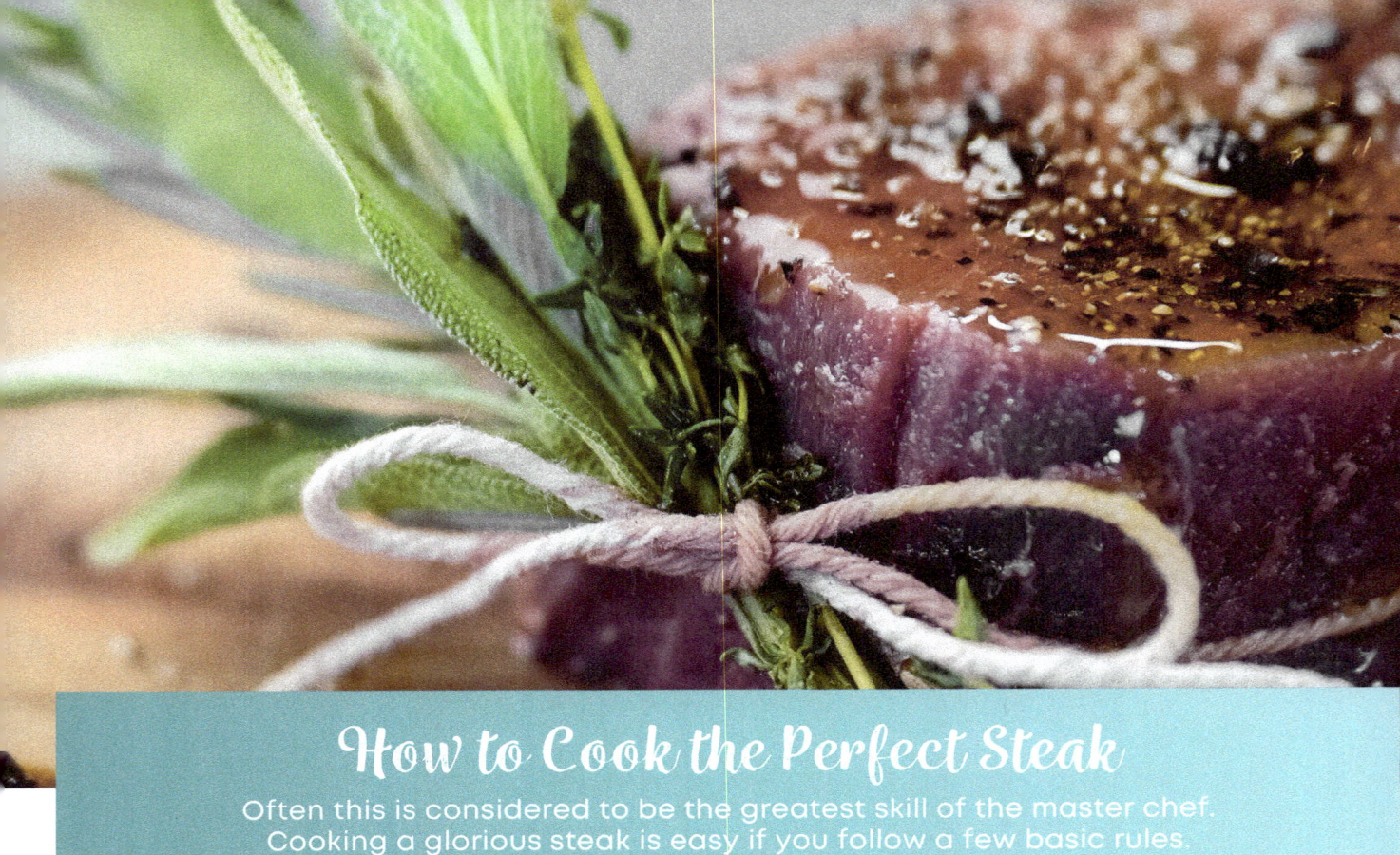

How to Cook the Perfect Steak

Often this is considered to be the greatest skill of the master chef.
Cooking a glorious steak is easy if you follow a few basic rules.

First of all, you need to choose the best steak you can afford for the occasion.
Stay away from steaks that are sinewy and fatty. Favourites are fillet, porterhouse, rump, sirloin or T-bone, these are all from the hindquarter and are considerably more tender than forequarter cuts.
Cook meat at room temperature.
Your pan should be heavy-bottomed so that it retains heat evenly and well.

Fry your steak in equal amounts of butter and vegetable oil: the butter will add flavour, while the vegetable oil will allow the right temperature to be achieved. Don't use one without the other. You can also just use canola cooking spray in a nonstick pan; it works just as well and has no extra calories!
Always heat the pan with the butter and oil until swear word hot BEFORE adding the steak. The steak, once added, should sizzle and hiss. DO NOT STIR OR MOVE THE STEAK, but simply allow the meat to seal on the side you have put down first. Only turn the steak over once the first side is perfectly brown, and this is the side you should present up on the plate, as it will be the best side.

Once the first side is done, you can then turn the steak over and cook to the doneness you prefer.
Never press, poke or fiddle with the steak! Rather, leave the juices inside where they belong!

*It's all in the sauce – I have included some funky
and glamorous ways to serve your perfect steak... enjoy!*

Steak Done-ness Test

Checking for doneness - this is truly the most important part, many steaks are ruined by overcooking, remember, the steak will continue to cook as it rests, very important or else the steak will be ruined. See my steak doneness test. A practiced poke with your finger and you will eventually be able to judge the approximate doneness of your steak. Use the list below as a guide, but experience is the best teacher.

VERY RARE STEAK
Feels soft and squishy, like touching your cheek.
Internal temp of 26-28 degrees C.

RARE STEAK
Soft and yielding to the touch, like poking your cheek with your finger.
Internal temp of 49-51 degrees C.

MEDIUM-RARE STEAK
Yields gently to the touch, like poking your chin on the fleshiest part.
Internal temp of 55-57 degrees C.

MEDIUM STEAK
Yields only slightly to the touch, beginning to firm up, again like your chin would feel if you pressed with your finger. Internal temp of 60-63 degrees C.

MEDIUM-WELL STEAK
Firm to the touch, like pressing your forehead.
Internal temp of 65-69 degrees C.

WELL-DONE STEAK
Hard to the touch, does not give way.
Internal temp of 71 degrees C and over.

Resting

Now, for the most important part, don't serve it right away. Let the steak "rest" for about 5 to 10 minutes, depending on the thickness. This allows the juices to move back into the meat. Resting should be done in
a place that is about room temperature and with only a loose covering over it. If you doubt me, try cutting a steak in half right off the grill. Let a second steak rest for five minutes, and then cut into it. See which one is juicier.

Porcini & Sage Cream with Dirty Black Fillet

SERVINGS: 4-6

INGREDIENTS

1 tablespoon canola oil to heat in the pan to sear the beef
200 g fillet or rump per person, thick cut to about 4-5 cm
season well with salt and pepper
4 cloves garlic, minced
4 shallots finely chopped
1 cup porcini or your favourite mushroom finely chopped
1 teaspoon freshly chopped sage or thyme
1 chicken/mushroom or vegetable stock cube
100ml cream
season well with black salt/flake salt and pepper to get the steak blackened

METHOD

This is how to easily and perfectly cook a successful steak.
Heat the oil in a saucepan over medium-low heat. Add the seasoned steak to the pan; it should sizzle!

Do not turn the steaks until the first side to hit the pan has made the sexiest crust. It should look brown and perfect with heaps of personality and flavour, not grey and dodgy.
Once cooked, you can turn over and do the next side, keeping that sizzle sound UP in the pan.
We want the same result for the second side, too!
Depending on how you like this cooked, if you are going for rare, you can now add the garlic and shallots and cook for 5 minutes, stirring, being careful not to burn them, but browning them will be perfect.
If you want a more medium style, I would turn the steak over, drop the heat and cook a further 4-5 minutes on the original side.

Now add the mushrooms, the sage, the crumbled-up stock cube and the cream and then stir through and let heat through and boil for about a minute. If you leave it for longer, it will reduce, which is sometimes good if the flavour wasn't deep enough to start with, BUT if you over-reduce you will be left with a salty sauce so please add a bit more hot water and taste again!
Serve with the steak and your choice of sides, either the butterbean puree, parsnip or sweet potato fries, or good old fashioned potatoes of your choice!

Steak served with Baked Camembert & Fragrant Garlic

SERVINGS: 3-4

INGREDIENTS

1 round Camembert

2 - 3 cloves garlic

sprigs of fresh thyme or rosemary, oregano or marjoram

METHOD

Place the Camembert in an ovenproof bowl or saucer which is more or less the same size as the cheese. Something with sides is ideal but not essential, you will serve the cheese from this bowl too to save extra work!

Peel the garlic and then cut it into slivers, make holes in the cheese by using the tip of your paring knife, bury the garlic slivers in the slits and follow with a sprig of herb.

Stud the entire cheese like this, it will look absolutely gorgeous!

Just before you are ready to serve, bake in a preheated oven of 200c for about 8 minutes until the cheese is oozy and the garlic fragrant, the smells will waft out of your oven door!

Serve as big dollops on your perfect steak...sublime!

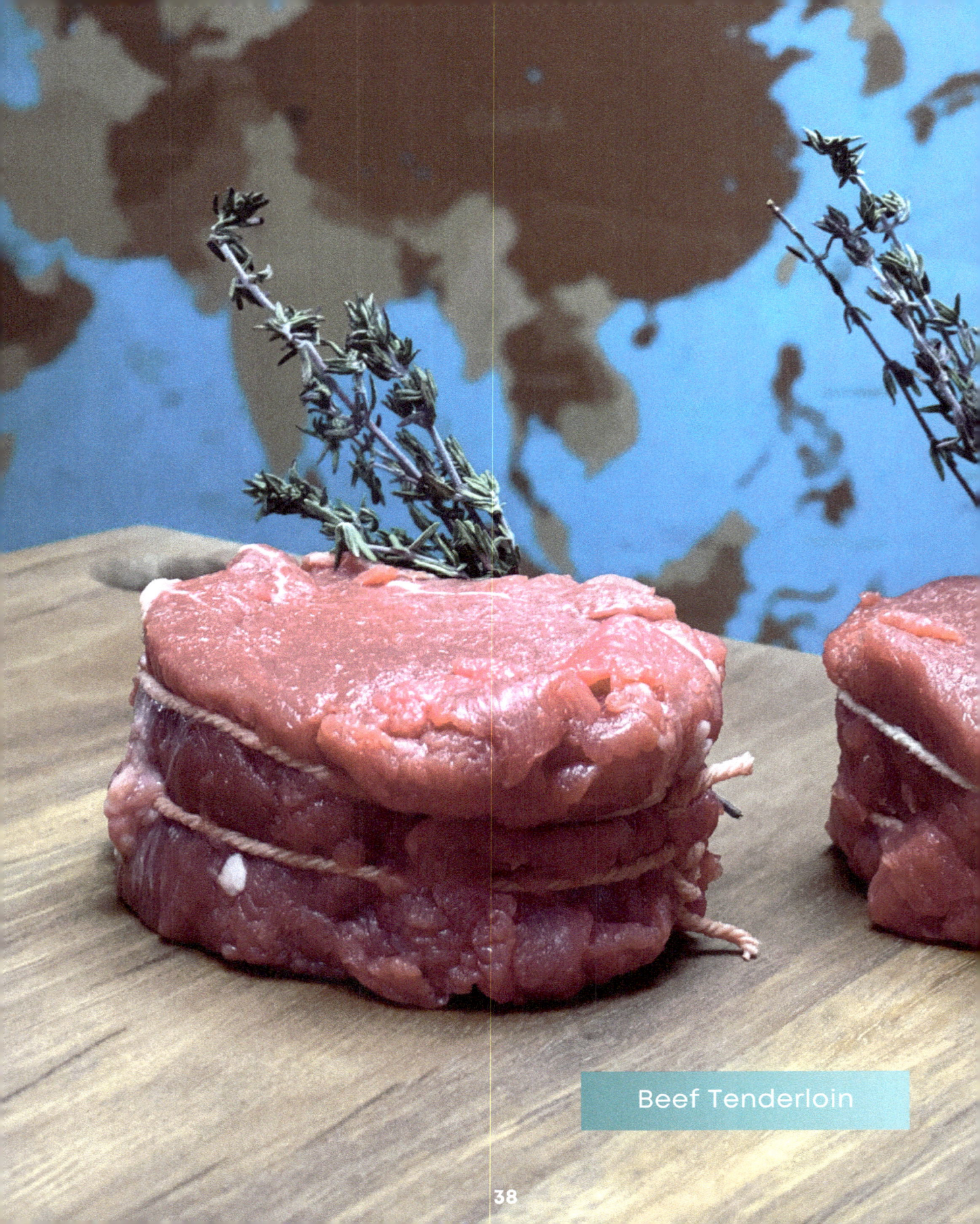

Beef Tenderloin

Beef Tenderloin with Burnt Basil & Black Pepper Butter, on a Baked Stack Mirepoix of Vegetables

INGREDIENTS

200g fillet or rump per person, seasoned with black salt and black pepper

25g butter per person

1 teaspoon fresh basil per person

A quarter teaspoon of black pepper per person

Roasted diced vegetables to serve

METHOD

Prepare tenderloin as per above.

In a pan heat the butter, basil and pepper.

Heat until the butter has melted and started separating into clarified butter underneath and white foamy milk solids on top.

The minute the white foam starts to go golden, shake through until the entire batch is golden and then remove from heat.

If you have just gone too far and you don't want any further colour, pour hot butter into a cold ceramic dish with a metal spoon or fork in it (so the bowl doesn't crack) and then serve on the delicious steak.

Serve on a dice of selected roasted vegetables.

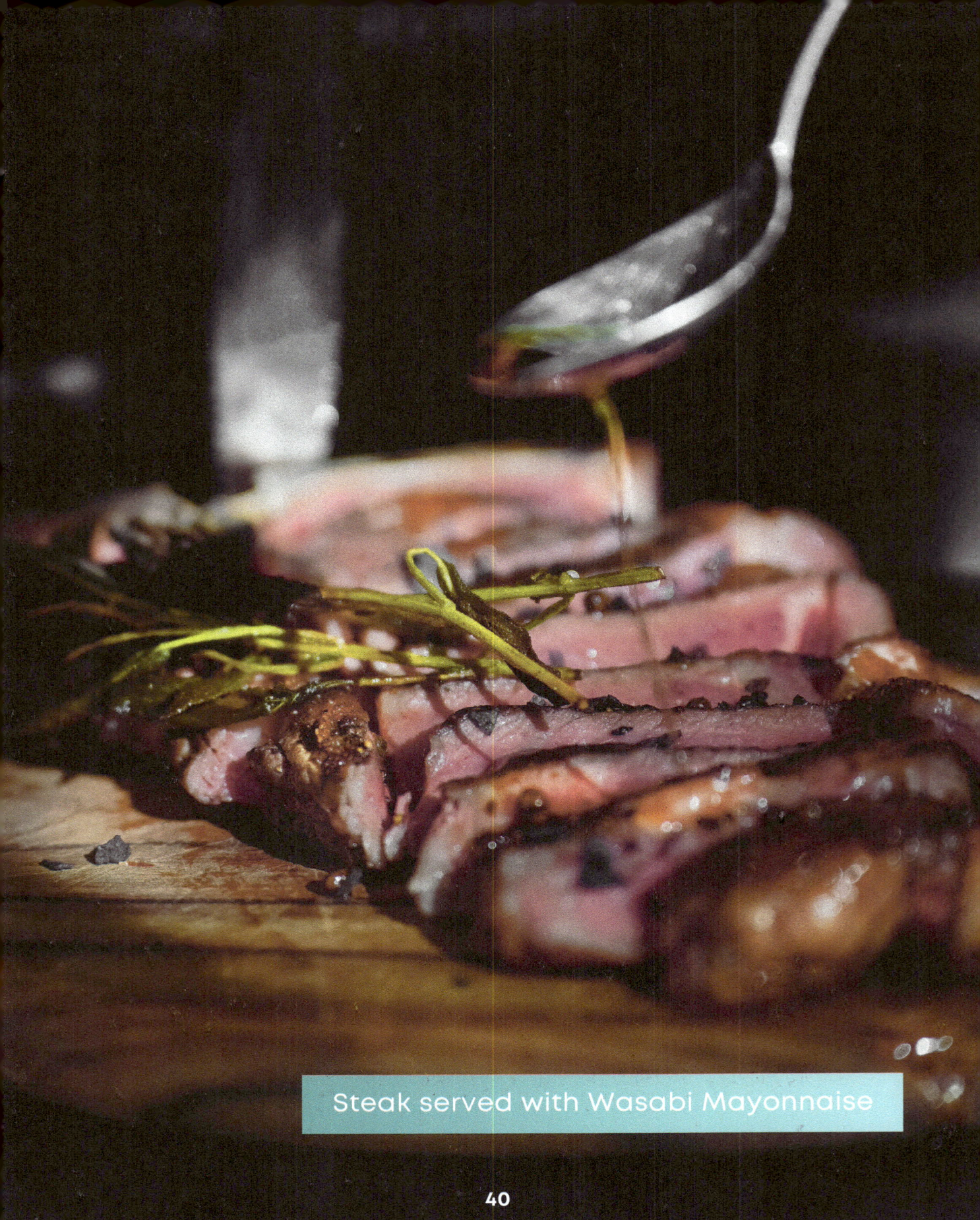
Steak served with Wasabi Mayonnaise

Steak served with Wasabi Mayonnaise

SERVINGS: 4-6

INGREDIENTS

2 cloves garlic, crushed to a fine paste
1 teaspoon grainy mustard
1 teaspoon wasabi or horseradish,
1 egg yolk (room temperature)
Juice of one lemon, at least 20 ml
280-300 ml sunflower/vegetable oil
salt and pepper to taste

METHOD

Wasabi is from the same family as horseradish and is the perfect funky accompaniment to the perfect steak. This can be made in advance and then kept in an airtight container.

Place the garlic, mustard, wasabi, egg yolk, lemon juice and seasoning into a processor, blend until smooth and then add the oil in a thin stream until the mixture thickens.
Do not overbeat; the minute it thickens, stop the machine!
This can also be done by hand with a whisk.

VARIATONS

Serve your steak with Oysters Kilpatrick = Surf and Turf/Reef and Beef.
Serve your steak with herb and chilli butter (soften butter, blend, place in the fridge)
Serve your steak with truffle oil or whipped truffle butter
Serve your steak with pesto and cream mixed together.
Serve your steak with grainy mustard mixed with a bit of cream
Serve with cooked prawns on a skewer with strawberries and lots of black pepper

Quickie & Perfectly Sexy Stir Fries

TASTY | HEALTHY | NUTRITIOUS | QUICK

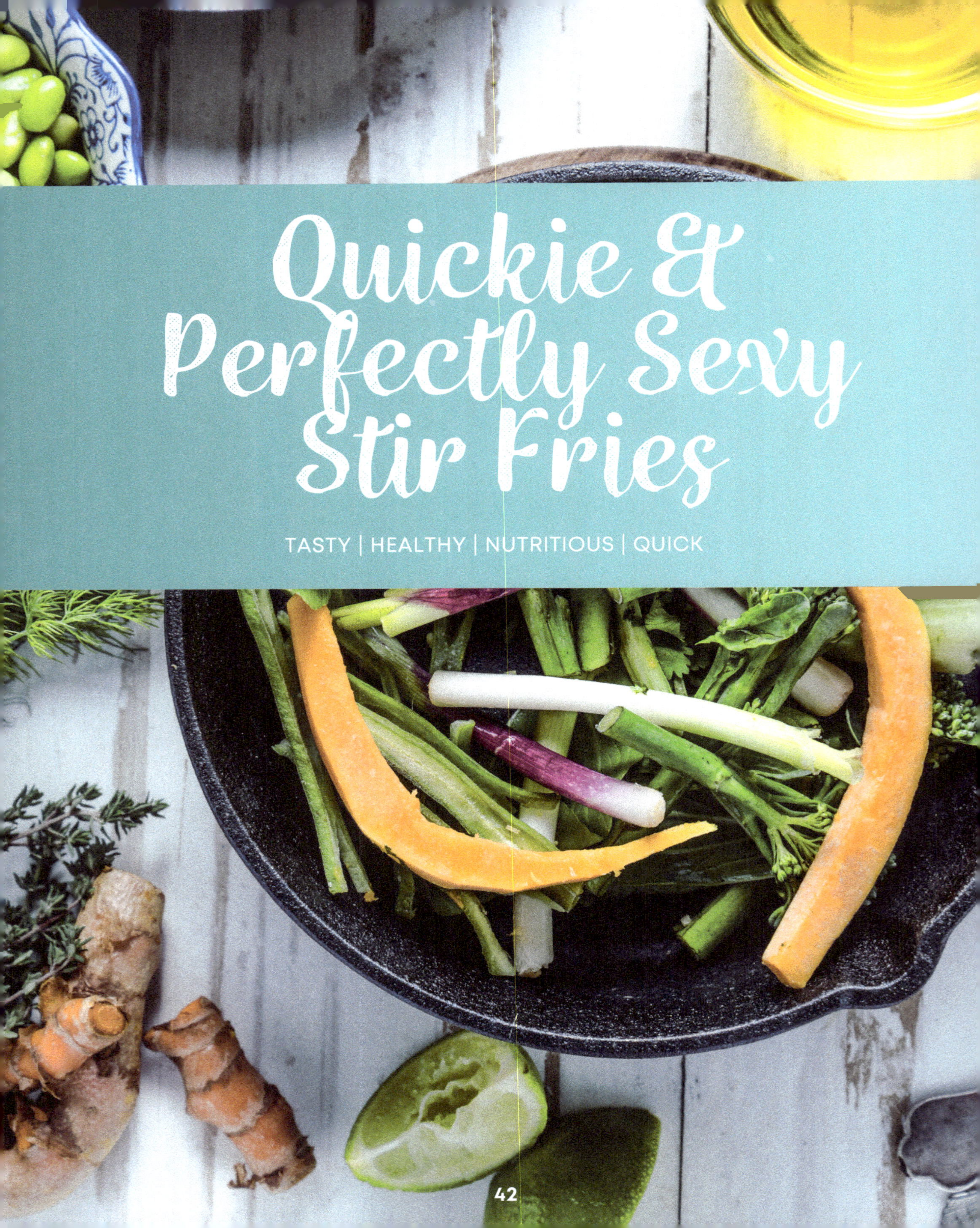

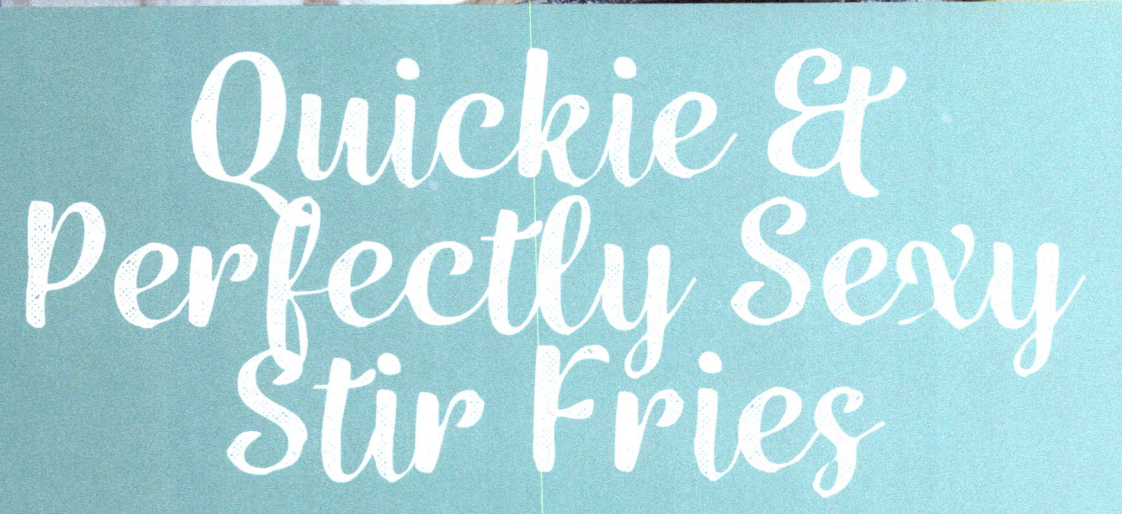

Stir Fry Ingredients

SERVINGS: 4-6

1-2 tablespoons peanut/canola/sunflower/rice bran oil
600g chicken/pork/beef strips

MARINADE:
3 tablespoons honey or plum jam
3 tablespoons soya sauce
2 cloves garlic finely crushed
2 tablespoons crushed ginger
1-3 chillies finely chopped
2 drops sesame oil (optional)

VEGGIES:
1 cup zucchini, finely sliced or spiralized
1 cup carrots, finely sliced or spiralized
1 cup red onion finely sliced
2 cups finely sliced red or wombok cabbage
1 cup finely sliced red capsicum/red pepper

TIPS

Stir-fries are a wonderful, healthy, economical family meal. Not only are they tasty, they are bursting with health and nutrition and are full of colour, flavour and personality.

BUT...are your stir fries soggy and full of liquid, or are they gloriously sticky like your favourite takeaway from your Asian restaurant? There are so many varieties of the good old stir fry so the only wisdom I can impart is how to cook it successfully every time! Get that wok out, guys and let's get cooking.
You don't have to have a wok; a good old frying pan will be just as good.
Sometimes woks are designed for gas, so if you are using yours and the base doesn't fully make contact with the stovetop, this could be an issue when trying to get that fabulous intense heat needed for ultimate stir fry success.

Remember, it's all about keeping the heat up, the sizzle sizzling, in the pan the ENTIRE time you cook the stir-fry. Once the veggies are in, it's okay to reduce the heat and even put the heat off; we only want those to 'wilt' or steam through anyway.
Always cut your meat and your vegetables super thin so that the cooking time is short and sweet. It's these little tricks and tips that will make your stir fry time happy instead of stressful.

Also, a sharp knife is a must. A blunt knife will make your slicing task tedious and time-consuming, and you'll get cranky before you've even started.

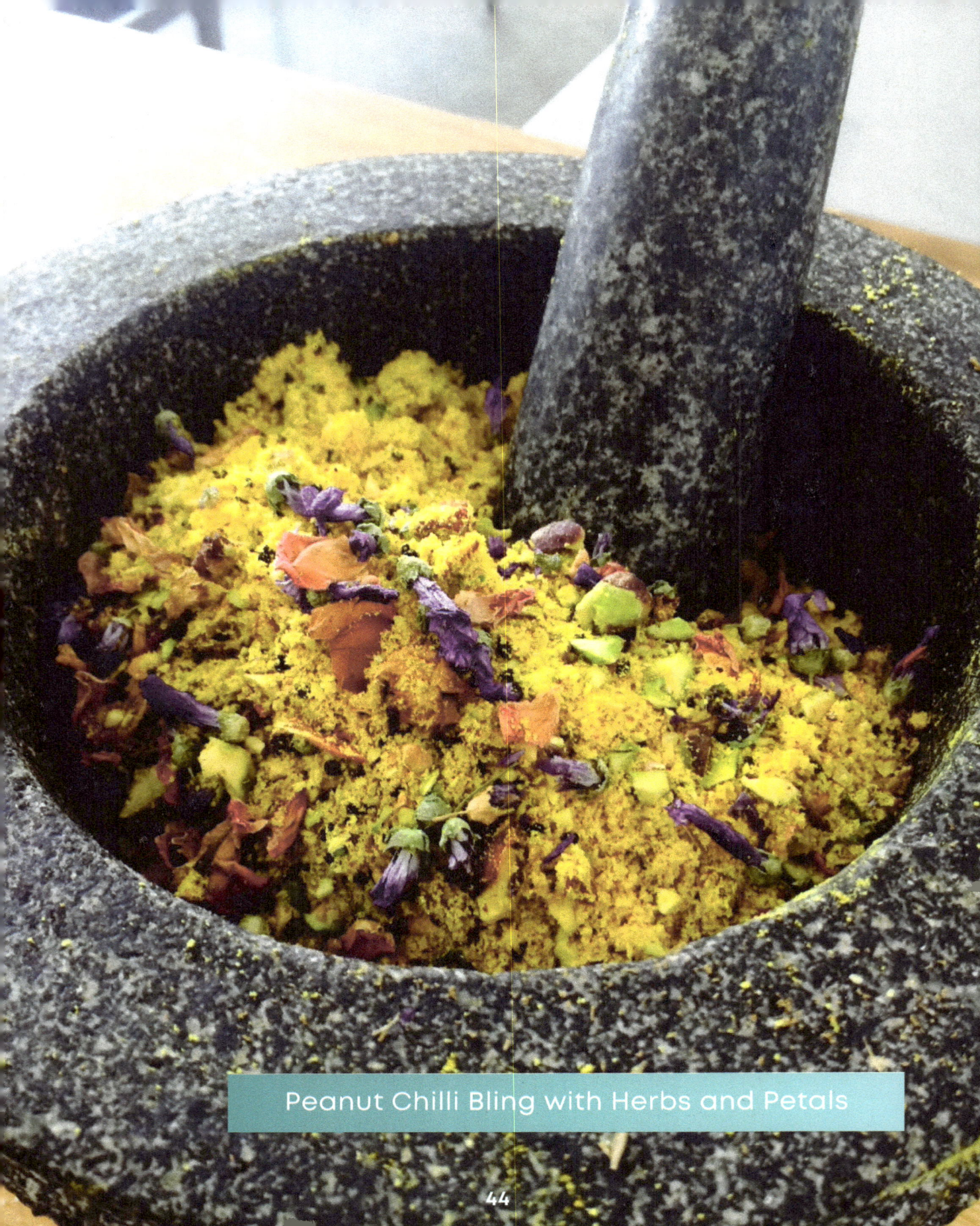

Peanut Chilli Bling with Herbs and Petals

Peanut, Chilli, Herb Bling with Petals for Crunch

SERVINGS: 4-6

INGREDIENTS

1/2 cup peanuts, crushed and pan toasted
1-2 chopped fresh chillies, or use about half a teaspoon dried
1/2 cup freshly chopped mint/basil/coriander...you decide!
Edible Petals like cornflower, saffron, dianthus, violet, snapdragon

METHOD

Remember. Your mission is to keep the sizzle up in your pan...if the pan goes quiet on you, you need to back away from the pan, get some of the pan naked, and then let the pan get back to temperature. HOT HOT HOT!

Put the marinade ingredients over the thin meat strips. Stir to combine.
Heat and grease the pan with the oil. When the pan is smoking hot, add the marinated chicken/pork/beef in a pile on one side of the pan. Please don't spread the meat over the pan; all that will do is smother the heat! Leave the meat in the pile until the first side of the meat that hit the pan is beautifully brown and sexy and, fragrant, and sealed. You must have a sneaky look underneath one of the pieces using your tongs. Move that meat around by jiggling it with your tongs, but don't stir too much. Don't burn this!
Keep checking!

ONLY when that meat is brown underneath do you do a half stir, so that some 'new' meat can hit the base of the pan. Keep doing this, keeping the sizzle high in the pan until all the meat has been perfectly browned. This way, your meat won't stew, and you can live happily ever after in the kitchen!

Once all the meat looks heavenly, sticky and brown do you start adding the vegetables on the top. You can remove the meat from the pan if your pan is too small for all this action. Stir as much as you like now to get those vegetables hot and wilted right through. Check the seasoning and serve with rice, noodles, or just like that in a bowl with the heavenly peanut bling on top for valuable flavour and crunch!

Why not try this Chinese-style sweet-and-sour marinade on your next stir-fry?
It's so simple - see it on the next page.

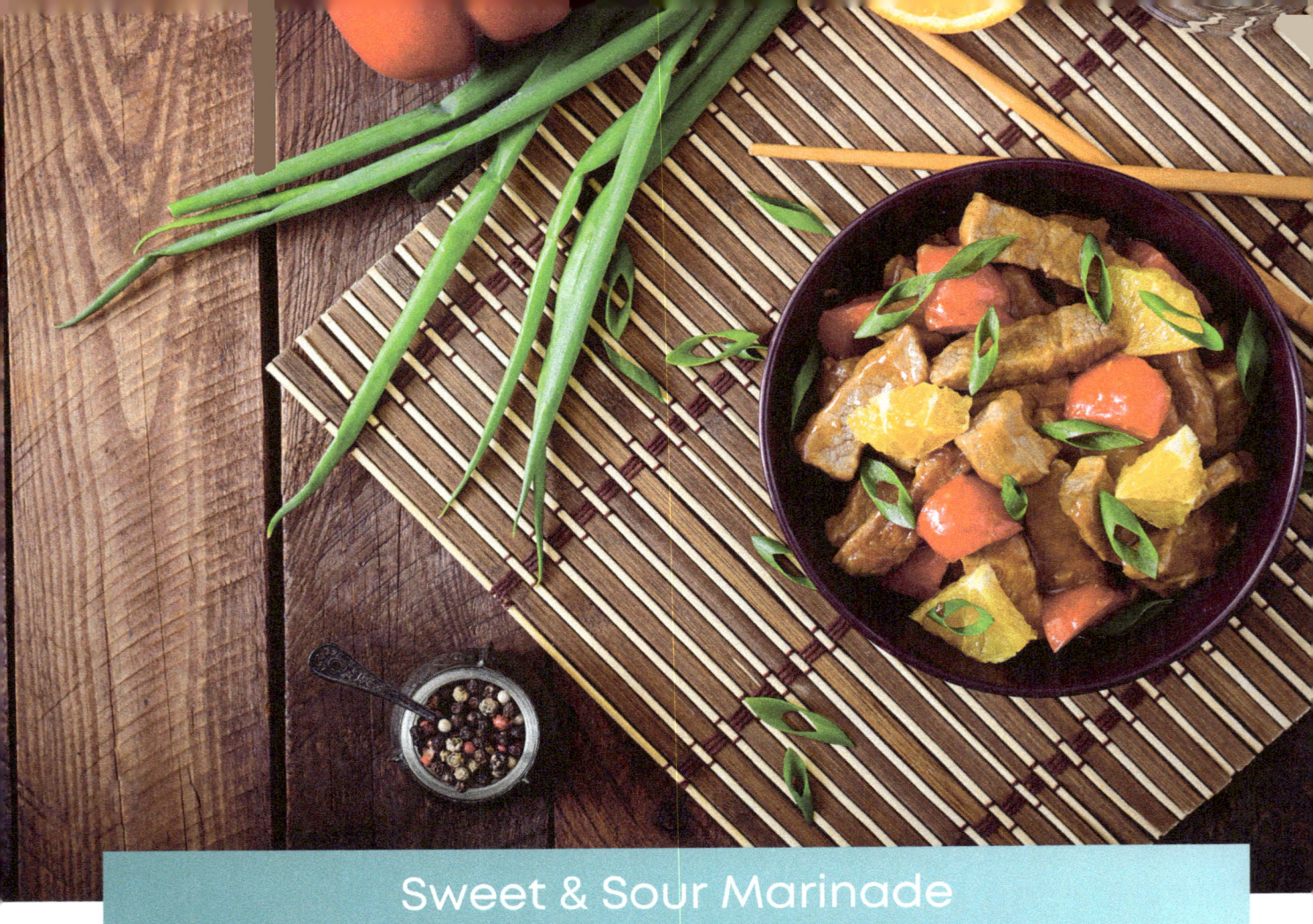

Sweet & Sour Marinade

SERVINGS: 4-6

INGREDIENTS

2 tablespoons tomato paste
4 tablespoons white wine or cider vinegar
3 tablespoons brown sugar
1 teaspoon Chinese five-spice powder
1/3-cup pineapple chunks blended to a puree (or just chop them up)
1 tablespoon Chinese Cooking wine
1 tablespoon soy sauce

METHOD

Simply mix together and then use as a marinade on approximately 400-600 g protein or vegetables, for your favourite stir fry using the cooking method prescribed for successful stir-frying!

Quickie Fish Dishes

SO HEALTHY AND DELICIOUS

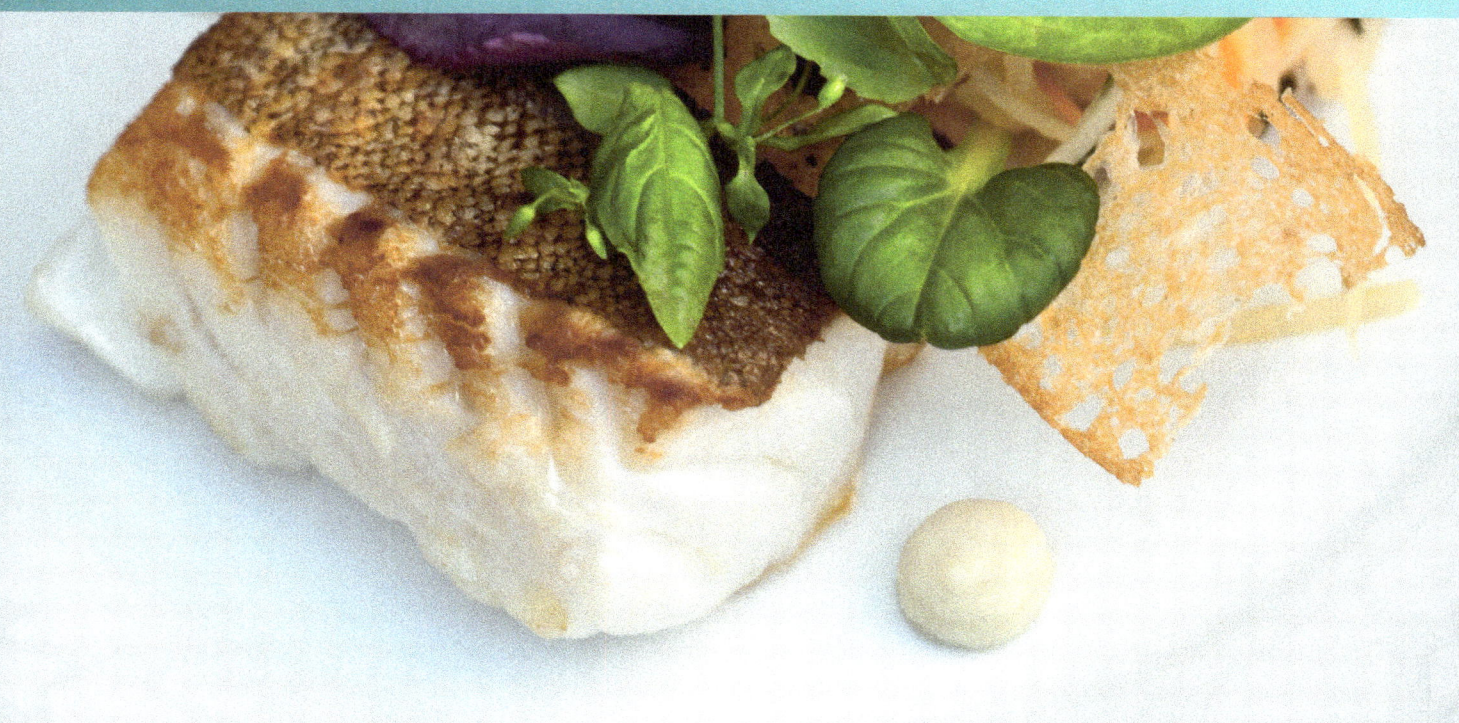

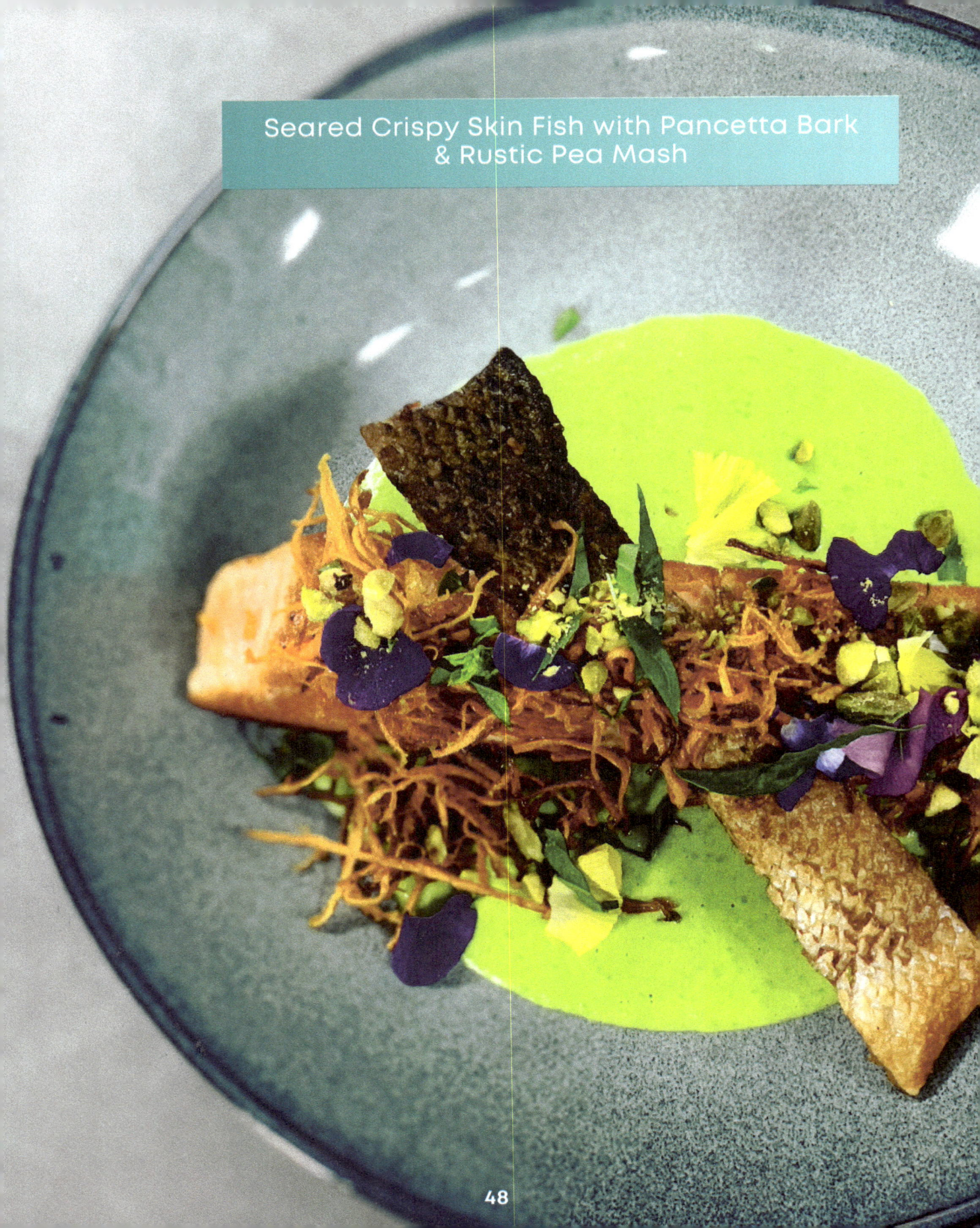
Seared Crispy Skin Fish with Pancetta Bark & Rustic Pea Mash

Seared Crispy Skin Fish with Pancetta Bark & Rustic Pea Mash

SERVINGS: 4-6

INGREDIENTS

600-800 g fish, skin on
Salt and pepper to season
Half lemon or lime per serving
4-6 strips Pancetta
placed on a roasting tray and then baked until crispy in a hot oven of 200C

METHOD

First of all, I want you to know that you, too, can get perfectly crisp fish skin every time! Here's how!

This is my favourite recipe for when I am entertaining because it is practically stress-free.
A beautiful piece of fish or salmon needs little masking and if cooked perfectly, will simply shine.
The trick is to cook the fish properly and get the skin sexy and crispy. You need to get your pan or BBQ SWEAR WORD HOT and greased with about 5 ml vegetable or rice bran oil in the pan just so that the fish doesn't stick.

When the pan is hot, place the fish (not skin side) presentation side down, and use your tongs to ensure it doesn't stick. Just give the piece a little wiggle to ensure it hasn't stuck, but it will create a sexy crust of flavour and colour.

When the first side is brown (simply look underneath and lift with your tongs), turn it over to do the skin side, too. After about a minute or two, you should be able to remove the skin using the tongs. Don't stress if it breaks or you have to strip-peel it off; it is all part of the rustic glamour of this dish.
Place the skin aside and turn the skin-free side down to brown it off. When the fish is cooked (check by placing a fork or knife in the centre of the thickest part, and if it flakes when you twist, it is done)

Remove from the pan and now lower the heat, and fry the skin nice and hot but not so hot that it burns in a flash…this will dry and crisp up the skin, and the best way is to remove the skin so you don't overcook the fish! NEVER serve soggy fish skin…it is just not glamorous and can be easily crisped up by just allowing it some alone time in the pan.

Serve with the amazingly versatile pea puree. (on the next page)
Don't like peas? Use butterbeans (drained out of a tin) instead.

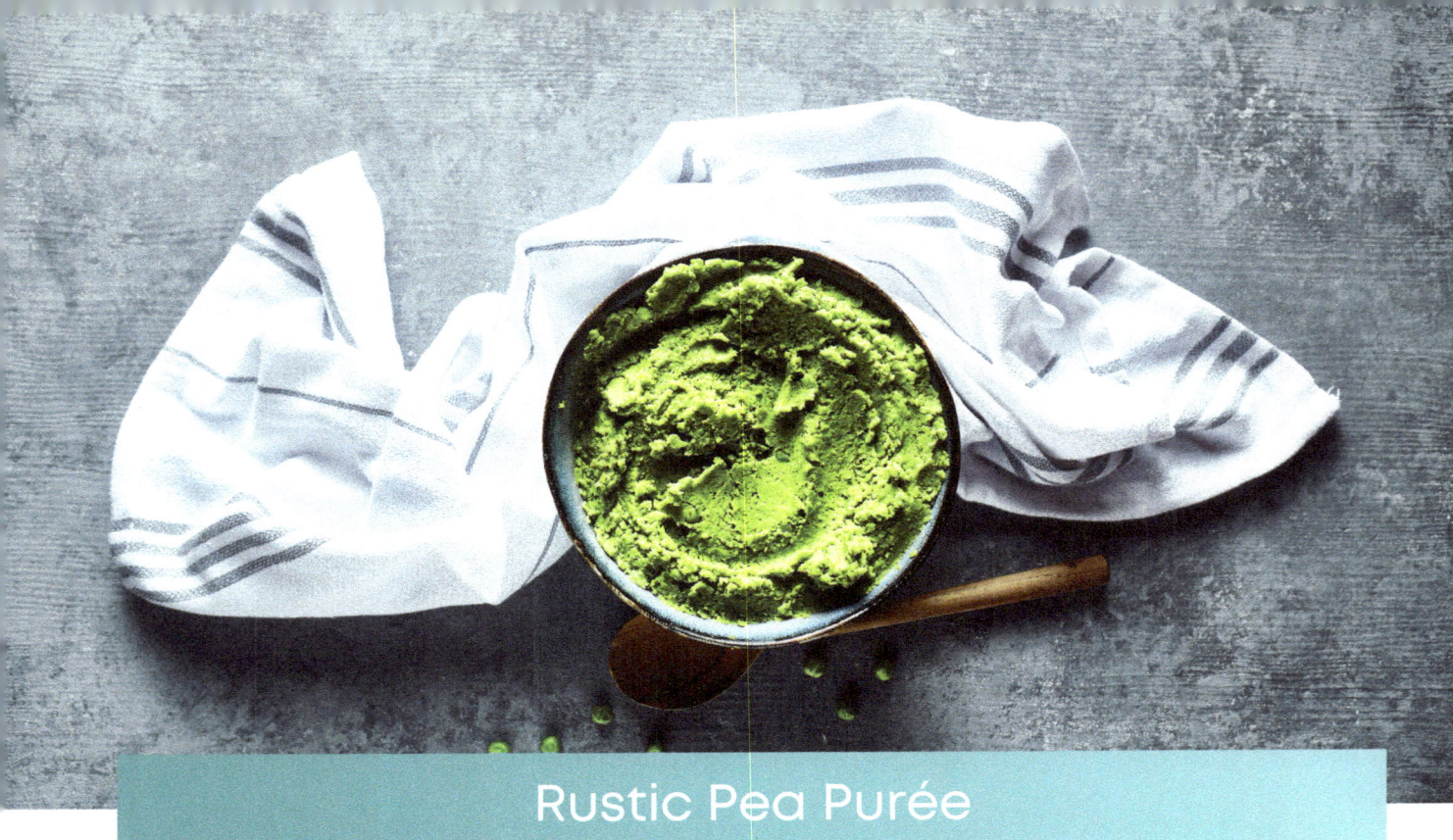

Rustic Pea Purée

SERVINGS: 4-6

INGREDIENTS

2 cups frozen peas
1 onion finely chopped
1 clove garlic minced
150-250ml chicken or vegetable stock
(depending on thickness required - please adjust)
20g butter
80-150ml cream

METHOD

Place all the ingredients into a medium saucepan and boil over medium heat for about 15 minutes. Remove from the heat and blend to a smooth puree with a stick blender or manual masher. Adjust the seasoning and thickness and then serve

SERVING IDEA

Place a sexy seared salmon or fish fillet and some cooked pancetta onto the pea puree, drizzle with olive oil, petals and micro herbs and fried carrot strips!

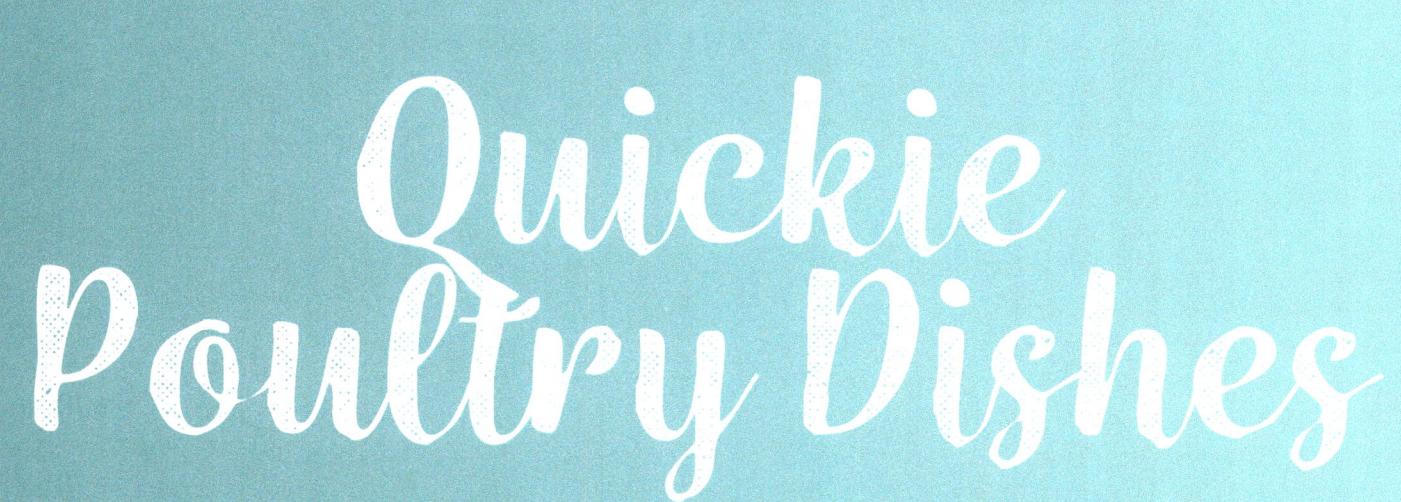

Quickie Poultry Dishes

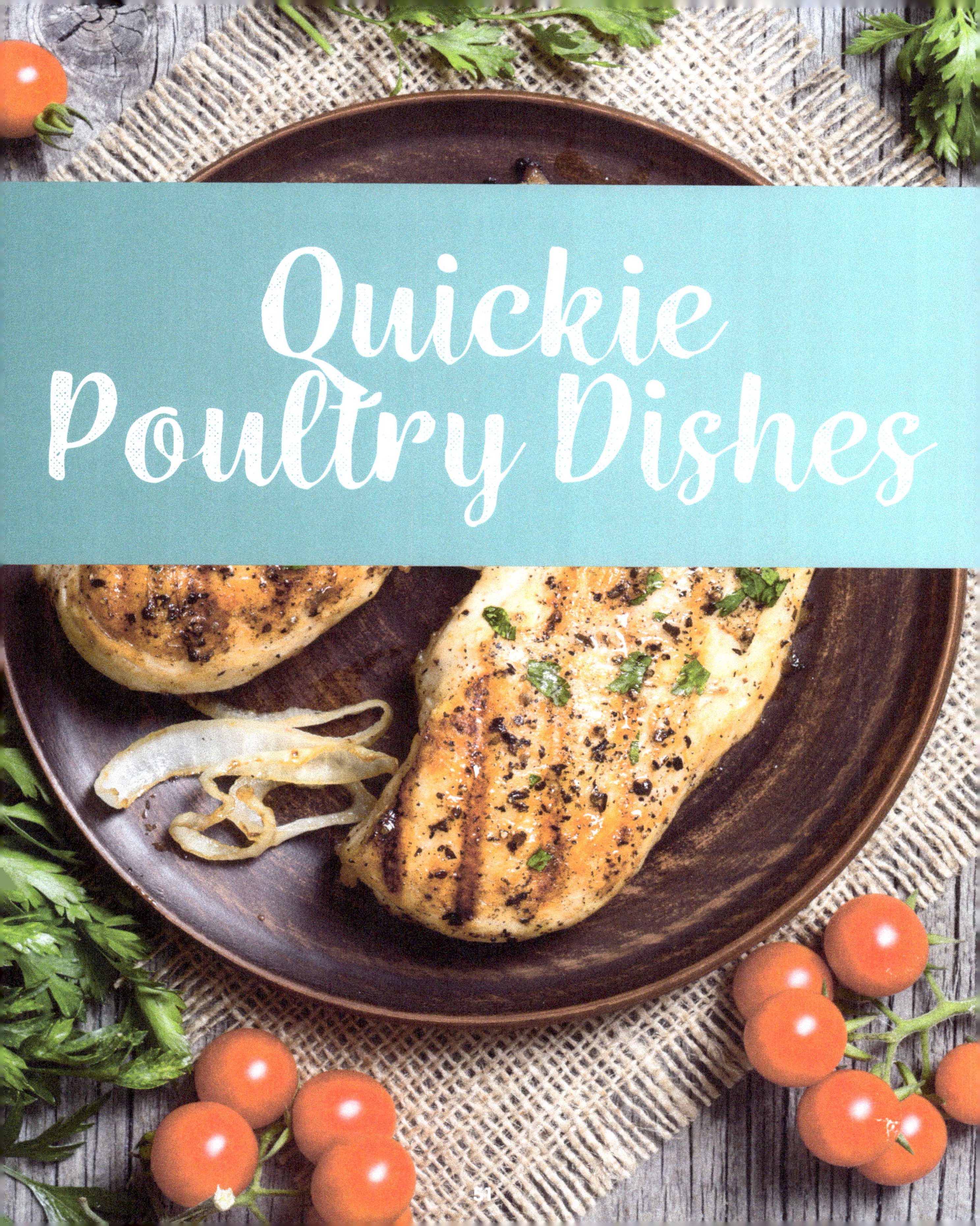

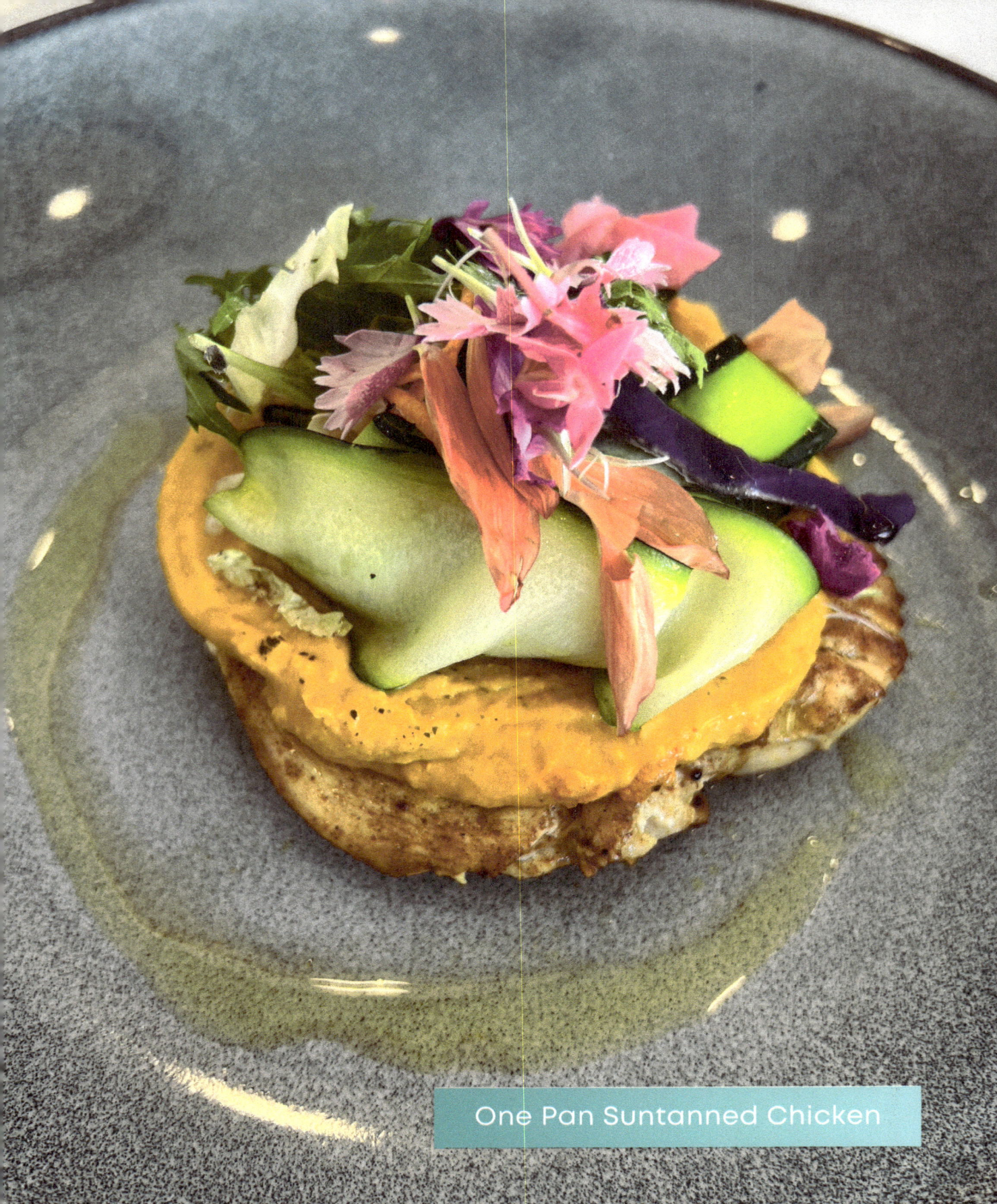

One Pan Suntanned Chicken

One Pan Suntanned Chicken

SERVINGS: 4-6

INGREDIENTS

600-800g chicken breast fillets

1 teaspoon turmeric

1-2 tablespoons of either curry powder, paprika, fajita spice, ras el hanout or Thai Curry paste

oil or water to bind, about 20-30ml

salt and pepper to season

1 cup sliced cabbage or a bunch/packet of sliced spinach

1 cup sliced leek

1 cup sliced capsicum

You can use ANY finely sliced vegetables you like!

2 teaspoons pistachios or peanuts or fried shallots for crunch!

METHOD

Okay, who's sick of washing pots and pans and millions of dishes? I certainly am. Join me as I show you the art of preparing a quick yet magnificent chicken breast in half the time and with half the fuss...but with all the sexiness and gorgeous flavour you've come to deserve. For those nights and days when you really just need to get a healthy, nutritious meal onto the table in under 15 minutes. I can't wait to hear about how you turned this dish into your own special design! It's so versatile that you can change the spices and the vegetables a hundred times...just like your favourite outfit. New earrings, new handbag, it's a new outfit! Gents, for you, it's new shoes, a new tie, a new outfit.

Slice the chicken breast in half lengthways. Now, use a nice sharp knife to cut slashes in shallow cuts into the chicken breast. This will open up the breast, helping it to cook faster AND helping that flavour to really get in there. Once you have your slashed chicken breast, blend your turmeric and your choice of spice with the oil or water until it forms a nice wet paste. Brush on with a pastry brush or simply combine with a spoon to coat, season well with salt and pepper.

Heat and grease a frying pan with a few sprays of canola or rice bran spray or a tablespoon of vegetable oil. When the pan is swear word hot, add the chicken...it should SIZZLE as it hits the pan! Let the first side get really nice and brown and fragrant, about 2-3 minutes, before turning over and doing the other side. Cook the second side until sexy and brown, and fragrant, and then turn it over again; you can reduce the heat at this stage.

Now add the vegetables on top and over the chicken, leave for a minute, and then stir through. Cook for just a few minutes, really just until the vegetables are wilted rather than overcooked, and then you're ready to serve. You can top it with a dollop of sour cream or yoghurt, depending on what spices you used, and then add a squeeze of fresh lemon or lime juice to freshen up the dish.

Voila! Too easy I know, but a really good one to know for those times that you have to get that food on the table. You can also use this method for pork chops and pork fillets. Please don't do this to a steak.

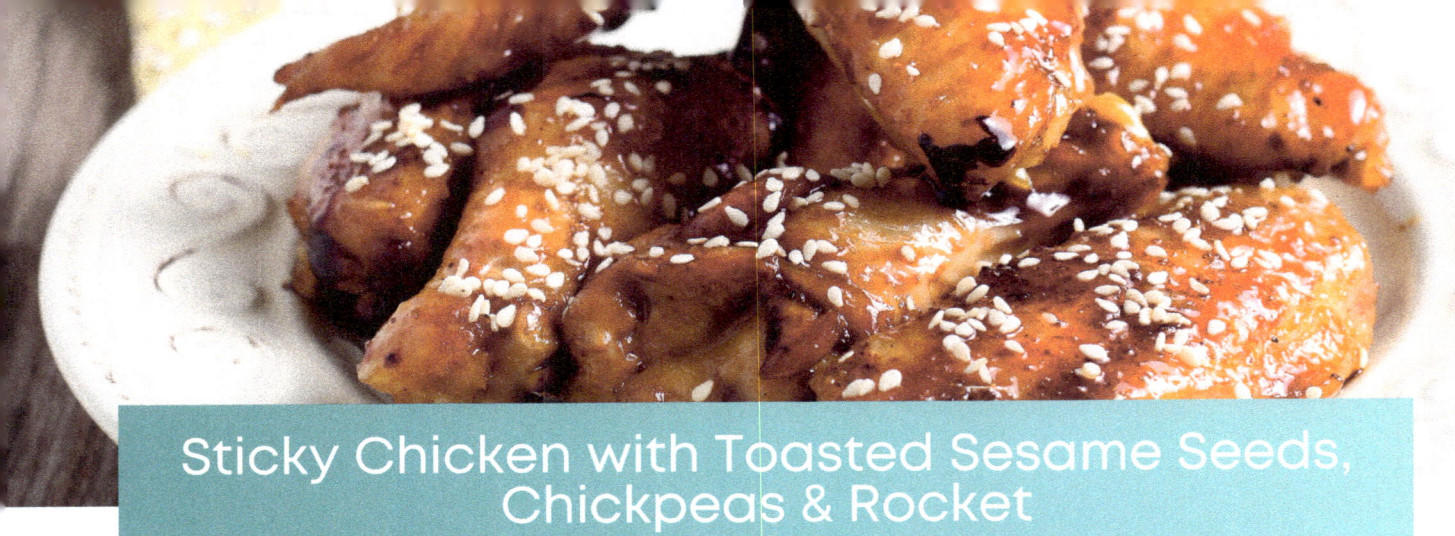

Sticky Chicken with Toasted Sesame Seeds, Chickpeas & Rocket

SERVINGS: 4-6

INGREDIENTS

2 tablespoons vegetable oil
750 g chicken breast fillets sliced across the grain
2 tablespoons tomato paste
2 tablespoons soy sauce
80 ml syrup or honey
1 teaspoon chicken stock powder
1 finely chopped onion
2 cloves garlic, finely chopped,
2 teaspoons fresh ginger,
Juice and zest of one lemon or lime
Salt and freshly ground pepper
1 tin chickpeas drained

METHOD

Prepare the chicken by slicing it across the grain or lengthways.
Marinade chicken with tomato paste, soy, honey, stock, onion, garlic, ginger, juice, zest and seasoning.
Heat the oil until swear word hot but not smoking, and then gently add the chicken, shaking off excess marinade. DO NOT STIR, but rather wait for the first layer you have put down to brown.
I know it is tempting to stir, but only do so when you are confident the chicken is perfectly golden; only then stir it through.

Stirring right in the beginning will cause the temperature of the oil to drop, and you will end up stewing the chicken, and it will never brown. Fry in hot oil until the chicken is brown and sticky.
Sprinkle with the toasted sesame seeds and serve on a bed of chickpeas, rocket and assorted salad leaves (or coriander!)

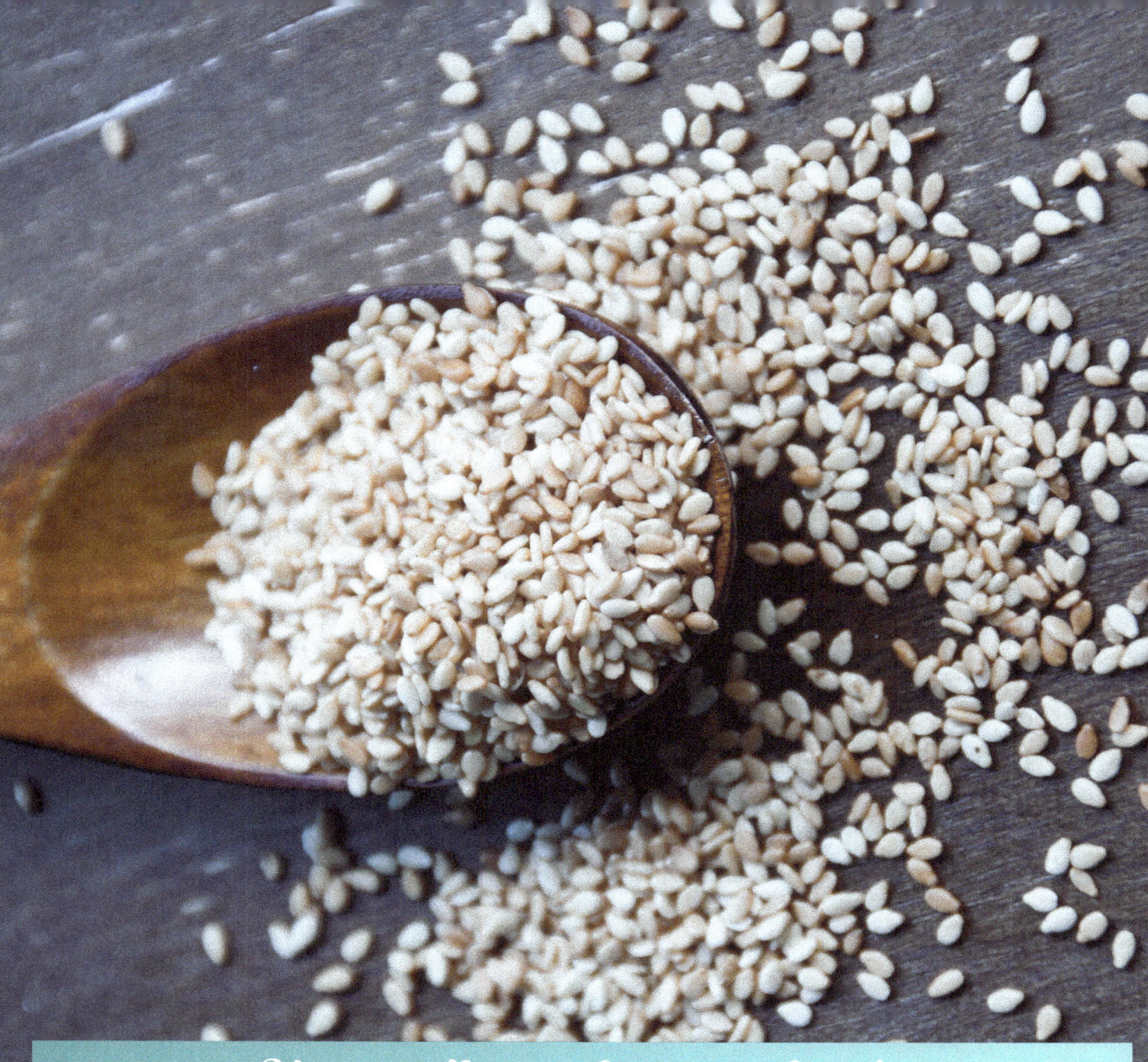

How to Roast Sesame Seeds

Place 3 tablespoons of sesame seeds in a clean and dry frying pan; make sure you have two minutes to do this because the minute you leave them alone, they will burn! Set the heat to moderate and allow the pan to heat up. Shake the seeds until they are golden and fragrant and just about to start popping. They should start smelling really good, and that's when they are ready!

By roasting them you increase their flavour profile by 100%

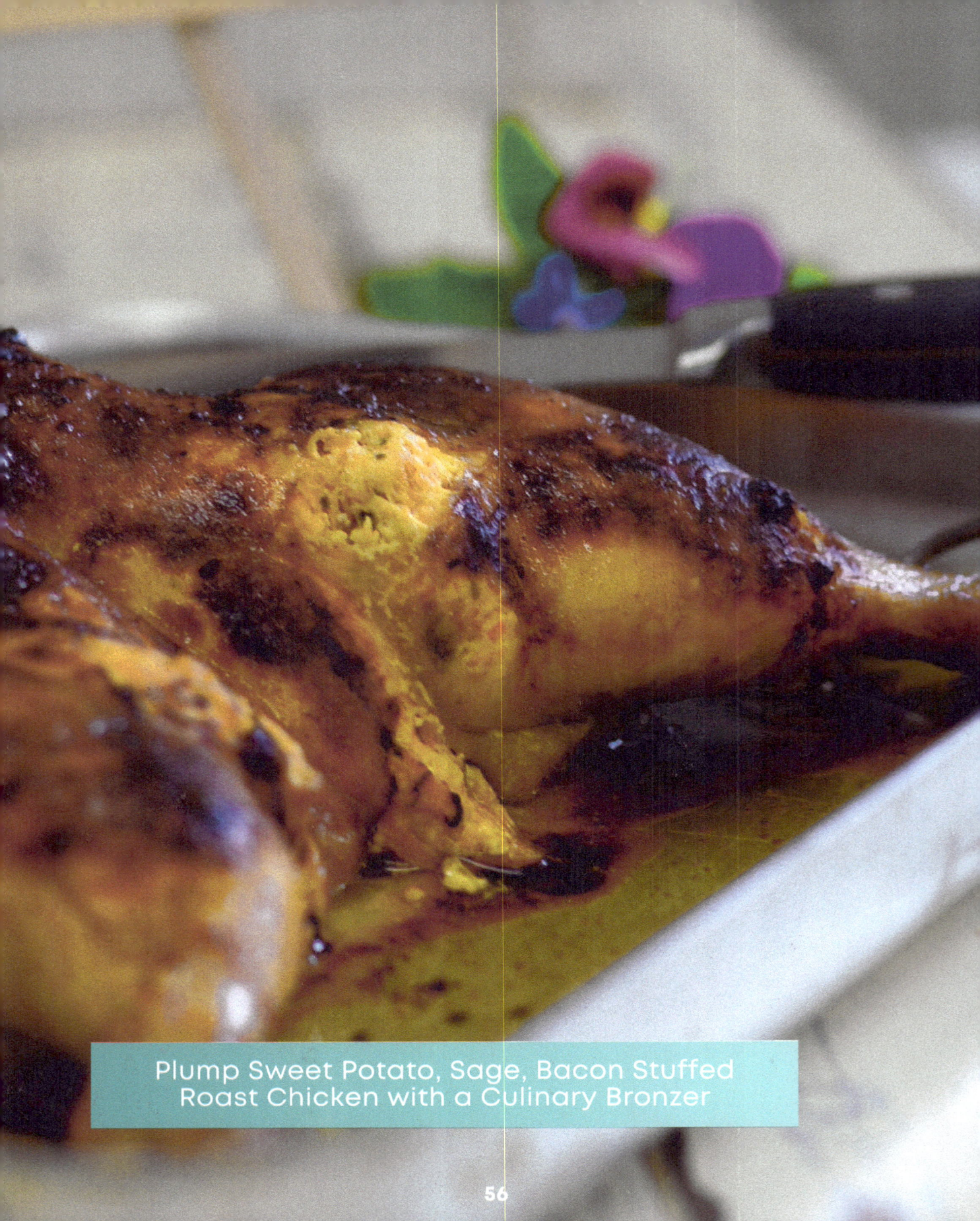

Plump Sweet Potato, Sage, Bacon Stuffed Roast Chicken with a Culinary Bronzer

Plump Sweet Potato, Sage, Bacon Stuffed Roast Chicken with a Culinary Bronzer

SERVINGS: 4-6

INGREDIENTS

CHICKEN

1 family-sized chicken
or use a few 500g spatchcocks instead
1 teaspoon turmeric powder
1 tablespoon curry powder or ras el hanout
50ml olive oil
1 teaspoon flake salt to season

STUFFING

100 g bacon, speck or chorizo
2 cloves garlic, finely chopped
1 onion finely chopped
1 teaspoon fresh or dried sage
2 cups sweet potato cooked
2 tablespoons feta or cream cheese or Parmesan (optional)
Combine together and season to taste; you can add a cup of breadcrumbs!

METHOD

Bling up your next roast with this fabulous 'spray-tanned' roast chicken.
Roast chicken is an all-time favourite. It's the definitive crowd-pleaser and will never go out of fashion. 'Bling' up your next roast with this fabulous turmeric and curry spray-tanned chicken stuffed with roasted sweet potato and chilli.

Prepare the filling by heating and greasing a frying pan until nice and hot (as I like to say "swear word" hot) so that when you add the bacon, it sizzles. Shake the pan, but do not stir too soon. Allow the bacon to brown, and then add the garlic, onion and sage. Reduce the heat and allow the onion to soften before adding the sweet potato mash. Season to taste and allow to cool.

Cut the chicken down the backbone and then open it up to make a chicken flattie. Once laying flat, loosen the skin from the neck side of the bird, loosening it from the flesh all the way down the breasts and down towards the thighs and drumstick as well, creating an envelope for the stuffing. Place spoonfuls of the filling onto the breast and then work it down over onto the drumstick. Keep filling the 'envelope' up until the skin is full all the
way down the drumsticks, thigh and over the breast. Reshape the bird.
Make a 'bronzer' paste with the oil, turmeric and curry powder and then brush all over the bird, giving your bird some fabulous colour and personality.
Roast hot and fast in an oven of 200c for about 20-30 minutes until the juices run clear.
Serve this gorgeous super-model of a bird with a lovely fresh salad, roast vegetables or anything you like!
What do you think of this idea? Would you like more recipes to bling up a simple roast?
Happy cooking, and make sure you put some personality on your plate and bling up every meal.

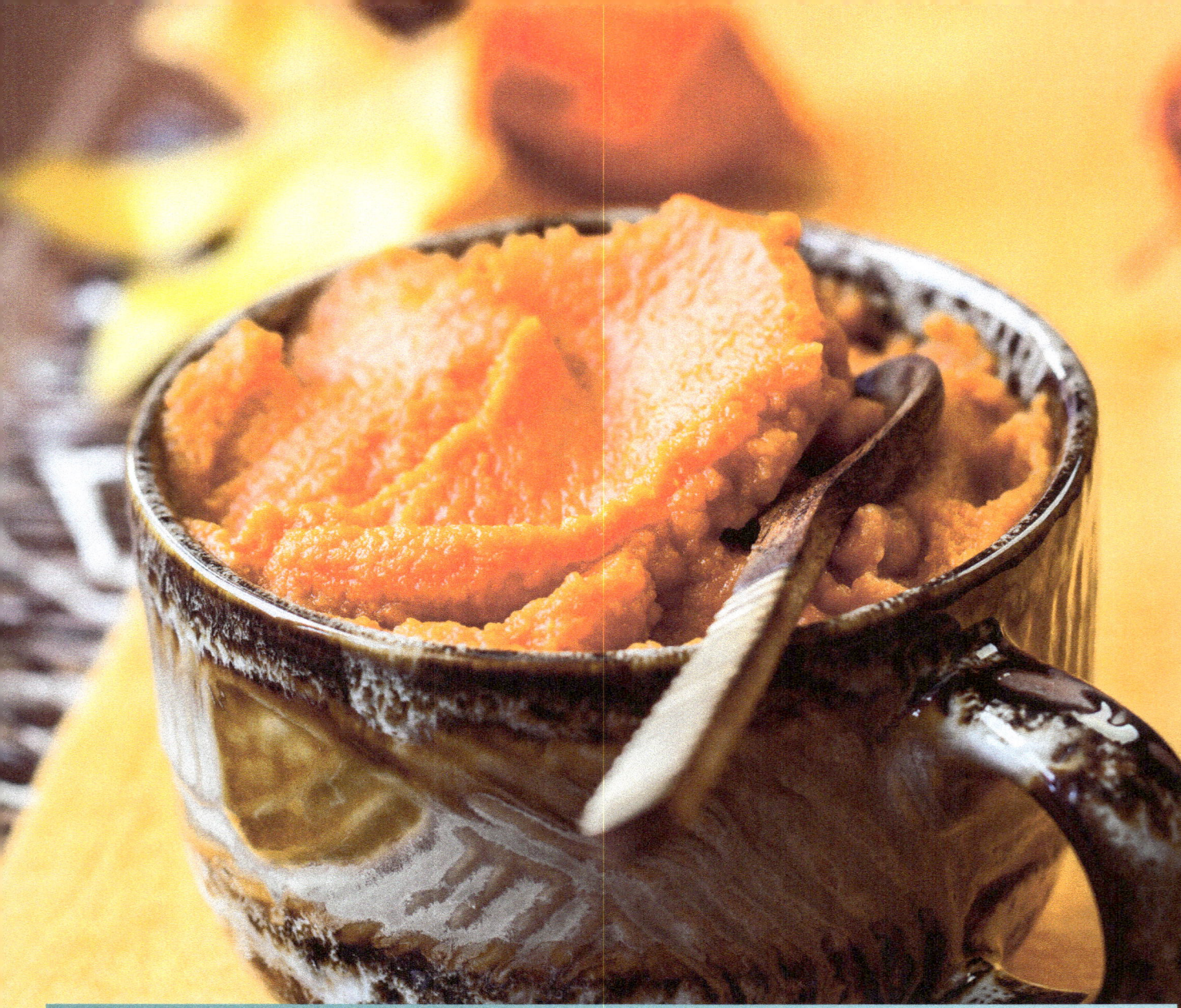

Here's a different stuffing for next time!

Chilli & Pumpkin Stuffing

1 onion finely chopped
1 teaspoon finely chopped chilli
1 teaspoon finely chopped sage
1 teaspoon finely chopped garlic
2 cups roasted/cooked pumpkin (or use butternut or sweet potato)
1 cup bacon bits/speck/chorizo finely chopped

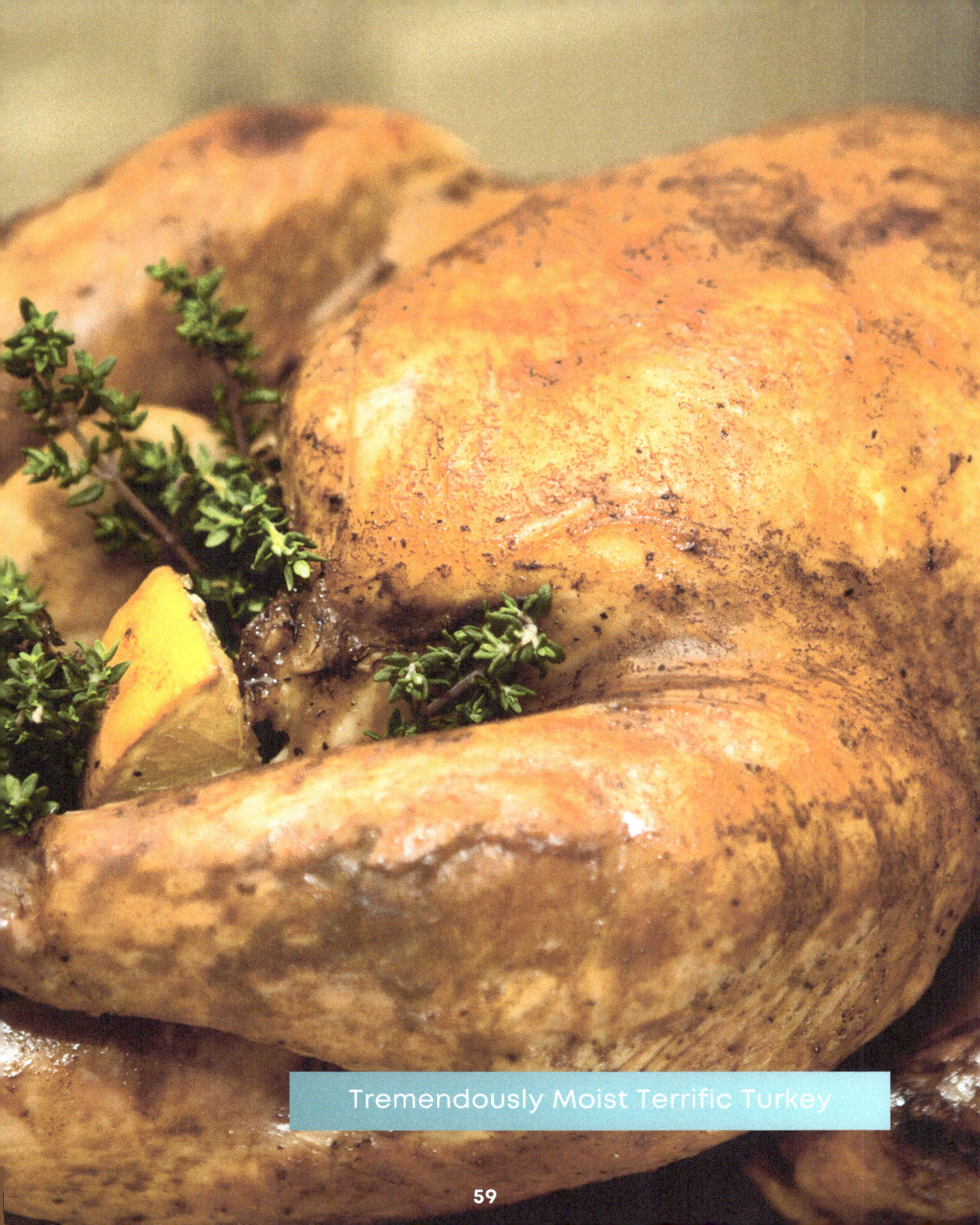
Tremendously Moist Terrific Turkey

Tremendously Moist Terrific Turkey

SERVINGS: 8-10

INGREDIENTS

TURKEY
1 turkey between 3 and 5 kilograms

STUFFING
200g streaky bacon finely chopped
400g pork mince finely chopped
2 cups onion finely chopped
2 cloves garlic (optional)
2 tablespoons freshly chopped sage
Zest and juice of one lemon (optional)
1 teaspoon turmeric (purely for colour)
3 tablespoons naughty butter (this will help give the turkey breast some moisture, personality and flavour)
1 cup fresh breadcrumbs/roast sweet potato /roast potato
Pinch salt
Pinch nutmeg

METHOD

I know this seems like a lot of onion, but you will thank me!
Start by heating a frying pan or large enough pan with a little spray of canola or vegetable oil. Add the bacon to the pan when the pan is swear word hot…it should sizzle and 'talk' to you. Don't stir straight away; let the first lot of bacon on the bottom brown deliciously before stirring. Lots of stirring will cool down the pan too quickly, and you don't want bacon stew. If you are worried, at any stage, about this burning, give the pan a good firm 'cheffy' shake.

Once the bacon is sexy and brown and the fat has rendered out the bacon, keep the heat high and add the pork mince. Let the pan get back to temperature and only stir to prevent it from burning. Using two forks to get rid of the pork mince lumps is a good idea, I also sometimes stab my mince with the base of a whisk… breaks it up really well! When the pork components are brown and beautiful, you can now add the finely diced onions,
garlic, sage, lemon zest, turmeric and nutmeg. You can now reduce the heat and allow those onions to cook down. When soft and it all smells like a little heaven, add the butter, breadcrumbs/roast sweet potato or cooked potato and the lemon juice. Stir and season. Allow to cool.

Now, while cooling, you can tackle the turkey. What we are going to do here is cut the turkey down the backbone and then open it out flat so that it cooks faster. We can get a 3.5kg bird to cook down in 1.5 hours by using this technique.

Continued on next page >>>

Tremendously Moist Terrific Turkey *Continued*

METHOD

You need a big board and a sharp knife. Place the turkey breast down on the board. Cut down the backbone either to the left or right of the spine (don't cut directly in the middle. It's just too difficult). Once the back is open, turn the bird over and break its breastbone with your palm and break it flat. Place on the roasting tray. Is your oven preheated to 160C?

Put the neck side facing closest to you and then loosen the skin away from the turkey all the way down to the drumsticks; you're basically creating a 'turkey envelope' to put your stuffing into.

Use a large tablespoon to feed the cool stuffing onto each breast and then push the stuffing down right over the drumstick. Refill on top of the breast and then reshape the bird. If you have stuffing left over, take a piece of foil, grease it well and then roll the remaining stuffing into a sausage. Seal the foil, and then this can be baked about half an hour before serving the bird.

Rub the skin with lots of olive oil and salt. I even add a bit of turmeric, just a sprinkle, to the skin and rub some oil in to create a turkey spray tan. Season with salt and then place in the oven for approximately 3 hours.

If you need to speed things up, up the temp to 190c, and the bird should be done in 1h45.

Check if juices are running clear; I always check in the breast down by the breastbone to make sure.

This turkey will be terrific to carve, too, and all that juicy goodness will cook into the usually boring turkey meat.

Quickie Lamb Dishes

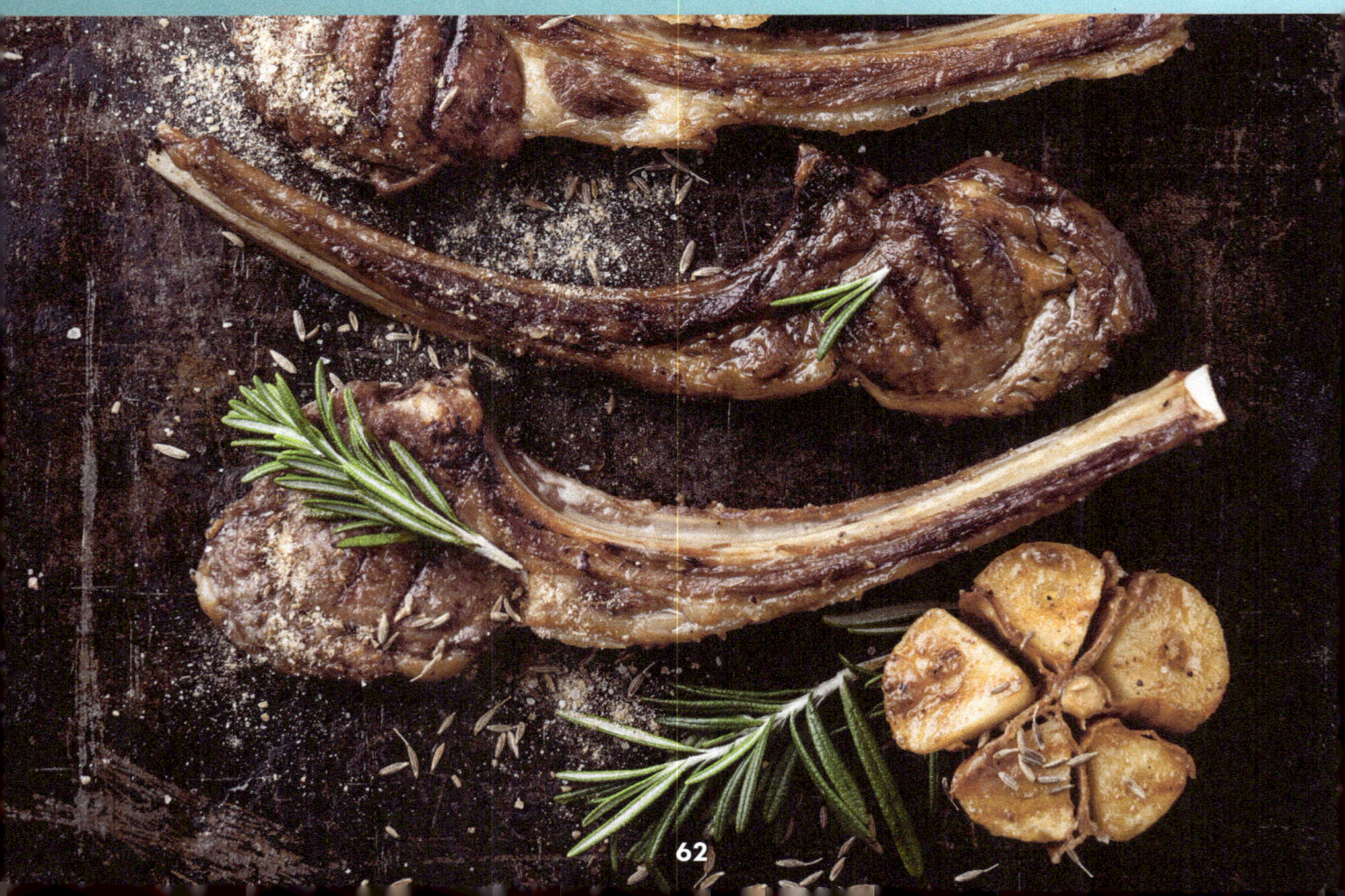

Fragrant Lamb Shoulder with Sticky Figs, Pistachio & Lemon Gravel

SERVINGS: 8-10

INGREDIENTS

LAMB

2-4 kg-lamb shoulder bone in
Salt and pepper to season
1-2 litres weak chicken stock
this will depend on the depth of the baking dish you use
1 teaspoon freshly grated turmeric (or powder)
1 tablespoon ground cumin/ras el hanout spice
1 cinnamon quill and three star anise

BLING

2 tablespoons chopped dried figs or pitted dates
zest of one lemon
1/2 cup almonds/pistachios/other nuts
roasted and chopped

METHOD

Season the shoulder with salt and pepper, some of the turmeric and spices and rub into the skin with a bit of water or oil to give the shoulder a nice suntan!

Now, you can place skin side up in a roasting tray with the stock, making sure the stock comes at least halfway up the shoulder so it is nicely submerged by half. If you have too much cooking liquid, reserve it for later, as you may need to top up the lamb during the cooking process.

Roast (actually, it's braising) in a hot oven of 220C for at least an hour, remove from the oven, turn the shoulder over, return to the oven for half an hour and turn over again.

Cook for another 15-30 minutes to get the skin nicely brown and crisp, and then remove from the oven. Make the bling by mixing the chopped dates, nuts and zest together.

Garnish the lamb with the bling, and then serve!

NOTE:

If you have more time, this benefits from a long slow cook, so reduce the heat to 160C and cook for 4 hours altogether! It will be falling apart with tenderness!

Sun-Tanned Pan-Lamb with Dates, Mint & Pistachio Bling

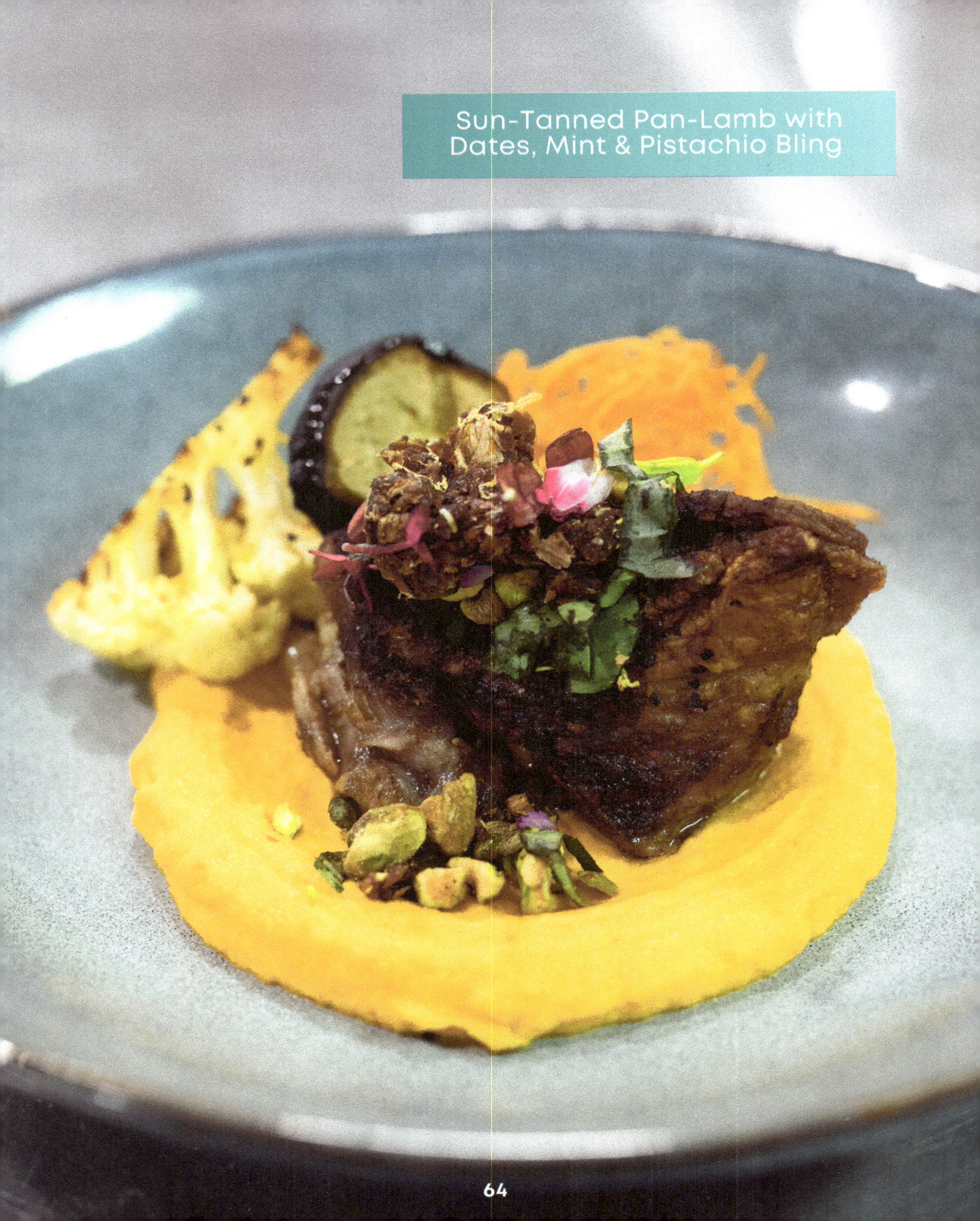

Sun-Tanned Pan-Lamb with Dates, Mint & Pistachio Bling

SERVINGS: 4-6

INGREDIENTS

1 – 1.5kg leg of lamb, deboned and sinews removed
(or use 600-800g lamb back strap)
1 tablespoon turmeric
1 tablespoon ras el hanout or cumin powder
Salt and pepper to season
2 tablespoons olive oil
1 cup dates, chopped. You can also use figs.
½ cup fresh mint leaves, loosely packed
½ cup nuts of your choice (I suggest almonds, cashews and pistachios)

METHOD

MEL'S NOTE:
Leg of lamb is fabulous for this dish but will take about 30 minutes to cook, first on the stovetop, then finish in the oven. The lamb back strap is twice as expensive, BUT you can cook those down in about 8 minutes, so you are practically paying for time and tenderness. Either way, this will be delicious, and try this with your next lamb loin chops as well for a fabulous tread.
Want to use shoulder...no problem; I have a recipe for that, too! See my previous post.

Preheat oven to 200°C only if you are using the leg. Debone the lamb (if required).
Make a rub with the turmeric, ras el hanout and oil. Rub this all over the lamb and allow it to rest while the pan heats. Heat a frying pan (that can go in the oven), and when hot, place the lamb in it.
Cook for about 4 minutes on each side – this is to seal the lamb. Place the lamb (on the frying pan you just used) into the oven for 10-15 minutes. The exact time required will depend on the shape of the meat, your oven and personal preferences.
Remove the lamb from the oven and allow to rest before slicing.
For the date accompaniment – combine the dates, mint and nuts together.

TO SERVE

Serve on a rocket salad with cumin and honey-glazed roasted carrots,
spiced yoghurt and with a butterbean mash.

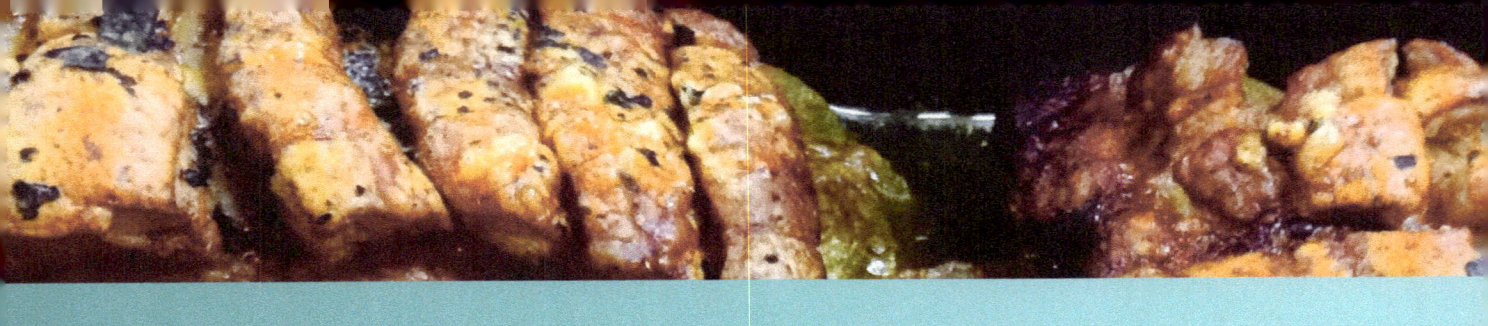

Quickie Pork Dishes

CRACKLING | BELLY | RASHERS | GLAZES

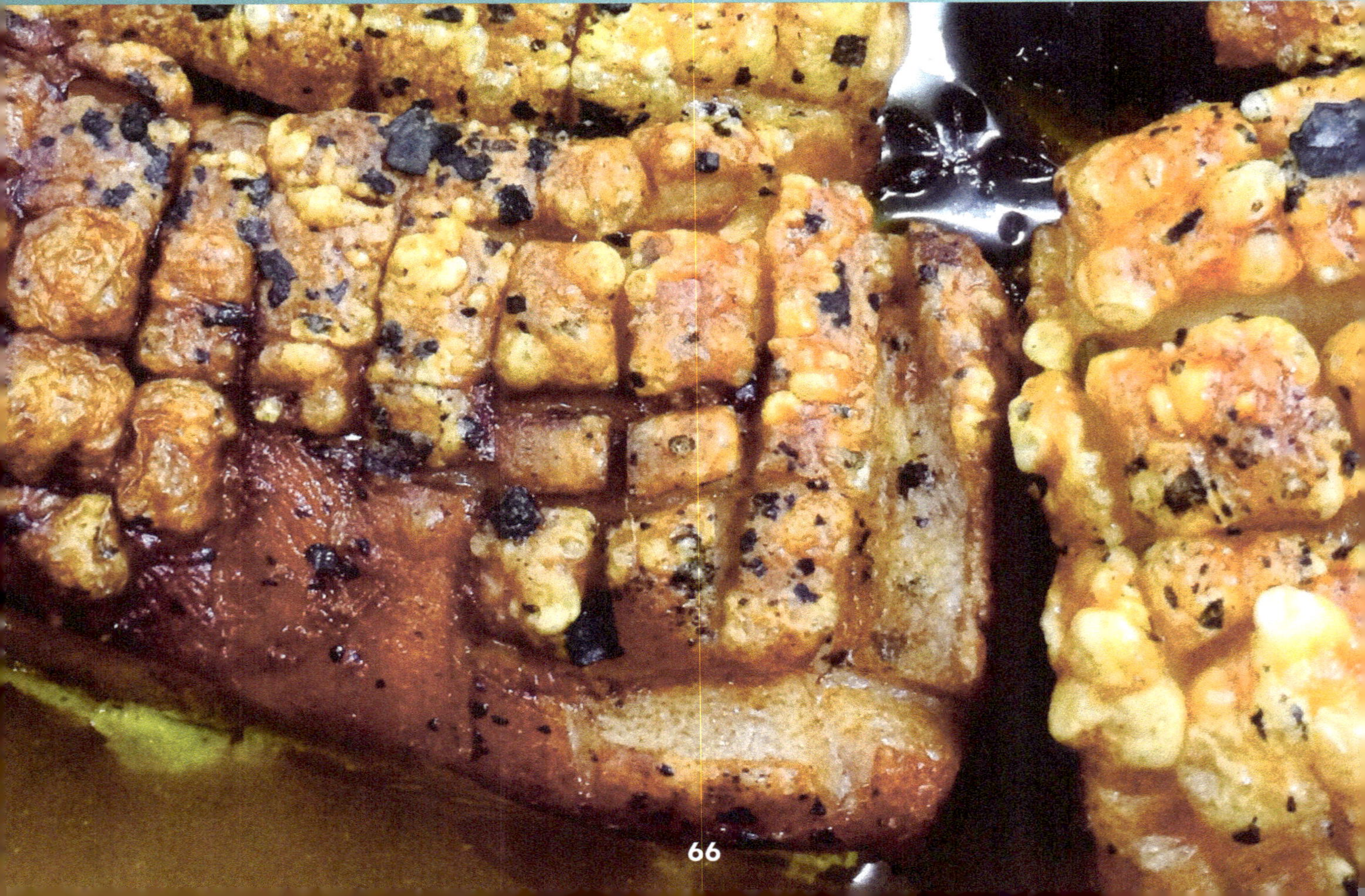

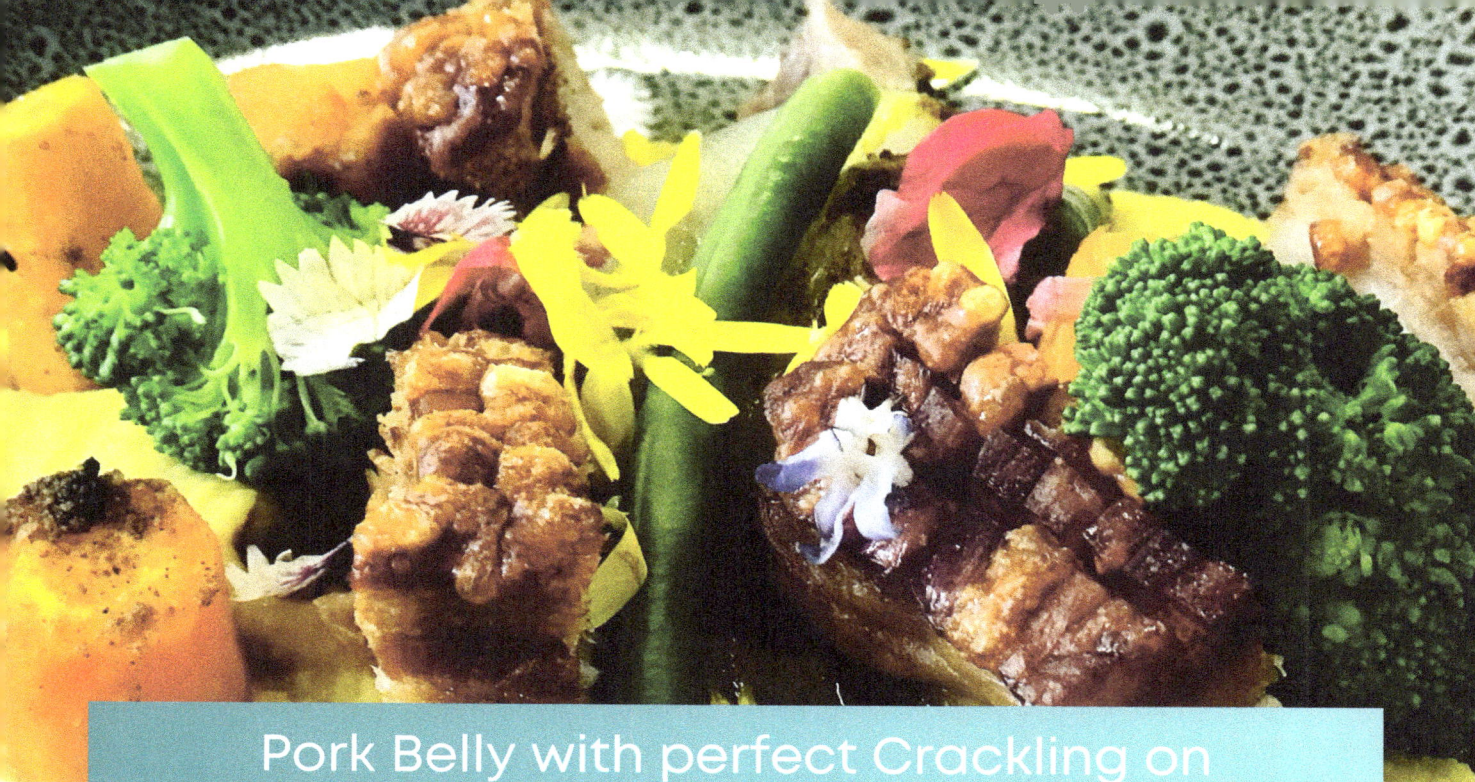

Pork Belly with perfect Crackling on Butterbean Purée

Pork Belly is one of my favourite things in the whole wide world. BUT, whatever I have done here with the belly, you can do with a pork loin roast or even pork shoulder.
I always remove the truss or the net and lay the pork out flat, though, as per that video on my YouTube to ensure you get the perfect crackling EVERY TIME.

I think over the years, it's become my speciality, and I really love this recipe so I had to share it with you. I couldn't be the only one having fun in the kitchen!

There are many myths and long-winded procedures to try and get that perfect crackling, but rest assured, it's easier than you think!

I must be one of the laziest chefs in the world. If I can put something in the oven and then leave it there for an hour and a bit and get a round of applause or a wow when it comes out, I'll do it! And that's exactly how this belly is prepared. It takes all the hard work out of being amazing in the kitchen, and you will be able to smile and feel free again!

Yes, it's decadent. No, you shouldn't wear your skinny jeans the next day. But life is short and decadent food, in moderation, with a balanced diet the rest of the time is okay. I call this one my 80/20 cheat treat and look here, I've served it with beautiful greens and a healthy pea puree, so it's practically a balanced meal!
Also, the belly is economical, and you can cater for many people without any stress.
Allow 250g of belly per person!

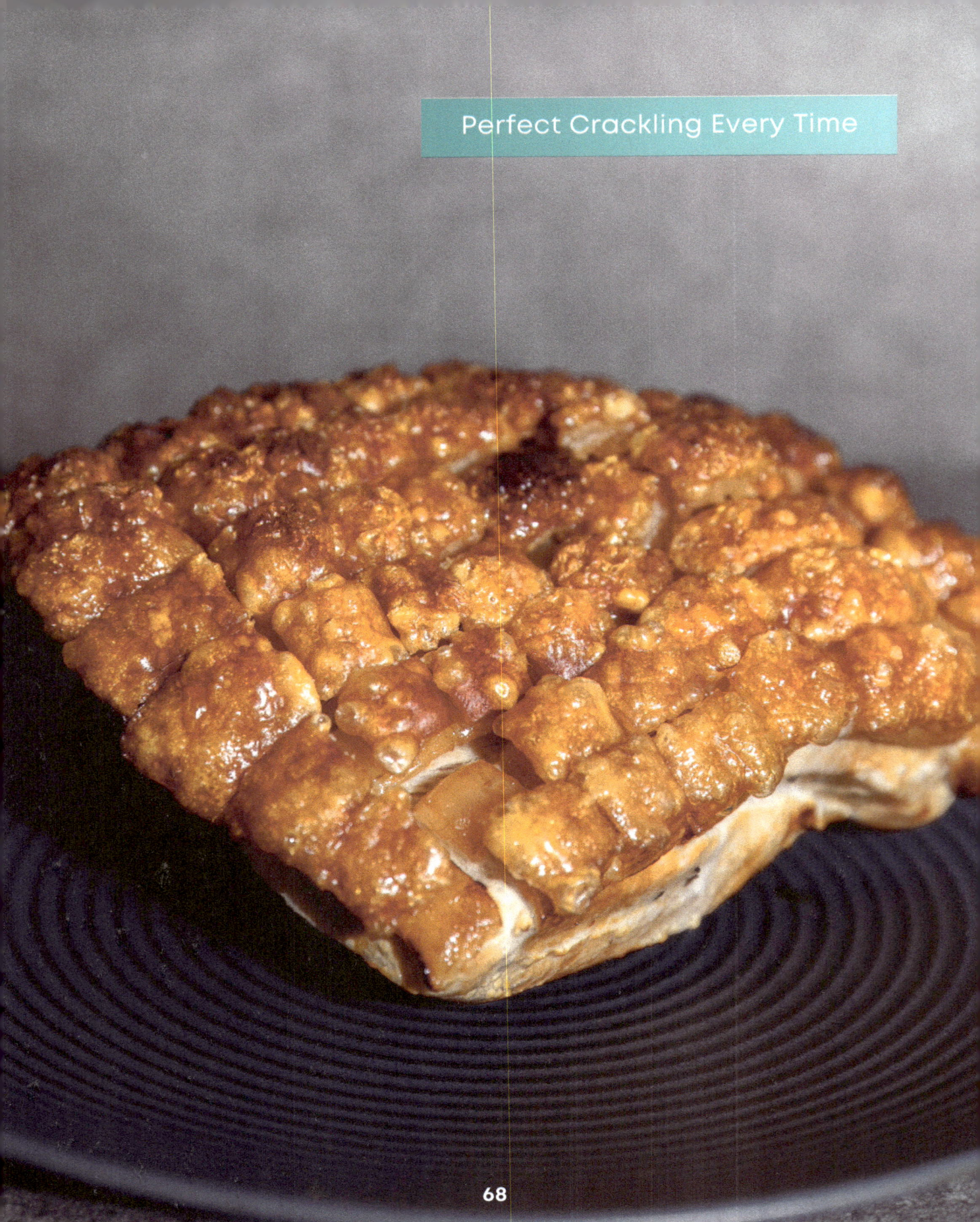

Perfect Crackling Every Time

Perfect Crackling Every Time

WARNING:
Every belly you take home is going to behave differently.
Different fat contents in the belly (lean or fatty), different levels of dryness/moisture in the skin (cryovac sealed or dried overnight skin), your oven/ equipment and your cooking method all have a part to play.
But DON'T PANIC; I'm about to reveal ALL.

BRAISING IS THE BEST COOKING METHOD FOR PORK BELLY WITH PERFECT CRACKLING

The meat is submerged in a tasty cooking liquid and the skin/rind is high and dry and exposed to extreme heat. The flavour AND colour of the cooking liquid will infuse into the meat and keep it perfectly tender and safe from drying out.

SCORING THE SKIN GIVES IT MORE SURFACE AREA SO MORE HEAT CAN POP OUT THE CRACKLING

Get your butcher to score the skin/rind to help that heat get right in there and help pop out that crackling. Most supermarket bellies are already scored. Of course, you can do it yourself, but don't bother if your knife is blunt you WILL end up in tears!

COOK THE BELLY IN A 'SWEAR-WORD' HOT OVEN

Yes, swear word hot so that you know how hot I want this oven. It's the ONLY way. You will not get a speeding fine if you go over 180C, which is the safe zone!
Crank the oven up to its maximum temperature of 220/250C

MINIMUM COOK TIME OF 1H 15MIN

Pork belly with crackling is not a midweek meal that you decide to cook when you've been stuck in traffic for an hour, the kids are screaming with hunger, and food needs to be on the table in 10 minutes flat.
I have recipes for that night, but this is not it.
Belly needs some alone time in the oven for at least an hour and 15 minutes. This is fabulous if you are having a dinner party, which means you can clean the kitchen, set the table, and get yourself all cleaned up and glamorous while the OVEN DOES THE WORK.
You might need to top up the cooking liquid once or twice, but that's about it.

GIVE THAT BELLY A SUNTAN UNDER THE GRILL

In most cases, after an hour in the oven, the belly might not have popped its crackling. Do not start crying, drinking excessively or panicking; there are ways and means to get your way.
Place the belly on the bottom shelf of your oven. It must be as far away from the grill as possible. Use a preheated grill. Stay close. Close the door.
The extreme heat or 'suntan' from the direct heat of the grill will blast that fat out and give you the perfect crackling, but BEWARE…if you get distracted or if something happens on Facebook and you forget about the belly it will burn. Stay close and monitor the crackling; you will be surprised what that long-distance relationship with the grill can do to your belly.
Once it's all popped out, remove it from the oven and get ready to get that round of applause.

Beautiful Suntanned Beer-Braised Pork Belly with Caramelised apples and onions

SERVINGS: 6-8

INGREDIENTS

1.5-2 kg Pork belly

2-4 cups weak chicken or vegetable stock

(The amount required depends on the size of your roasting dish)

1 can beer or cider

1 tablespoon turmeric (this is the secret to the belly suntan!)

1 tablespoon cumin/curry/ras el hanout powder

2-star anise

1 cinnamon stick

2 onions, thickly sliced

2 pears or apples, thickly sliced

Salt to sprinkle the rind

METHOD

To prepare the belly, first ensure that you have dried the skin as much as possible using a paper towel or a tea towel. Score the skin of the belly and cut the belly into serving-sized portions.

Place pear/apples and onion in a roasting dish and put the pork on top – the intention is to ensure that the pork skin will stay dry while it is being cooked. Essentially, we are using the onions and the apples/pears as CULINARY HIGH HEELS.

Mix the stock, beer/cider and spices together in a jug and CAREFULLY pour into the roasting dish – making sure not to wet the skin of the pork. You want the liquid to come about halfway up the side of the pork.

Pat the pork skin dry again and then dust liberally with salt and immediately place into a swear word hot oven (220 - 250C).

Cook for at least 1 ¼ hrs., checking regularly to ensure the liquid doesn't dry out. If the skin is not crackling, turn the grill on for 5 minutes at a time, place the belly on the bottom shelf, and then put it back in the oven, watching closely until that lovely skin pops out into perfect crackling - heaven.

TO SERVE

Turn the pork upside down to carve if needed – this makes cutting the crackling easier. But turn it back over quickly so it doesn't go soggy. Serve the cooking liquid, pears and onions as part of the dish. Make sure you taste it first and adjust the seasoning if necessary. If the liquid has cooked down too much, simply add more water and heat through. There is no need to thicken. You can serve this as a broth or thicken to make a gravy; just take some of the fat off first! A paper towel on the surface is the easiest, or you can plunge ice cubes into the liquid, and the ice will solidify the fat, and you can scoop the fatty ice cubes off and discard them.

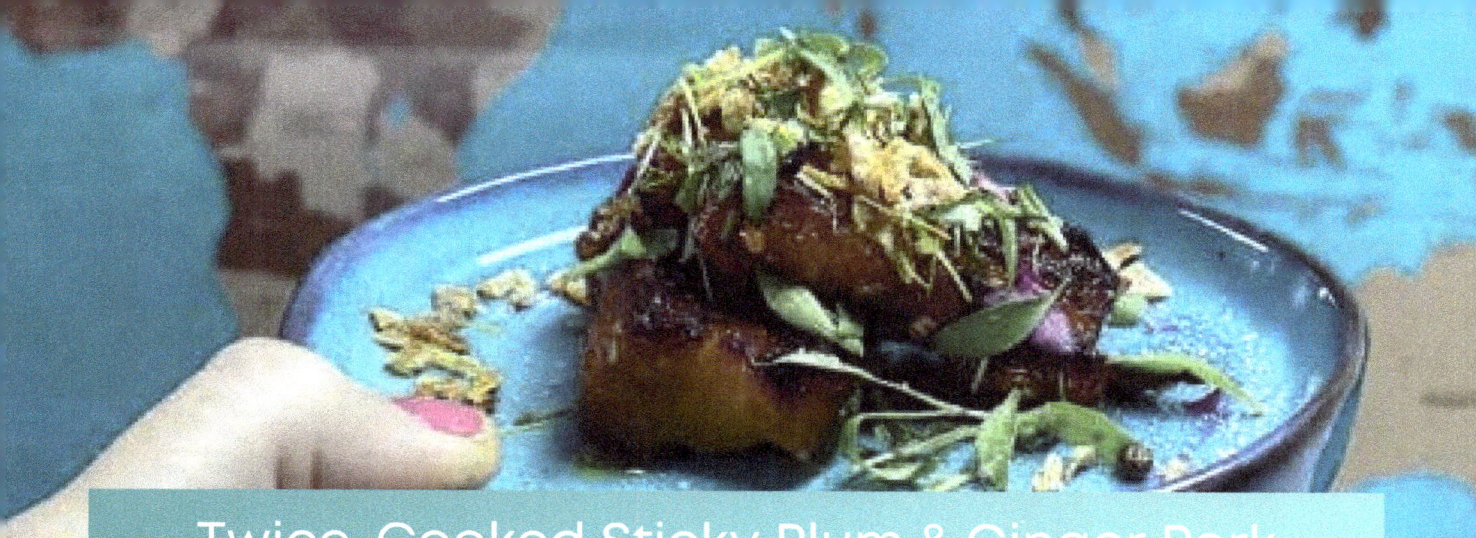

Twice-Cooked Sticky Plum & Ginger Pork Rashers

SERVINGS: 6-8

INGREDIENTS

PORK RASHERS
800g-1kg pork rashers
2 litres water
1 tablespoon salt
2 star anise/cardamom pods
1 teaspoon cinnamon
2 teaspoons turmeric powder

PLUM & GINGER GLAZE
3 tablespoons plum jam,
2 tablespoons crushed ginger
1 tablespoon crushed lemon grass
1 tablespoon crushed garlic
1 teaspoon turmeric

METHOD

The perfect BBQ or midweek entertainer.
Decadent and sticky pork rashers are the ultimate indulgence, and don't let the twice-cooked bit make you think these are difficult; they are reliably easy and well worth a try.
They will become your 'signature' dish for many years to come.

Place the water, salt and spices in a large pot and then boil the pork rashers hot and fast over a high heat for at least 20 minutes. Do not be alarmed! These will not look very appetising once they are boiled, but this will soon be rectified once we add our delicious culinary glaze.

Remove the rashers from the boiling liquid and then drain. Place in a large bowl. Mix the jam with the crushed pastes and then stir through the rashers to coat them. Place the rashers, single layer, in a greased roasting tray/baking dish and roast in a preheated oven of 200c for about 10-15 minutes until the rashers are golden and sticky. You can turn them over halfway, but if the oven is hot enough, they should seal from the heat of the tray as they roast. Serve hot. Delicious.

Quickie Sides & Accompaniments

CURRY PASTE | SAUCES | MASH | PURÉE

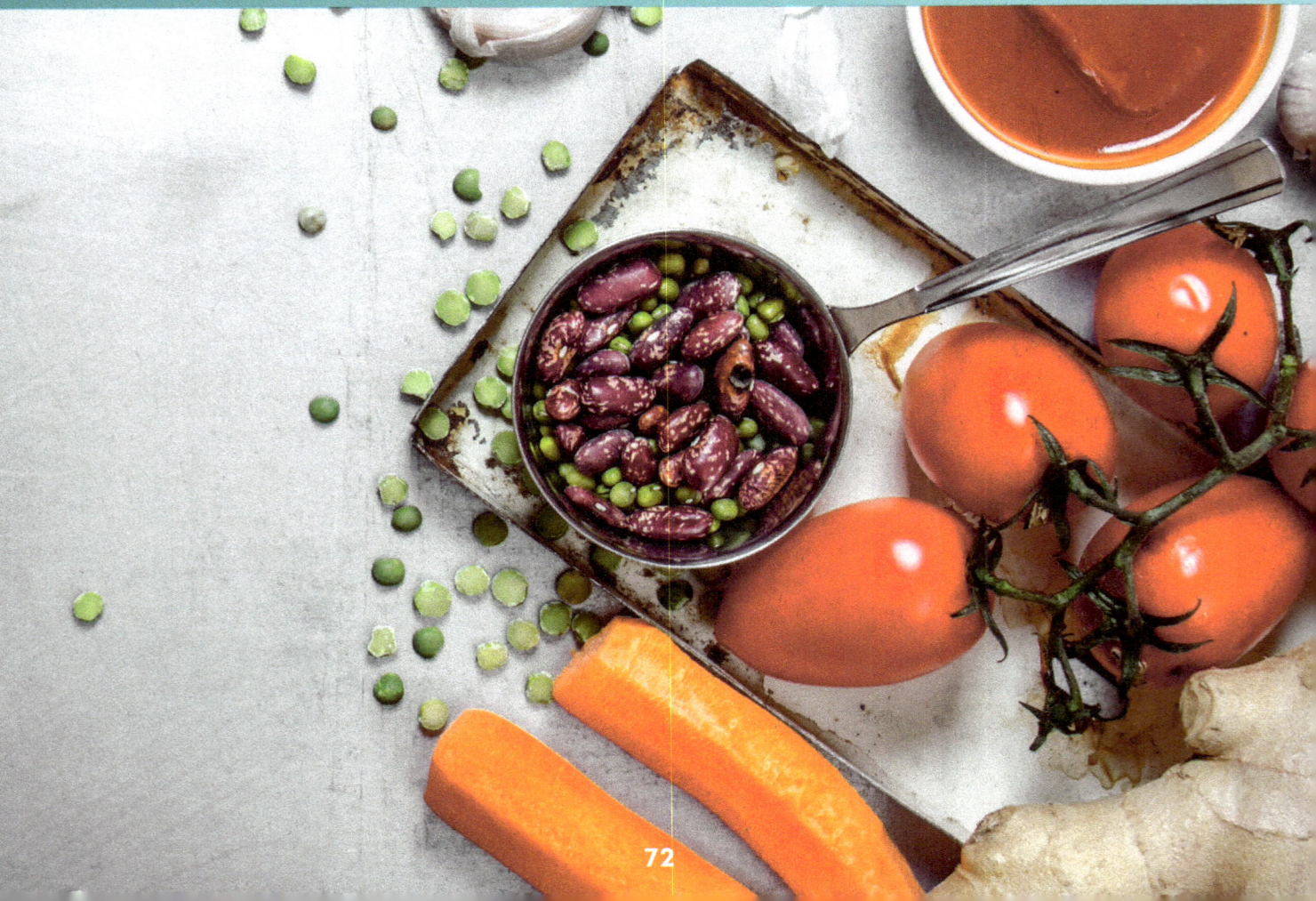

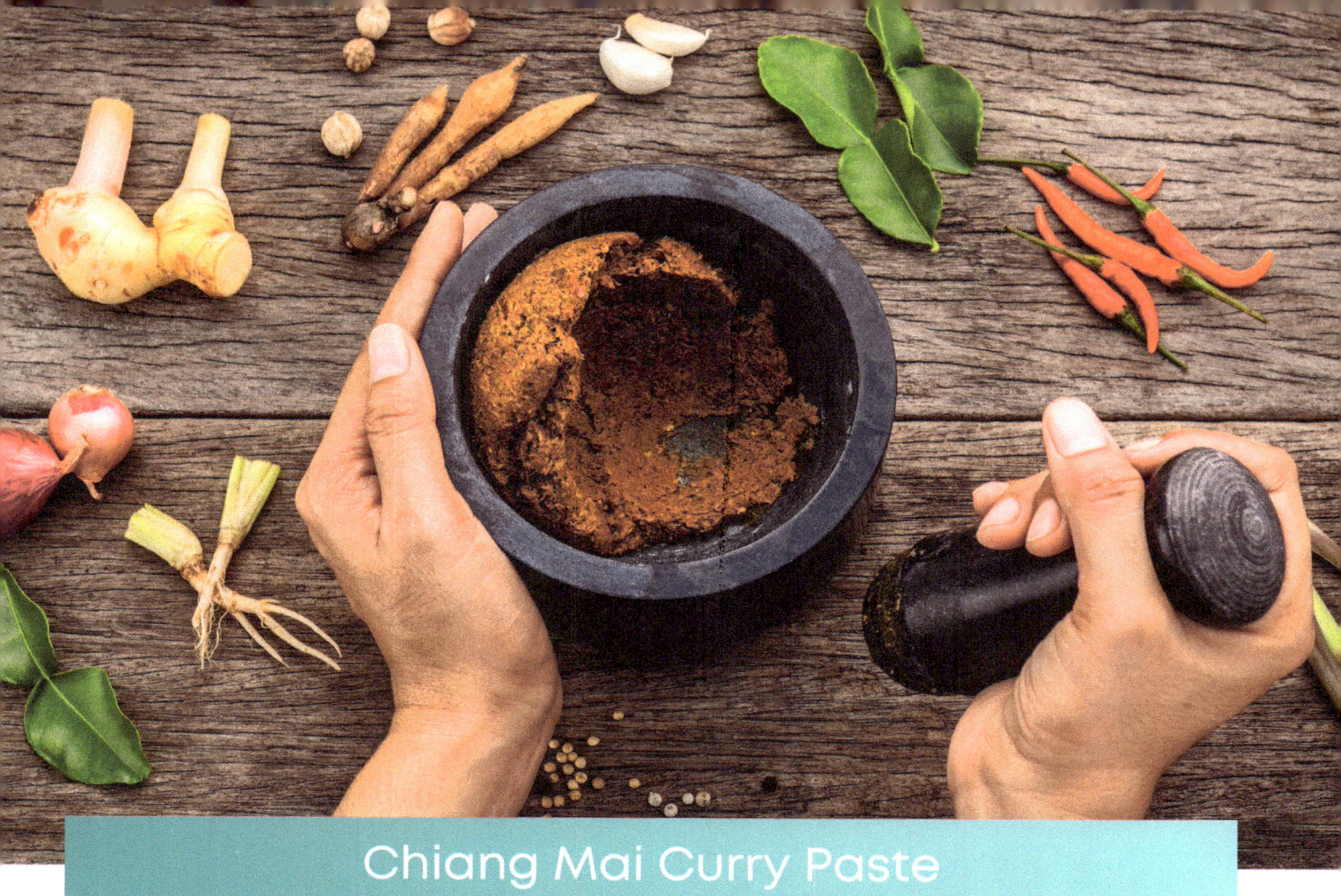

Chiang Mai Curry Paste

SERVINGS: 2-4

INGREDIENTS

½ teaspoon salt
3 big red chillies (or as you prefer)
2 tablespoons Ginza (ginger) skin removed, chopped
2 tablespoons lemongrass chopped
6 Asian shallots chopped
1 garlic clove chopped
1 teaspoon shrimp paste
1 tablespoon turmeric, fresh or dried

METHOD

Put all the ingredients in a mortar and pestle or a stick blender until it forms a smooth thick paste. Use on chicken, fish, beef, pork or vegetables.

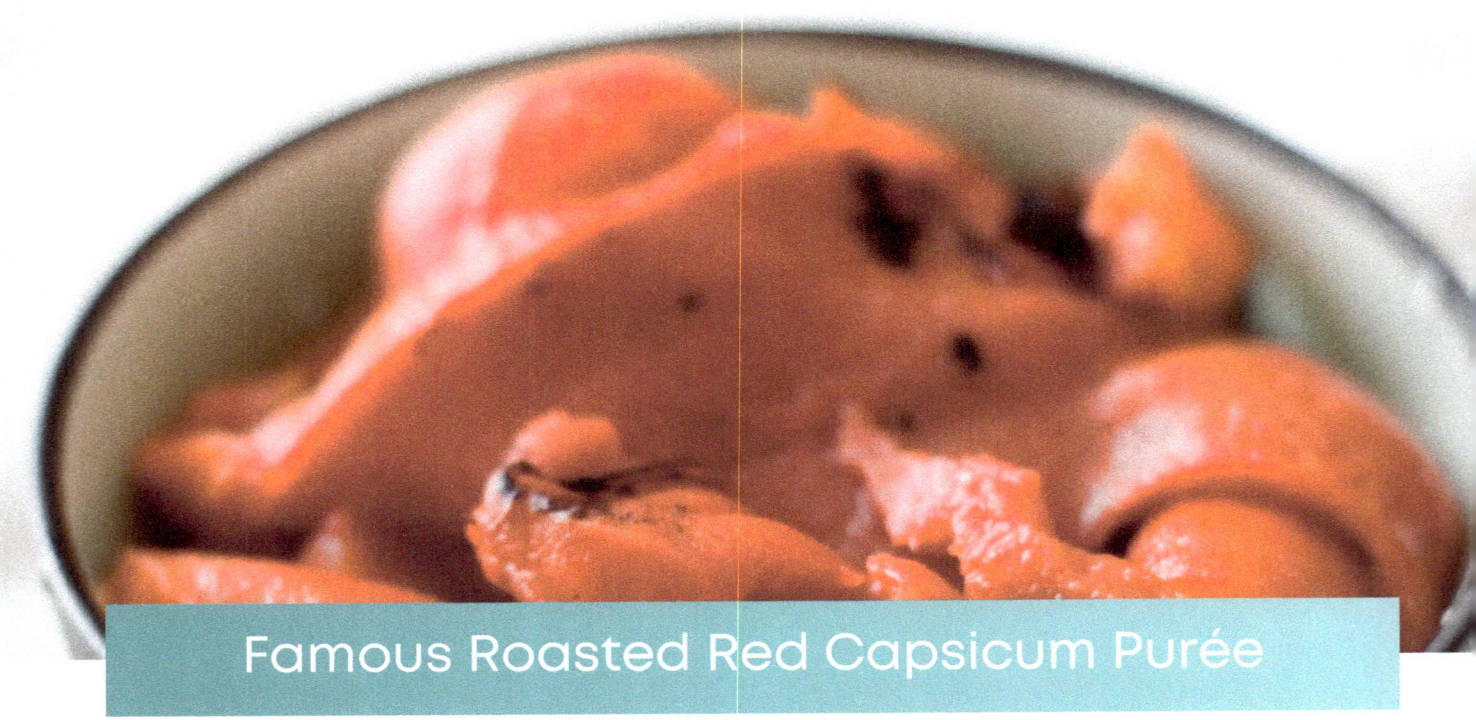

Famous Roasted Red Capsicum Purée

SERVINGS: 4-6

INGREDIENTS

Olive oil to fry

1 onion finely chopped

2 cloves garlic

1 cup roasted red capsicums

(cut in half, place under the grill until the skin goes black, cool, and then remove skin)

500ml tomato passata

Salt and pepper to season

Half a teaspoon of turmeric freshly grated or use powder

1 pinch cumin or Ras el Hanout OR Chilli

METHOD

As requested by so many. The most fabulous sauce EVER. Famous Roasted Red Capsicum Puree. I used this with the Moroccan Mince recipe but you can use it with pasta, chicken, steak or as a gravy replacement. Add a little sugar if you need to.

Fry the onions and the garlic in the oil until just soft. Add the cooked capsicum, the tomato passata/puree and the seasoning and cook through. Place these gorgeous ingredients in a food processor or use a stick blender and blend until smooth.

A fantastic accompaniment to a wide variety of dishes and salads, and heaps of fun to garnish with.

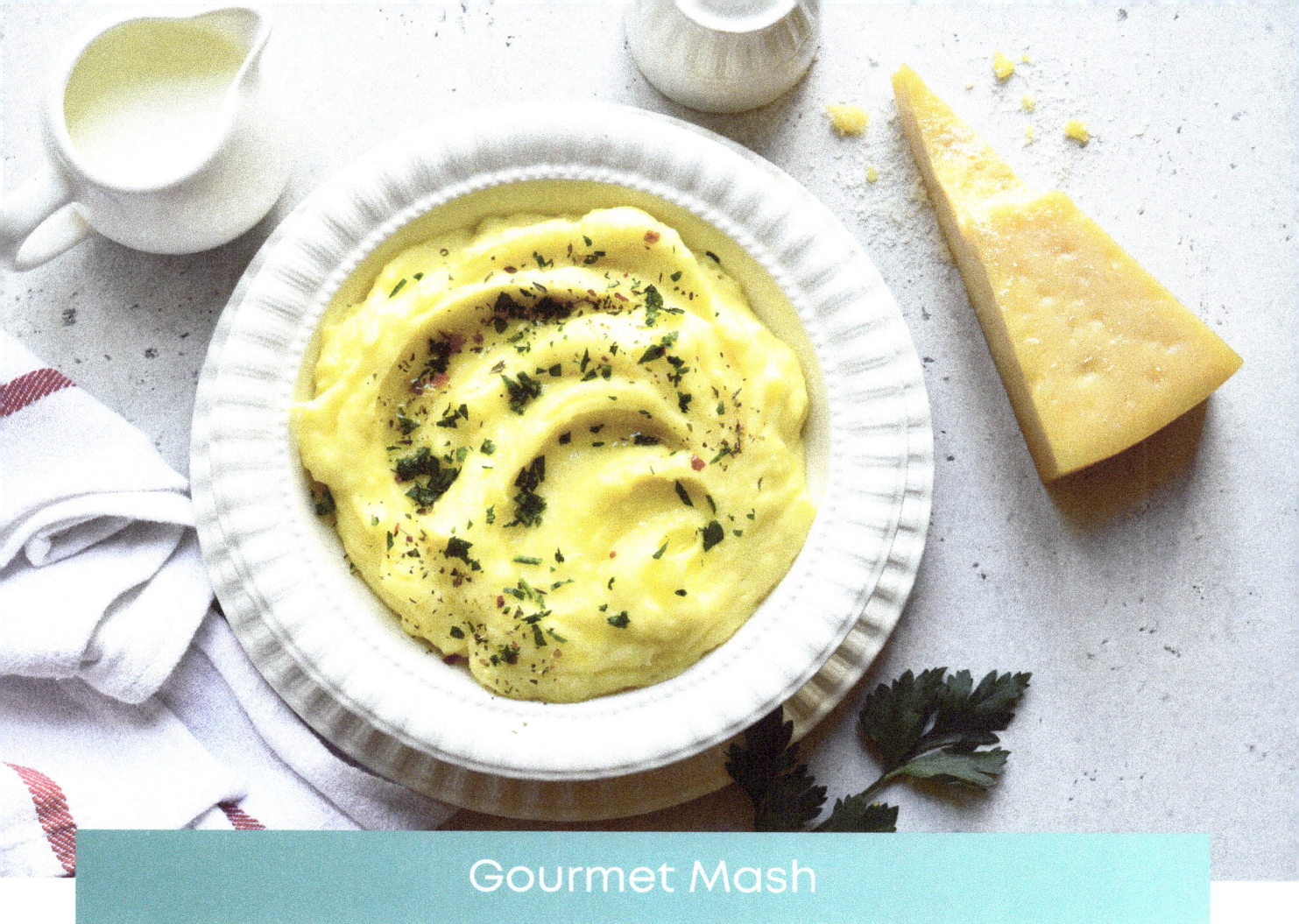

Gourmet Mash

SERVINGS: 4-6

INGREDIENTS

6 medium potatoes boiled until cooked in salted water
100 ml milk or cream
50 g butter
15 ml grainy mustard
15 ml chopped chives or parsley or herb of your choice
50 g grated Parmesan or Cheddar cheese
Salt and freshly ground pepper to taste

METHOD

Once the potatoes have cooked drain and then mash until free of lumps.
Now add the milk/cream and the butter as well as the remaining ingredients.
Season to taste and then serve in hot dollops with your main!

Quickie Desserts & Cakes

CAKES | PUDDINGS | PIES | MUFFINS | SCONES | BROWNIES

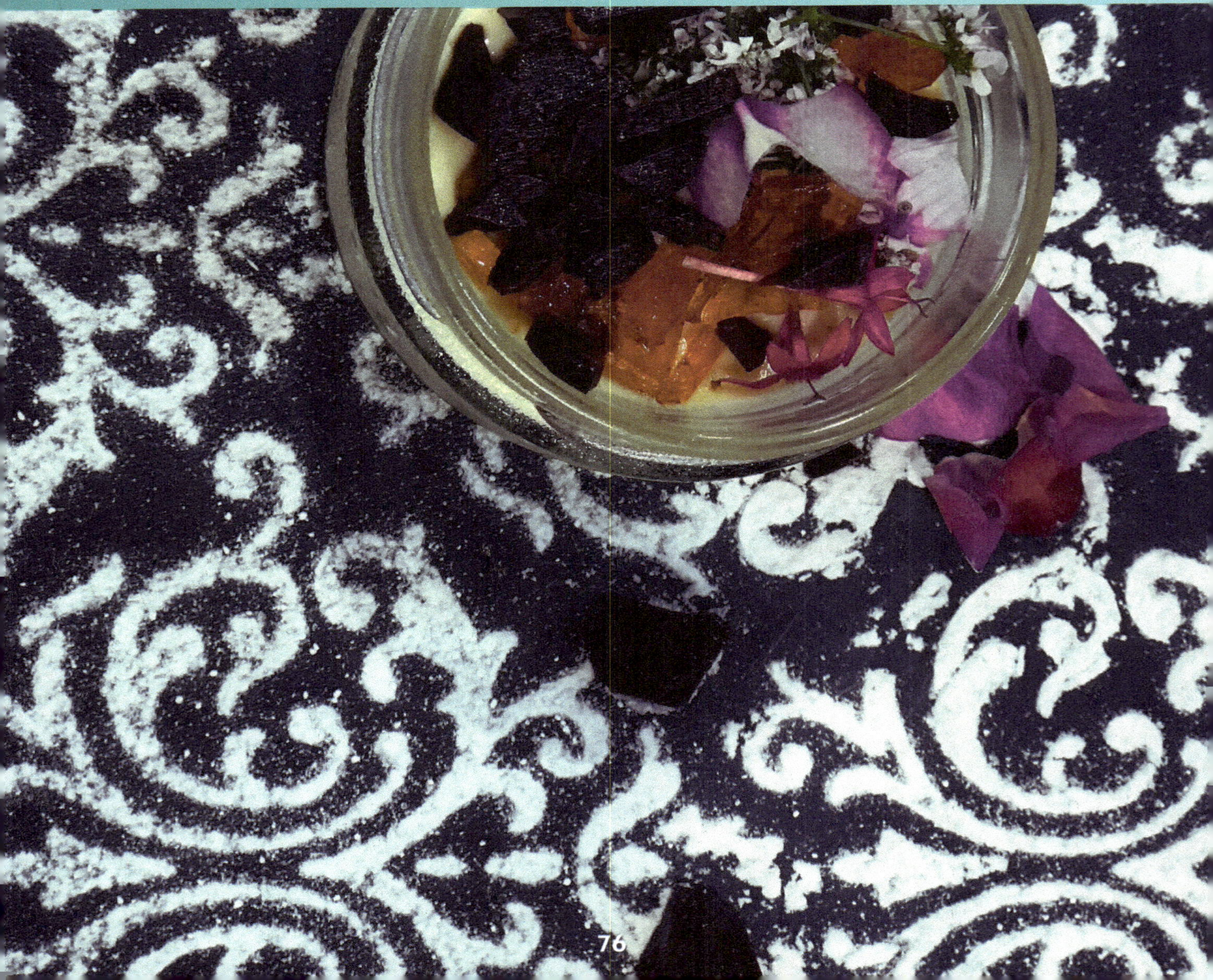

Easy Panna Cotta

SERVINGS: 6-10

INGREDIENTS

200ml full cream milk
800ml thickened cream
140g white, raw sugar, honey or maple syrup
1 teaspoon vanilla paste
4 sheets of gold gelatine soaked in cold water for 1 minute
(it will look like a wet tissue when you pick it up, then squeeze it out and add to the hot liquid)

METHOD

Try my tested recipe, and once you've mastered the basics, imagine how many different flavours you could make. Once you make your peace with the fact that leaf gelatine is EASY to use, you will literally live happily ever after! Please try to use leaf gelatine instead of powder gelatine; the quality and flavour are heaps better. Quick to make, but you do need 4-6 hours for this to set or even make a few days in advance. This recipe is on my YouTube channel.

Simply place the cream and milk in a saucepan and heat until just about to boil.
Make sure you stir so the bottom doesn't burn; the only flavour we want is beautiful creamy milk and cream; if you do burn it start again! Add the sugar and vanilla and stir until dissolved, and then add the softened and prepared gelatine and mix until dissolved. Pour into glasses, ramekins, dariole moulds or similar, cover with cling film and then place in the fridge. Depending on how large you have made them, they could take up to 6 hours to set, so these are perfect made in advance! Enjoy!

VARIATIONS

Flavours: These can be added to the cold milk and cream and will infuse into the cream when it heats.
Add 200g chocolate
Add 1 tablespoon lemon zest
Add 1 teaspoon edible lavender
Add a cinnamon quill
Add 2 star anise

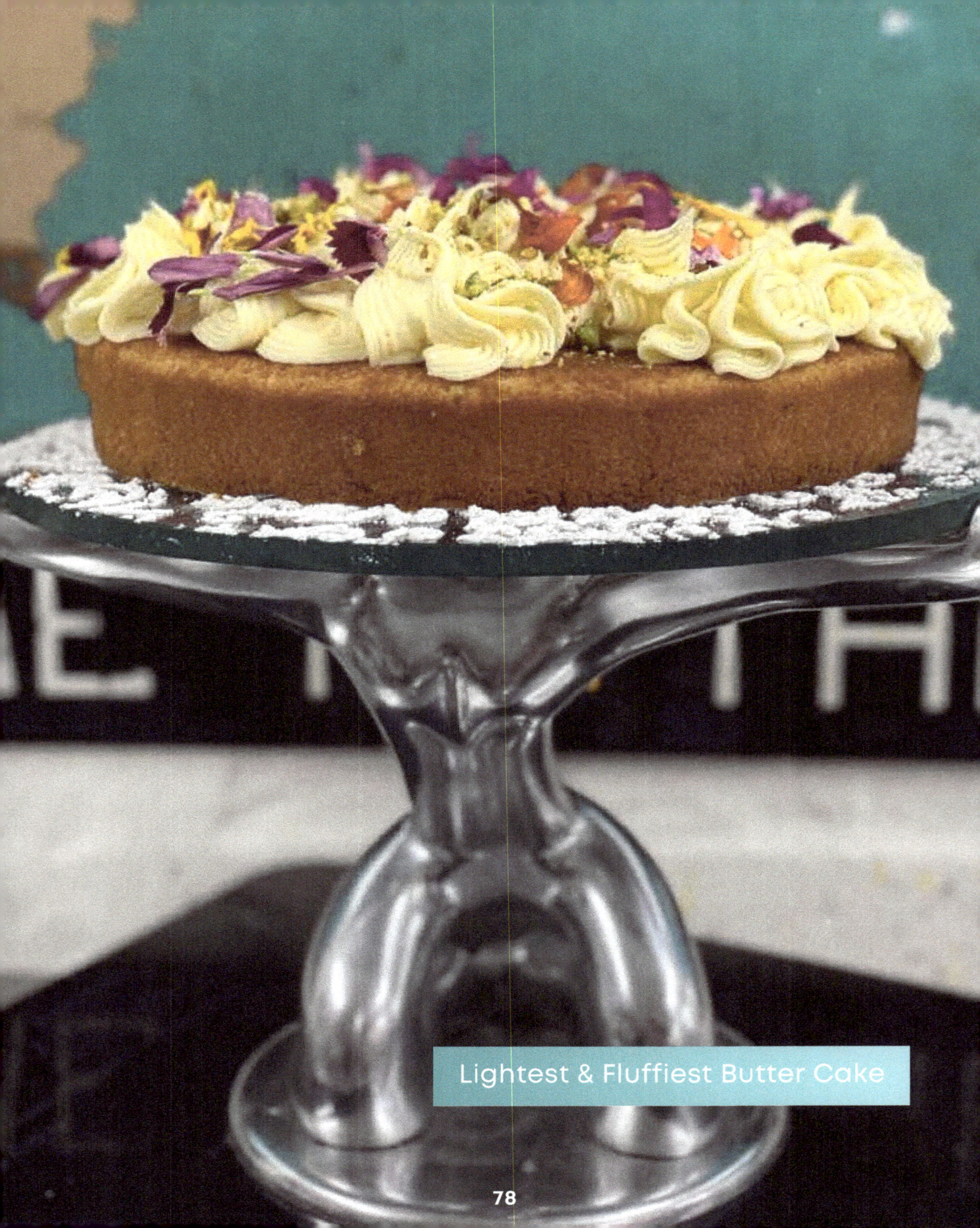

Lightest & Fluffiest Butter Cake

SERVINGS: 6-10

INGREDIENTS

CAKE

- 4 large room-temperature free-range eggs
- 225 g salted butter
- 1/4 cup white sugar AND 3/4 cup white sugar
- 200g self-raising flour
- 60ml milk
- 10ml vanilla extract
- 1 teaspoon grated lime or lemon

ICING

- 250g butter
- 3 cups icing mixture
- Milk on the side, about 30-60ml *to get the consistency you like*
- 10 ml vanilla paste

This is the cake I made when I married the man of my dreams. I knew this was his favourite cake so I perfected it. And I just can't wait to get old together. I'm always so grateful to get to the next year, I don't mind the wrinkles, I am just lucky to still be here so that I can spend more time spreading culinary happiness.

And, for those who know me, do I ever like to share happiness? So the best way for me to do that is to share this amazing recipe with you so that you too can join in the good vibes that will surely arise the minute you put this amazing light fluffy delicious ridiculously easy cake on your taste buds. I don't often bake, because I can't be trusted not to eat the entire cake myself, but this one is worth it. I would do 100 burpees or sit-ups just to have ONE slice of this deliciousness…and like they say…life is short so EAT THE CAKE!

METHOD

Firstly, separate the eggs. Beat the 4 egg whites until just about to hit peak stage, and then add the 1/4 cup white sugar and beat until thick and looking like meringue.

In a separate bowl, beat the 3/4 cup sugar and butter with the whisk attachment until light and pale fluffy. The sugar must be dissolved right through, and the mixture should look like a little bit of heaven…all light and fluffy! Now put the mixer on to really low and add the egg yolks, self-raising flour, milk, vanilla and zest. Mix well to form a smooth batter.

Using a plastic spatula, fold in the meringue mix gently to incorporate it with the batter, but don't over-mix; you want to combine the two mixes lightly. Now pour into a greased baking dish or cake mould.

Bake for about 45 minutes at 170c, until a skewer comes out clean from the middle.

Always check at the 15-minute mark to make sure the temperature is perfect; if it's going too dark too quickly, drop the temp to 160C! Once cooked, remove from the oven and cool.

Beat the butter with the whisk until very light and very fluffy. Add the icing mixture to the vanilla paste and then mix again till smooth. At this stage, you can add the milk slowly, slowly, to get the consistency you need! Once the cake is cooled, ice as required and decorate with fresh flowers, chocolate shavings or sugared lemons.

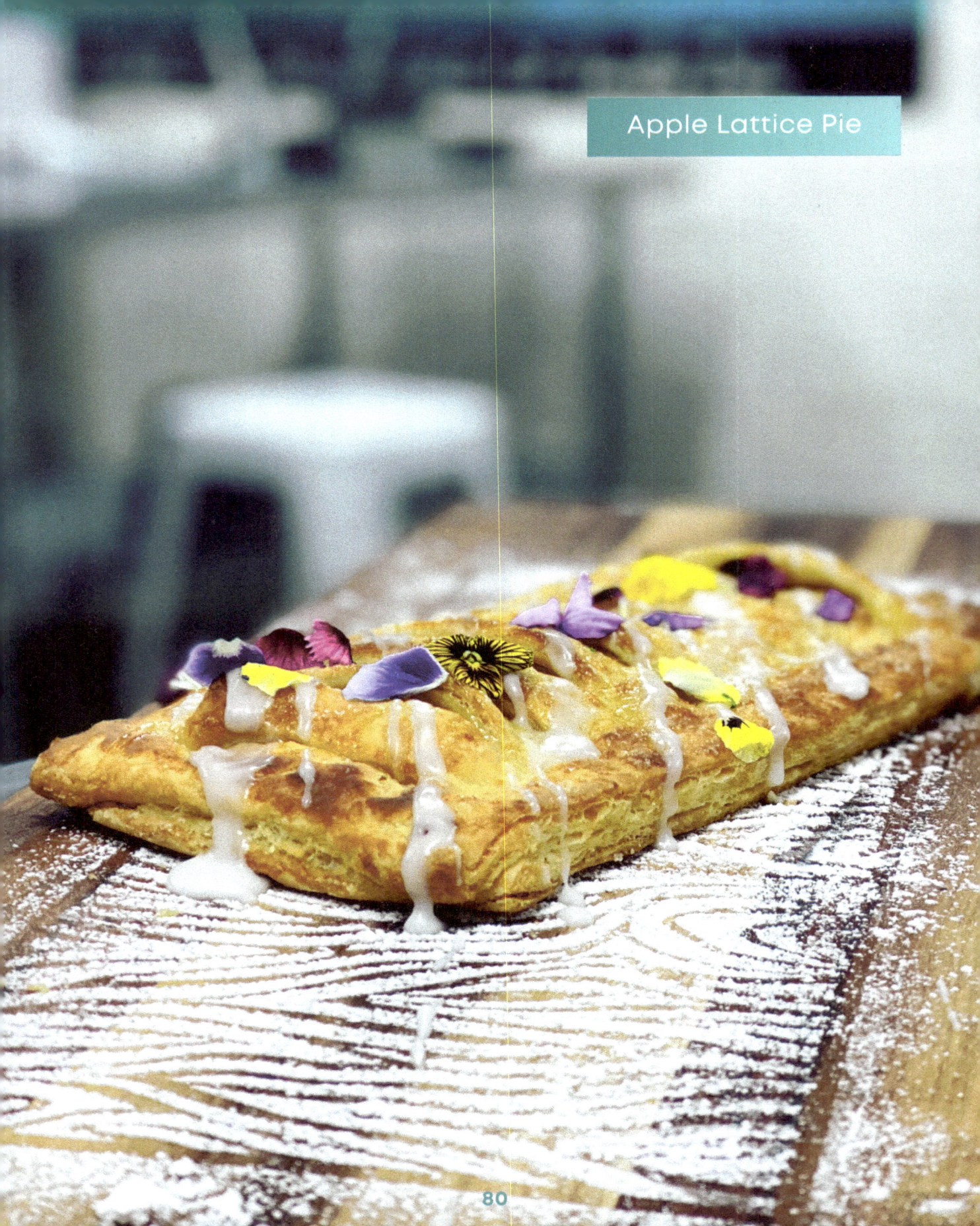

Apple Lattice Pie

Vanilla Apple Lattice Pie

SERVINGS: 6-8

INGREDIENTS

PIE
2 sheets of puff pastry
2 large apples cored and then sliced
(can also use pears, mangos, nectarines and peaches)
3 tablespoons apricot jam
50 ml milk to brush pastry
250 ml really thick custard blended with 100 ml cream
2 tablespoons white sugar to dredge over pastry

ICING
1 cup icing sugar mixed to a paste with
Hot water (to bind, about a tablespoon)
1 teaspoon vanilla extract or essence

METHOD

Cut the pastry in half lengthways.
Place the apricot jam onto one half of the pastry, taking care to leave a border of about 2 cm.
Dollop the cup of thick custard on top of the apricot jam, and take care to leave the border clean.
Place the sliced apples neatly on top of the jam.
Fold the remaining piece of pastry in half lengthways and slice on the fold to create a lattice, taking care to leave a border of about 2 cm.
Brush the filled pastry on the border with the milk and then top with the second piece of pastry.
Brush again with the milk and then dredge with sugar.
Bake in a preheated oven of 200c for about 15 – 20 minutes until golden.
Remove from heat and then drizzle with the glaze icing.
Reserve a little of the glaze icing and mix with a teaspoon of cocoa powder, mix until smooth.
Drizzle over the white glaze as a delectable contrast.
Serve hot or cold with ice cream or cream… deliciously simple.
It will slice into at least 8 slices, but you can make them smaller.

Carrot Cake

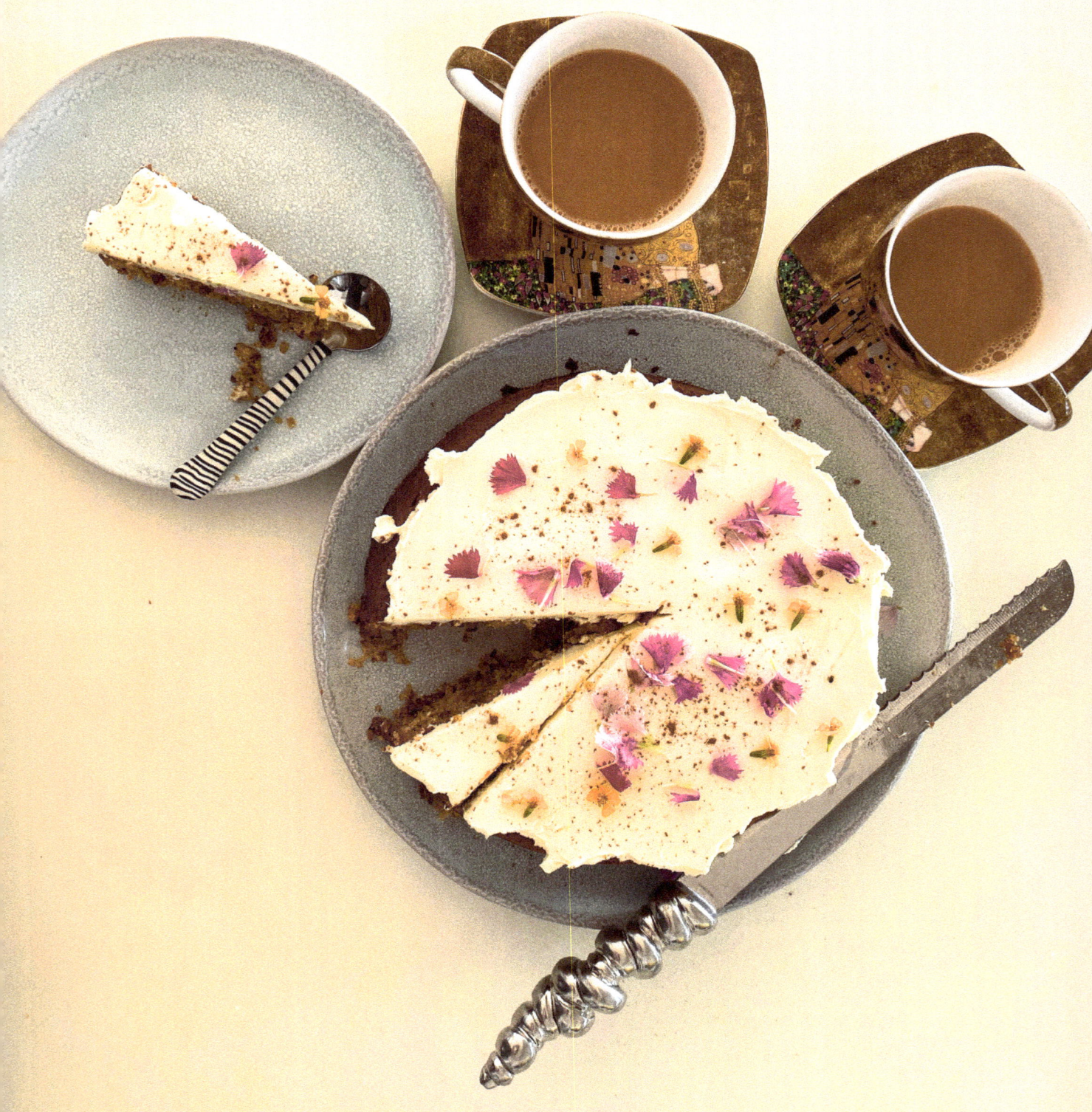

Carrot Cake

SERVINGS: 8-12

INGREDIENTS

CAKE
- 185g softened butter
- 3/4 cup brown sugar
- 5ml vanilla extract or paste
- 2 eggs
- 2 medium-sized purple or normal carrots
- 1 cup self-raising flour
- 1/2 a teaspoon cinnamon
- 1/2 a teaspoon mixed spice or ras el hanout
- 1/2 teaspoon bicarbonate of soda
- 1 cup of pecans and/or pistachios.

ICING
- 1 small tub of ricotta or cream cheese
- 2 tablespoons icing sugar
- 2 ml vanilla paste
- juice and zest of one lime

I'm afraid to say that this is one of my favourite pastimes. Eating and making cake. It reminds me of my mother and my aunts and how we always used to bake and create together.
Now I live in Australia, and my mother and my aunts are scattered all over the world.

And although we Zoom and call and Whatsapp all the time, nothing can beat a cup of tea and a chat over a plate of something decadent to really appreciate mother and daughter time TOGETHER.
My mother has always been a very keen and accomplished baker. We used to live miles and miles away from the closest tiny towns so our 'entertainment' was not going to malls and movies or restaurants as there simply weren't any around. No, our entertainment was ripping out recipes out of magazines and sticking them into our recipe folders. Or pouring over recipe books booked out from the library (no Google search in those days, lol). We also grew most of our own vegetables and produce so there were always fresh eggs, fruit and ridiculously good milk from our cows. We used to have a stainless steel milk separator, spinning off the rich and delectably thick cream to be used on scones, churned into butter, or baked into cakes and cookies. Oh, the sweet memories.
The carrot cake was always a firm favourite, and although I've adapted this to be a little more glamorous essentially, it's just a jolly fabulous carrot cake.

METHOD

Beat together softened butter with brown sugar in a mixer until light and fluffy and until the sugar is dissolved. Add Vanilla Extract or Paste and eggs and mix together. Grate the purple carrots into the mixture. Sieve in self-raising flour and spices, bicarb and nuts. Mix together until combined, and then pour into a greased cake or loaf tin. Bake in a preheated oven of 170c for about 20-25 minutes until the cake is cooked; test with a skewer like they do in the movies.
Allow to cool. While the cake is cooling, you can whip up this delicious but ridiculously easy icing!
Take the ricotta or cream cheese, and into add the icing sugar, vanilla paste, lime juice and zest. Mix well, and then dollop this onto the cake! I cut the cake into portions first and arranged them on a platter before decorating each square with a dollop of the sweetened ricotta and a gorgeous little organic rose bud (available from my online store or at your local Indian spice shop)
Enjoy, and let me know what you think!

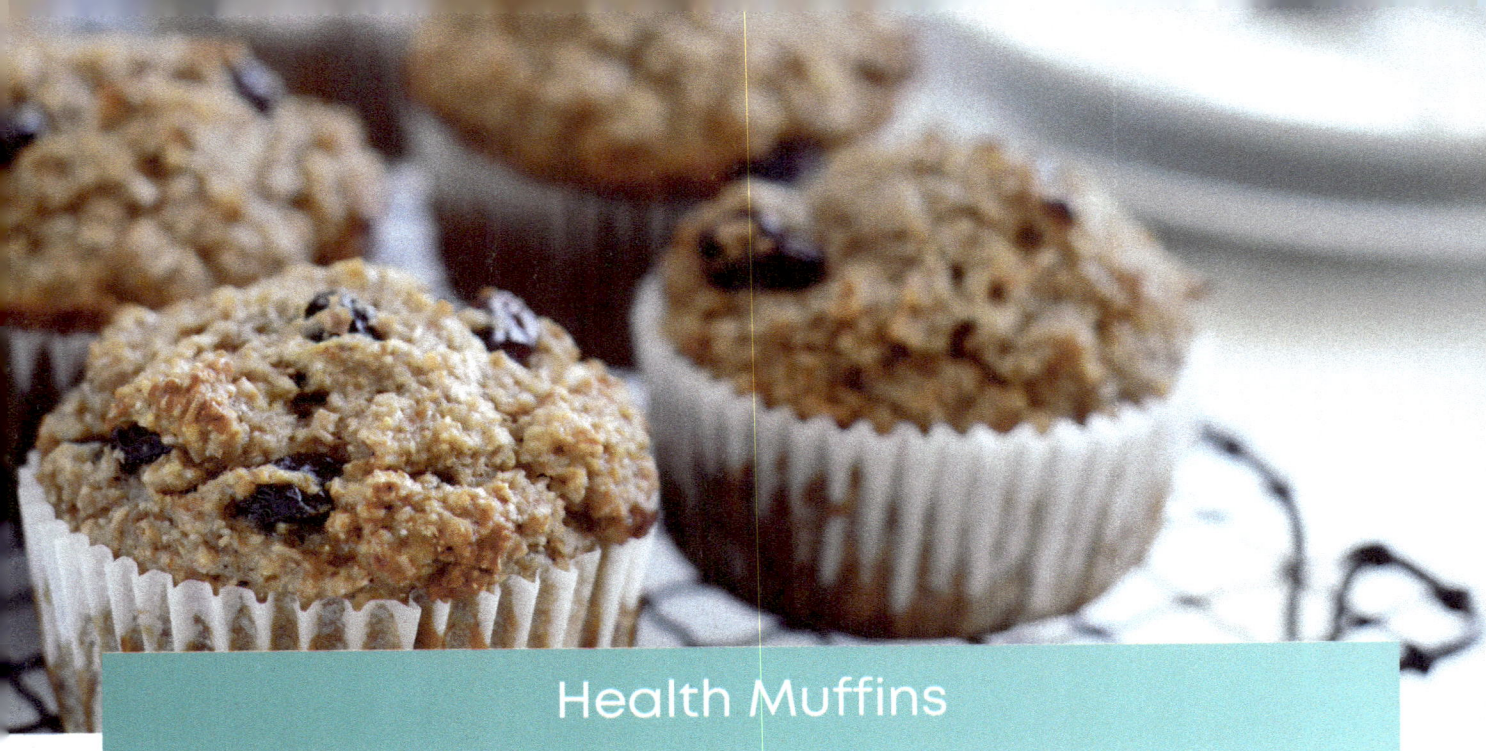

Health Muffins

SERVINGS: 8-12

INGREDIENTS

2 eggs

1 teaspoon salt

1.5 cups brown sugar

2.5 cups cake flour sifted

2.5 teaspoons bicarbonate of soda

2 cups milk

2 cups digestive bran

125 ml melted butter or vegetable oil

1 cup filling (see below method for ideas – do YOUR thing!)

METHOD

Simply mix all the ingredients together until you have a smooth batter, then spoon or pour into greased and floured muffin tins or terracotta pots and bake for about 10- 15 minutes in an oven of 180C until brown and golden.

You can then make them more special by adding a teaspoon of any of the fillings into the centre of the mixture in the muffin tin and mixing it in slightly. Then bake.

FILLING IDEAS:

Strawberries, Marmalade, Assorted Seeds, Lavender and Honey

Blueberry, Apple and Cinnamon, Peaches and Cream, Banana Poppy ripple

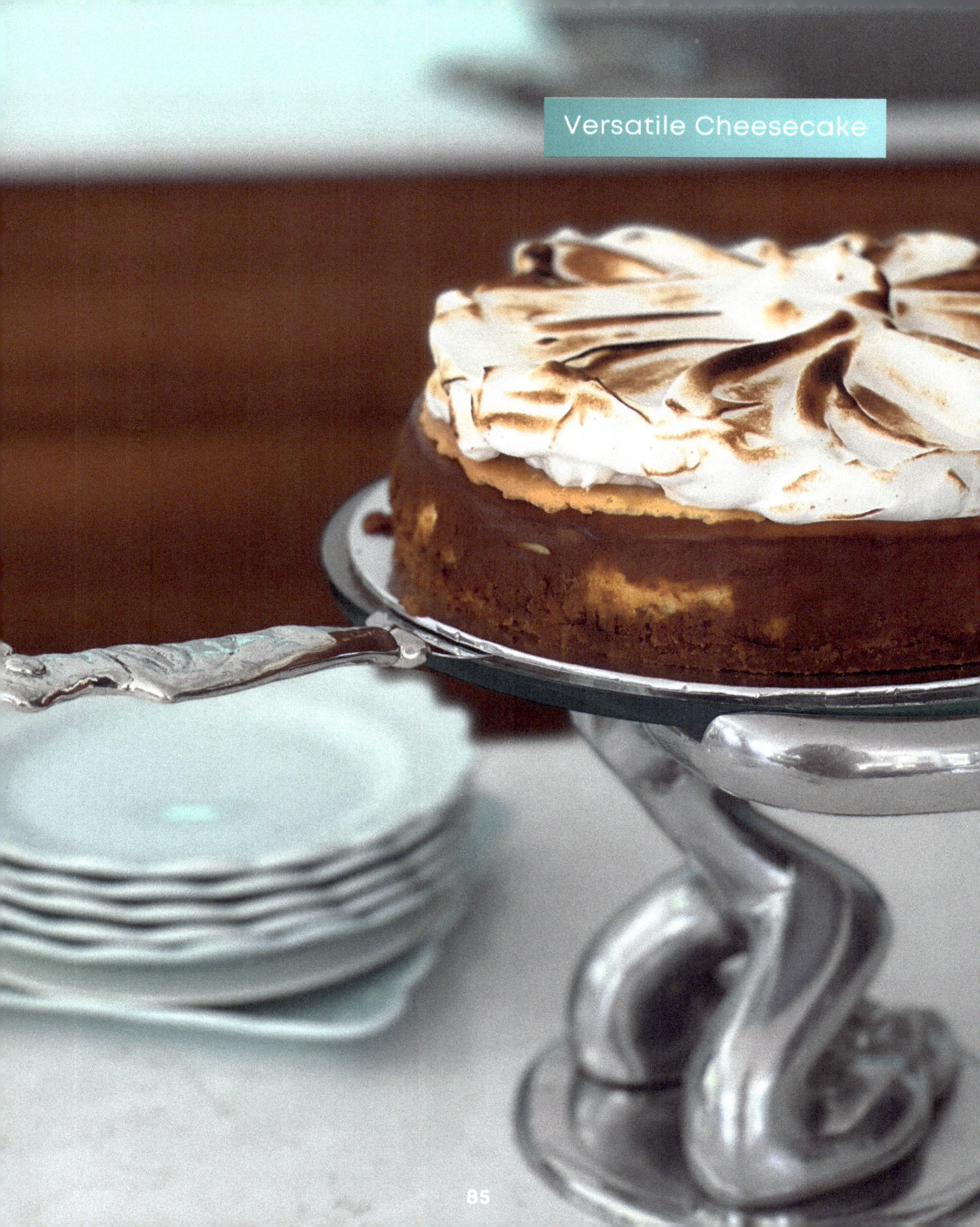

Versatile Cheesecake

Versatile Cheesecake

SERVINGS: 8-12

INGREDIENTS

BASE
200 g chocolate/vanilla sponge or biscuits crushed in a food processor then add 50 ml melted butter

FILLING
4 eggs
100 g sugar
1 tin condensed milk
750 g cream cheese
Hot water (to bind, about a tablespoon)
1 teaspoon vanilla extract or essence

METHOD

Beat the eggs, sugar and vanilla together until thick and fluffy.
Soften the cream cheese until it looks spreadable. Now add the cream cheese and condensed milk to the egg mixture and mix only till smooth; do not overbeat!
Place the biscuits in the base of the greased baking tin (cheesecake-friendly) and then top with the egg and cream cheese filling and bake for 30-40 minutes until set in the centre. The best way to tell is if the surface of the cheesecake looks MATT and not GLOSSY. You can also put your finger gently onto the surface, and if it comes away 'dry' the mixture has set and is cooked! Remove from the oven and allow to cool.
Now, it is time to decorate your cheesecake with anything you want.

This is where you can be creative. Any of the following will do.
100g chocolate melted with 100 ml cream to thin
250 g berries boiled up with 100 ml sugar and 250 ml fruit juice to make a thick jam
Lemon Curd
Chopped fudge
Meringue (add lemon zest to filling, top with meringue and then blow torch to brown)

To almost more than half the cooking time, why don't you bake individual cheesecakes in little ramekins, those will cook in about 10 minutes!

Mel's Family Recipe Telephone Pudding

SERVINGS: 8-10

INGREDIENTS

PUDDING

250 ml white sugar

125 ml soft or just melted butter

1 egg

375 ml plain flour, sifted

1 tsp baking powder & 1 teaspoon bicarbonate of soda dissolved in a 250 ml cup of milk

1 cup almonds or pecans blended to resemble breadcrumbs (optional; feel free to omit)

1 tsp powdered ginger

2 tablespoons apricot jam

Pinch of salt

SAUCE

250 ml cup of white sugar dissolved in 500 ml cup of boiling water

**A very old and dear family recipe passed for generations from one sweet tooth to the next.
We all have a copy of this recipe in our well-worn recipe folders and will often get a desperate call from a family member or a guest who has attended, BEGGING for the recipe.**

This decadent, delicious and world-famous recipe is known as TELEPHONE PUDDING. Yes, telephone pudding. As I said, you are guaranteed to get a phone call from a guest or a relative begging for the recipe over the phone once they have tried it. It remains, to date, my favourite all-time dessert.

Not only does it conjure up precious memories of family get-togethers and of my childhood, but it is now my quick fix for any homesickness that I feel.

Perhaps we should rename it EMAIL PUDDING or FACEBOOK PUDDING, but either way, I have decided to share it with you and spread the love. Enjoy.

With much love from my family to yours xxx

METHOD

Beat the sugar and the butter together until light and fluffy and then add the egg. Mix until smooth.

Add the remaining ingredients and mix through. Spoon into a greased baking dish.

Now make the sauce by mixing the sugar and the boiling water together. Use the back of a spoon to pour over the batter… DO NOT MIX.

Bake in a pre-heated oven of 160C for 25-30 minutes depending on how deep your baking dish is.

Check for doneness and then serve hot and sticky with a big dollop of whipped cream.

Family-friendly comfort food.

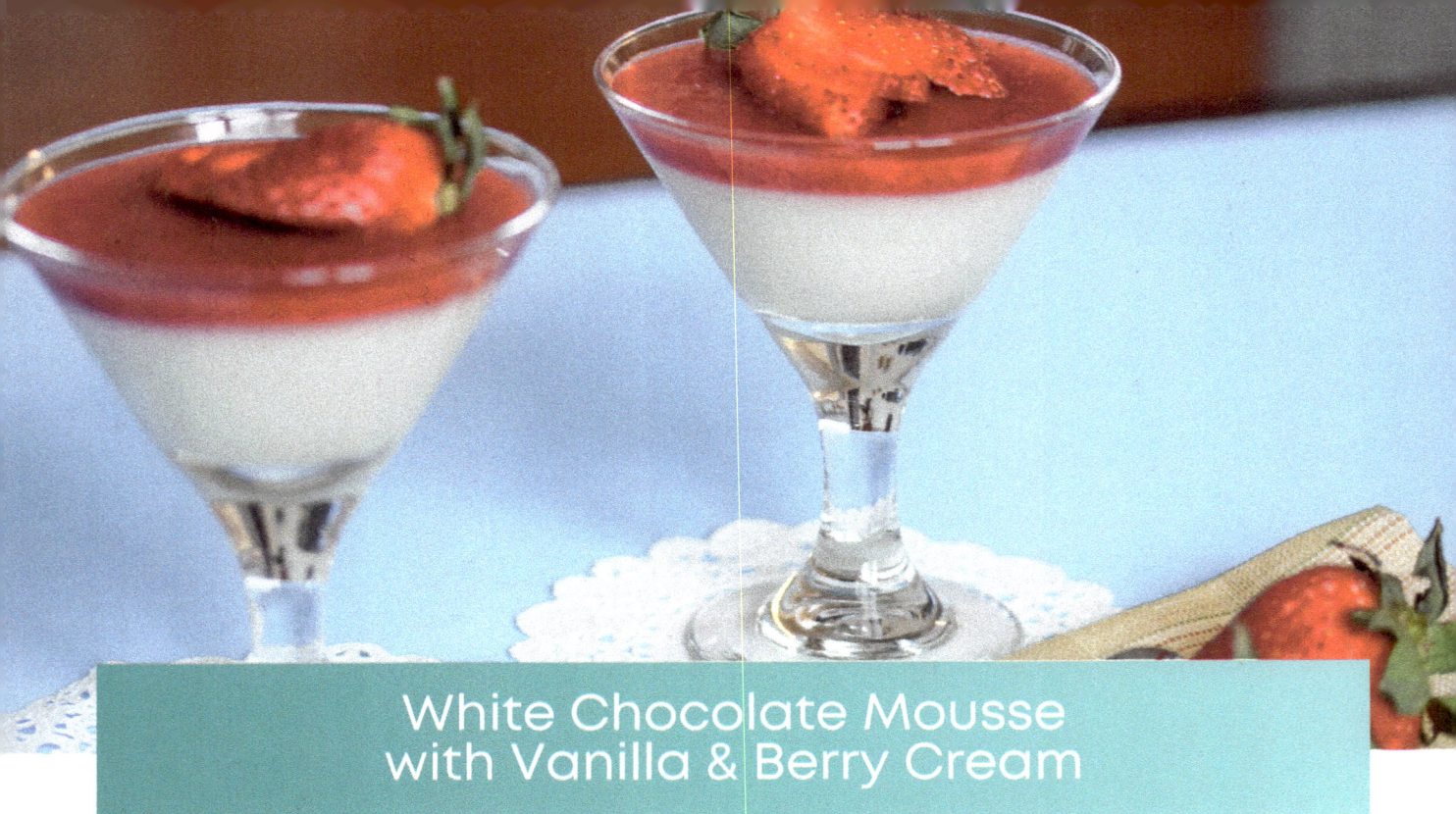

White Chocolate Mousse with Vanilla & Berry Cream

SERVINGS: 4-6

INGREDIENTS

200g white chocolate (or 100 g white, 100 g milk)
250 ml cream
50 ml strawberry juice or preserve
(you can use a good quality jam here)
250 g fresh or frozen berries blended to smooth in a processor
with 5 ml vanilla extract or essence

METHOD

Place chocolate, broken up, into a glass or ceramic bowl and drizzle in about 50ml of the cream.
This will ensure that the chocolate melts but doesn't scorch!
Melt chocolate for one minute on high in your microwave.
Whisk until smooth and free of any lumps.

Allow to cool and then fold in whipped cream, jam and blended berries with a plastic or metal spoon/spatula.
Place into ramekins, espresso cups, tea cups or yogurt tubs, or even a loaf tin. Freeze.

Mix the vanilla and the blitzed berries together and serve over the frozen mousse!
You can serve using your ice cream scoop for mousse balls, in a wine glass or similar.

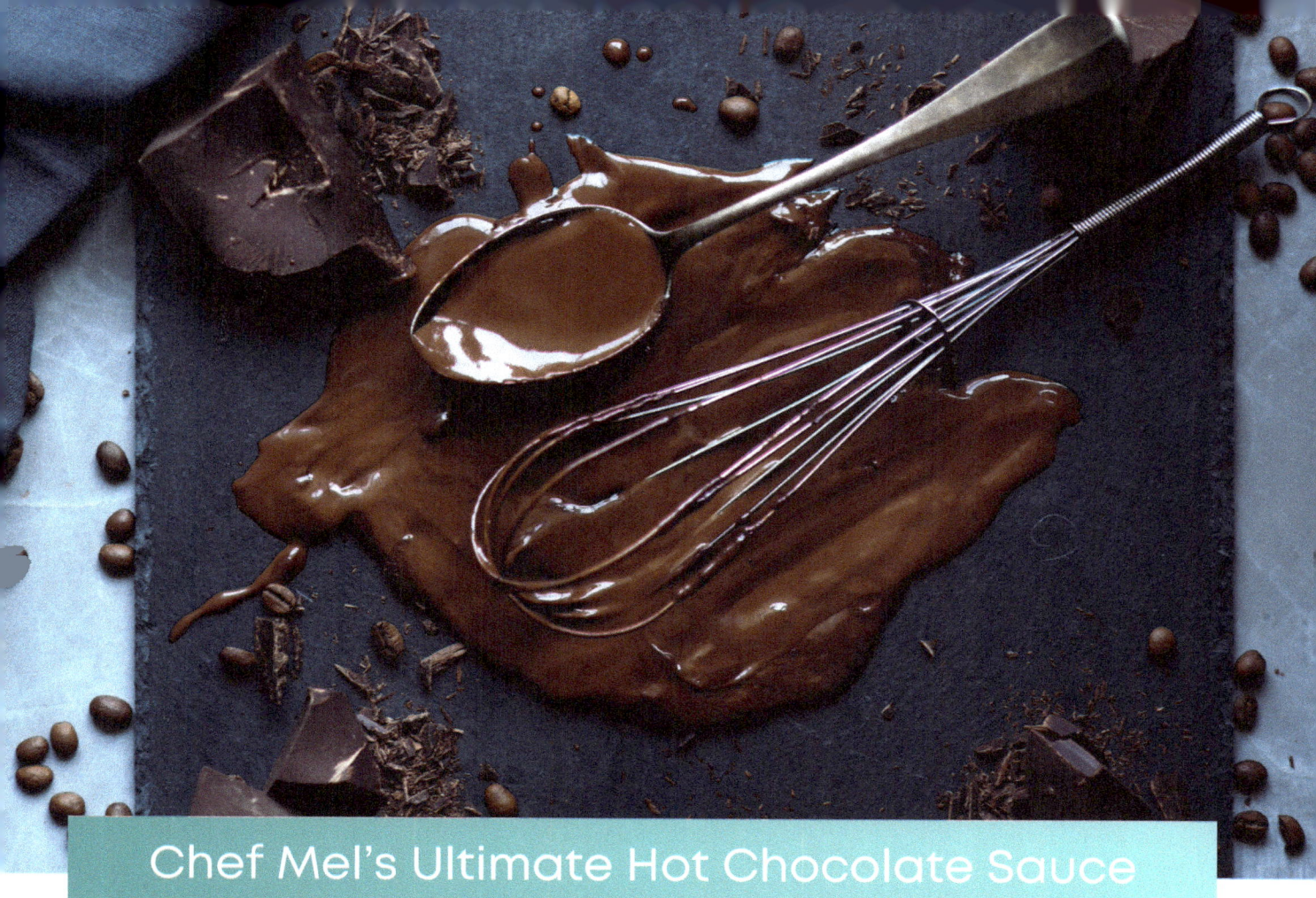

Chef Mel's Ultimate Hot Chocolate Sauce

SERVINGS: 4-6

INGREDIENTS

100g good chocolate *70% or milk chocolate*
125 ml cream
25 – 50 ml of your favourite liquor

METHOD

Nothing beats ice cream and chocolate sauce.
But it's got to be really good chocolate to be a really good chocolate sauce.

Break the chocolate into smaller pieces, place in a glass or ceramic bowl and cover with the cream.
Microwave on high for a minute until the cream is hot.
This will allow the chocolate to melt, so don't be tempted to overcook!
Whisk until smooth, add the alcohol and then serve with delicious ice cream, strawberries and pistachio nuts…
It's all in the presentation.

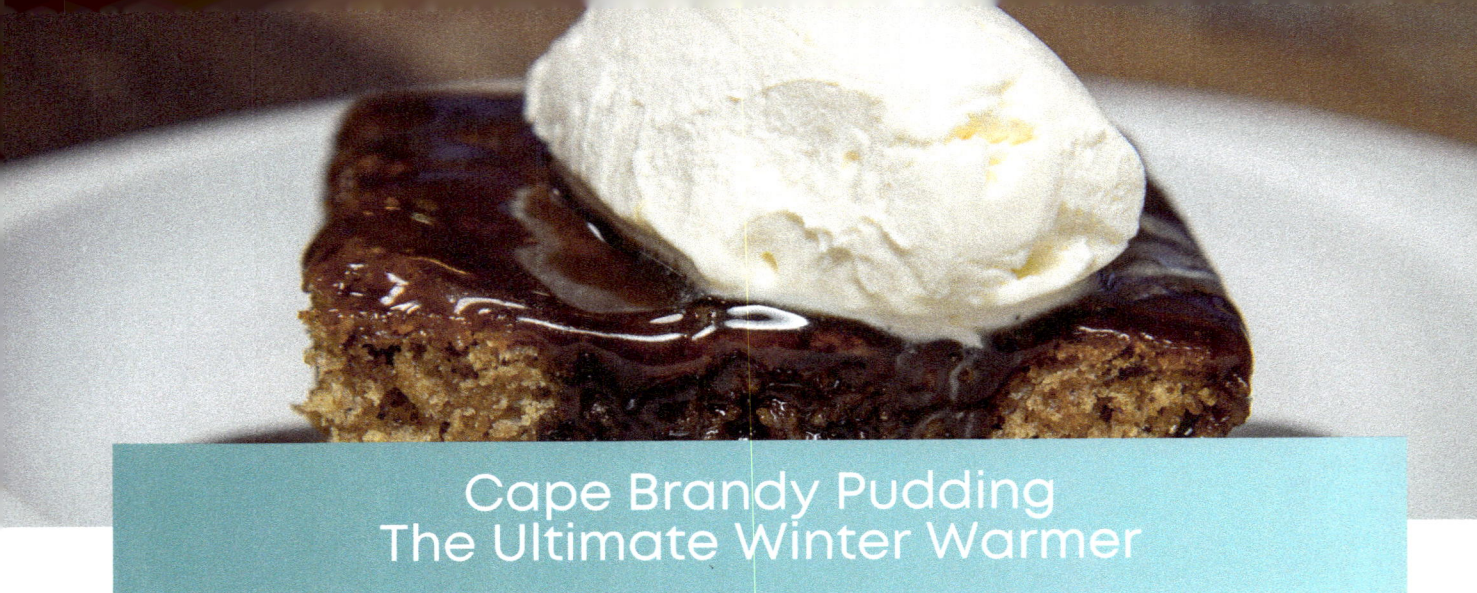

Cape Brandy Pudding
The Ultimate Winter Warmer

SERVINGS: 8-10

INGREDIENTS

250g stoned dates, chopped, soaked in 250 ml hot water
3ml bicarbonate of soda
140g butter
400g white sugar (200g for cake and 200g for sauce)
2 large eggs
250g flour
2 teaspoons baking powder
2ml salt
100g pecan nuts, chopped
125ml brandy
200ml water

METHOD

Soak the dates in the 250 ml hot water and mix well.
Beat the butter and 200g of the sugar together until light and fluffy; now add the eggs and beat.
Stir in the sifted flour and salt. Add the dates and nuts and mix until well combined; spoon into a greased baking dish. Make the syrup by mixing the remaining 200g sugar with the 125ml brandy and 200ml water and pour gently over the cake mixture using the back of a spoon.

NOTE:
Make sure the mixture only reaches halfway up the side of your baking dish, or else the sauce will boil over and ruin your oven!

Bake for about 25-30 minutes in an oven of 180C until done.
Serve hot with custard, whipped cream or ice cream! It's decadently simple, and everyone's favourite.
It can be baked in individual ramekins at a reduced cooking time of about 8 – 10 minutes.

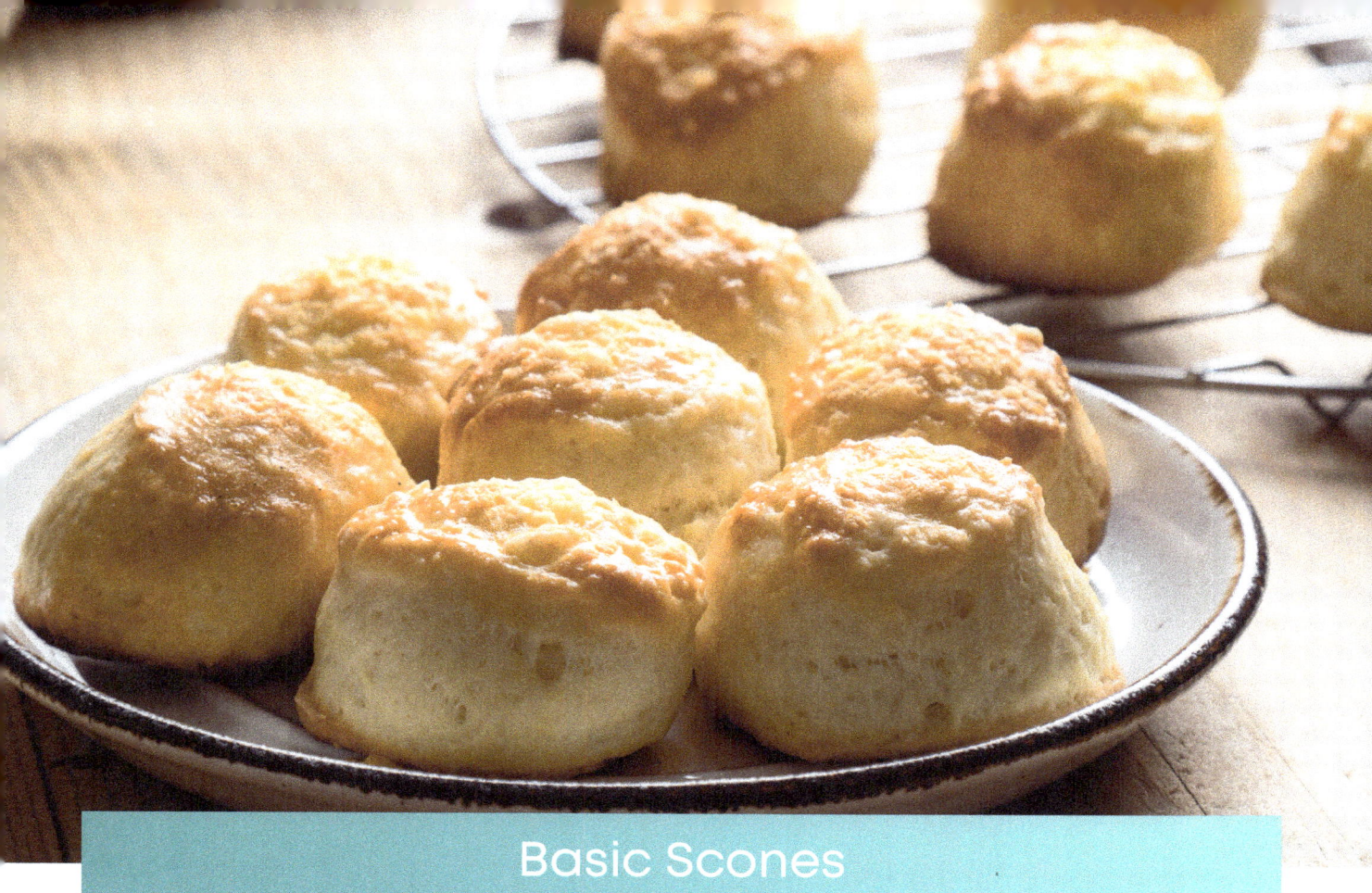

Basic Scones

SERVINGS: 6-8

INGREDIENTS

2 cups cake flour sifted = 500ml
2 teaspoons baking powder sifted
2 pinches salt
2 eggs beaten and placed in a 250ml cup measure
top to the 250 ml mark with milk or sour milk or even plain yogurt
125ml butter, melted or very very soft
or grate into dry ingredients and rub

METHOD

Mix all the ingredients together until a nice thick batter is formed; try not to over-mix, as these will become tough if overhandled. Less is more in this case.
Drop tablespoons of the mixture into greased and floured muffin tins, paper cups, terracotta pots, or just dollop onto a baking sheet. Bake at 180C for about 15 minutes until golden brown and cooked. Check for doneness. Serve with delicious butter.

Sweet Options for Scones

Add 2 tablespoons white sugar to the dry ingredients,
as well as a teaspoon vanilla or almond essence to make them sweet scones.

CHOCOLATE SCONES

Grate in 100g milk chocolate to make delicious chocolate muffins or chop up your favourite chocolate bar

BLUEBERRY SCONES

Add 2 tablespoons strawberry, blueberry or fig jam to the mix for fruity muffins,
serve with dollops of vanilla and whipped cream

LEMON & POPPY SCONES

Add the zest of one lemon or lime and a tablespoon of poppy seeds

Savoury Options for Scones

Simply add this to basic recipe, no need to adjust quantities.

FETA, PIQUANT PEPPER & CHIVE SCONES

Crumble 100g Feta. 2 tablespoons chopped piquant peppers and 2 tablespoons chopped chives into the mixture. You can use parsley, sage or similar instead (nice for colour)

WASABI & SALMON SCONES

Add 1 tablespoon wasabi and 100g chopped smoked salmon to the mixture

SUNDRIED TOMATO PESTO SCONES

Just add 2 teaspoons or a little more tomato pesto to your mixture

BASIL PESTO SCONES

As above, just add 2 teaspoons basil pesto

MUSTARD & SAGE SCONES

Add 2 teaspoons grainy mustard and 1 teaspoon chopped sage to the mix

Other Varieties to Mix & Match

CHOPPED OLIVES, CHOPPED SUN-DRIED TOMATOES
ONION, SESAME OR POPPY SEEDS
GRATED ONION AND GARLIC
CHEDDAR, BLUE, PARMESAN OR PECORINO CHEESE
HAM, COOKED BACON, COOKED MUSHROOMS

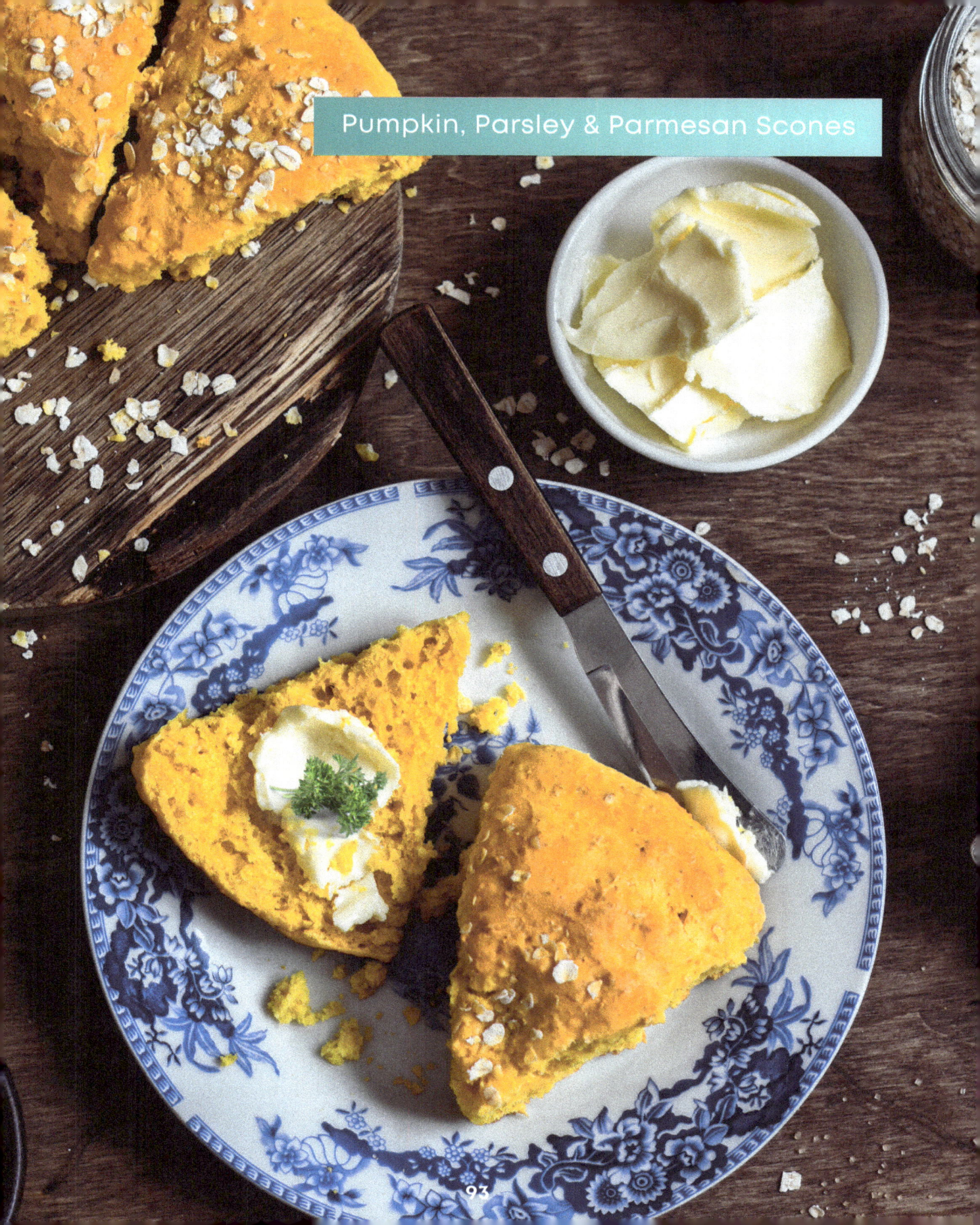

Pumpkin, Parsley & Parmesan Scones

Pumpkin, Parsley & Parmesan Scones

SERVINGS: 6-8

INGREDIENTS

2 cups plain flour sifted = 500ml
2 teaspoons baking powder sifted
2 pinches salt
2 tablespoons grated parmesan cheese (or cheddar)
2 tablespoons freshly chopped chives or parsley
2 eggs beaten– place in a 250ml cup measure
top to the 250ml mark with milk/ricotta/sour cream/ sour milk or plain yogurt
1/2 cup pumpkin, butternut, zucchini or carrot finely grated
– *place in a bowl with 125g grated or diced butter and 'melt' in the microwave for about a minute, this will melt the butter and soften the vegetable!*

RICOTTA PARSLEY & PEPPER DOLLOP

125g light ricotta
1/4 teaspoon lemon zest finely grated
1 teaspoon freshly chopped parsley
Lots of black freshly ground pepper/pink pepper
1 tablespoon parmesan cheese grated

METHOD

These are not just ANY old scones.
Behold - these are my old faithful's. They have never let me down, never not worked, and they are magnificently quick. The best part is that you don't need a scale; you don't need to fuss. Simply mix and bake.
I have 'blinged' up the humble scone; I think it was well overdue for a makeover, don't you? To add colour, personality and flavour, I have added grated pumpkin, or you could use carrot, zucchini or butternut instead! That, teamed with the herbs and the sexy ricotta spread, will give your next scone-serving session guaranteed *'ooh's and aahs.'*

Mix all the ingredients together until a nice thick batter is formed; try not to over-mix, as these will become tough if overhandled! Less is more in this case.
You can either drop tablespoons of the mixture into greased and floured muffin tins, paper cups, or terracotta pots or just dollop it onto a baking sheet OR, with floured hands, shape the dough into a square with your hands and simply cut it into 9 squares. Place squares on a baking tray.
Bake at 180C for about 15 minutes until golden brown and cooked.
Check for doneness. For the spread, mix all ingredients together in a bowl.
Serve with a delicious spread or just some lovely butter.

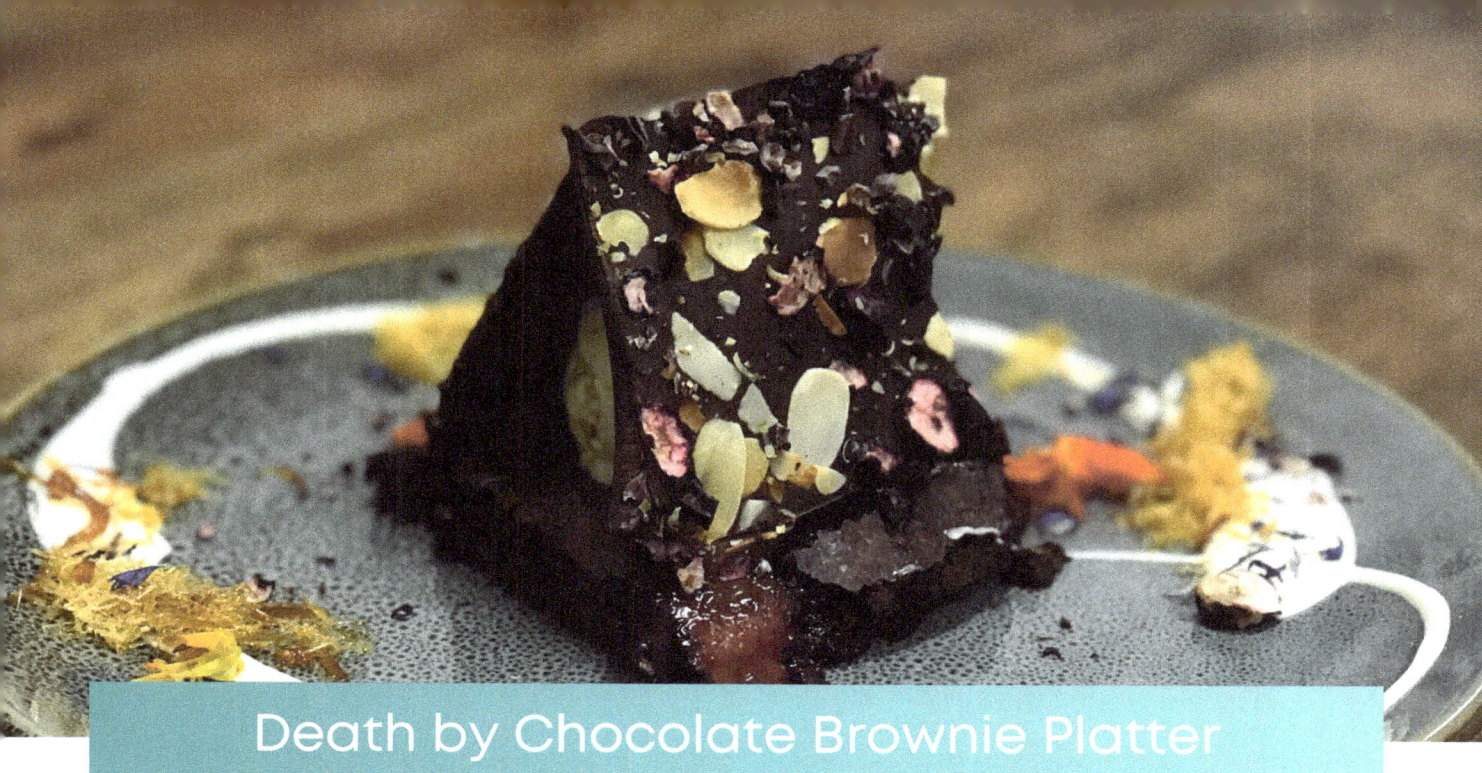

Death by Chocolate Brownie Platter

SERVINGS: 8-10

INGREDIENTS

250g unsalted butter
200g dark chocolate
4 large eggs
360g castor sugar
65g plain flour
1tsp baking powder
5g Ras el Hanout or vanilla paste
80g cocoa powder
100g chocolate chips/roasted nuts

METHOD

Melt butter and dark chocolate together. You must break the chocolate into pieces to help it melt more quickly. Once melted, stir through until smooth and allow to cool slightly.

Beat eggs and castor sugar together until pale and fluffy.

Sift plain flour, baking powder, Ras el Hanout and cocoa powder together. Mix all of these to make a smooth batter, and add chocolate chips or roasted nuts of your choice.

Spoon into a greased baking sheet and then bake in a moderate oven of 180C for 20-25 minutes until firm on the outside but still very gooey on the inside- do not be tempted to overcook these; they are best when extremely gooey.

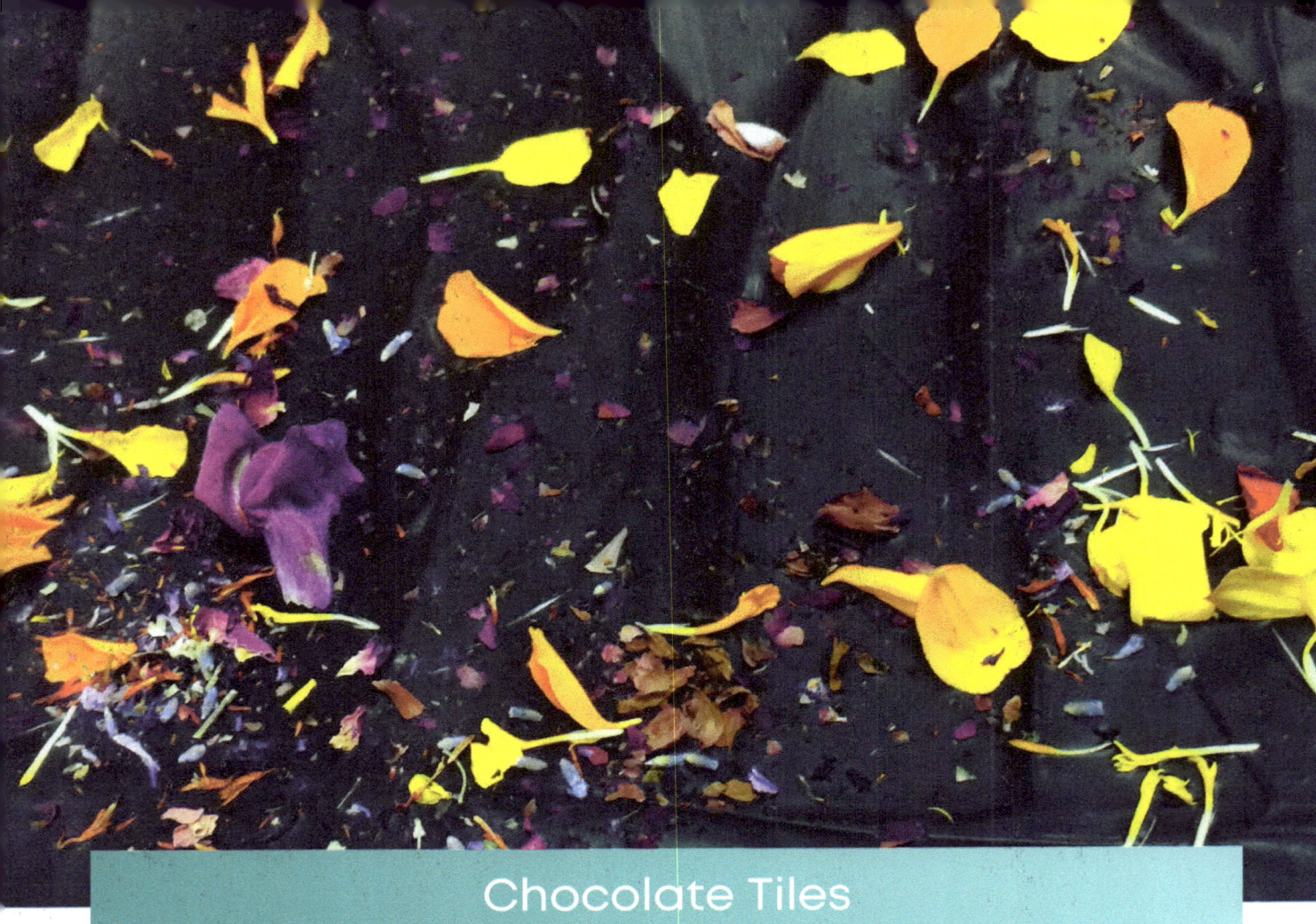

Chocolate Tiles

SERVINGS: 6-8

INGREDIENTS

200g chocolate buttons
Pistachios, Berries or bling for toppings

METHOD

Melt the chocolate buttons in a microwave bowl for 1 minute. Stir till smooth with a spatula. Grease a baking tray, some greaseproof paper, or a silicone mat. Pour the chocolate onto the prepared surface and 'paint' out to an A4 size using your spatula or spoon. Keep it nice, even and neat and then grate pistachios, berries or bling on top before it sets.
Allow to set in fridge or freezer and then cut into 'chocolate tiles'.

Pop a sexy scoop of ice cream on top of your chocolate brownie, then place the tiles on either side of the ice cream. You'll be sure to get a round of applause for this creation.

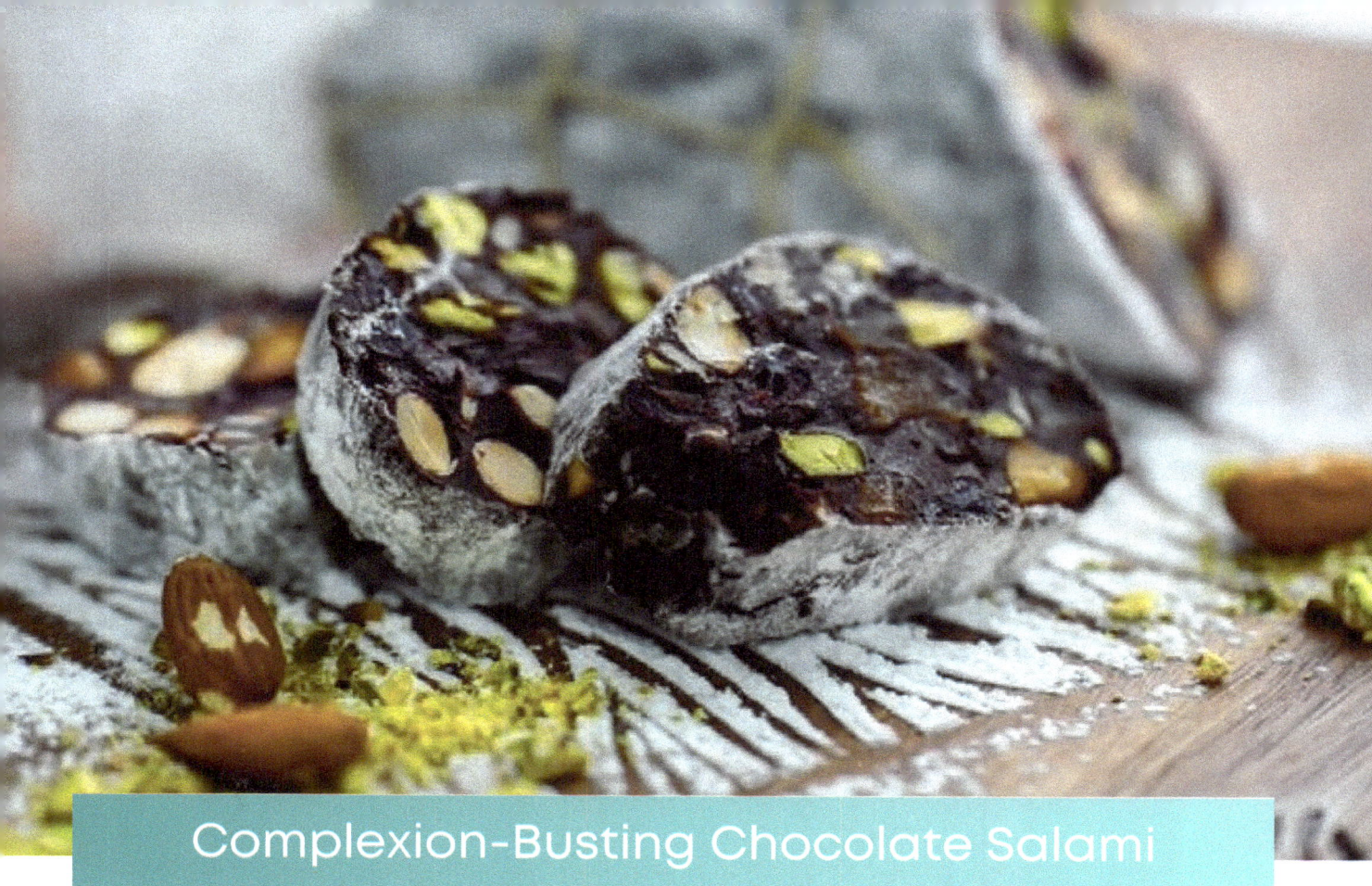

Complexion-Busting Chocolate Salami

SERVINGS: 6-8

INGREDIENTS

200g good quality chocolate (75% cocoa)
100ml coconut cream
1/2 cup toasted coconut, shredded
1/2 cup toasted cashews (unsalted)
1/2 cup pistachios or other nuts; almonds *are cheaper*
1/2 cup of dates or dried fruit
1 teaspoon vanilla bean paste
Nuts, biscotti or toasted coconut, ground to a 'dust'

METHOD

Melt the chocolate in the microwave for about 1 minute until it has softened, and you can stir it into a smooth paste. Add the remaining ingredients and place on a piece of parchment paper, then roll up as a 'salami', coating it in either nut dust, biscotti dust or coconut, and then chill before slicing or even rolling into 'goodie' balls… check your skin for a healthy glow soon after eating these!

NOTES

NOTES

This book is about taking the everyday meals you are already cooking, and transforming them into extraordinary, colourful and exciting dishes by learning the art of culinary bling and presentation.

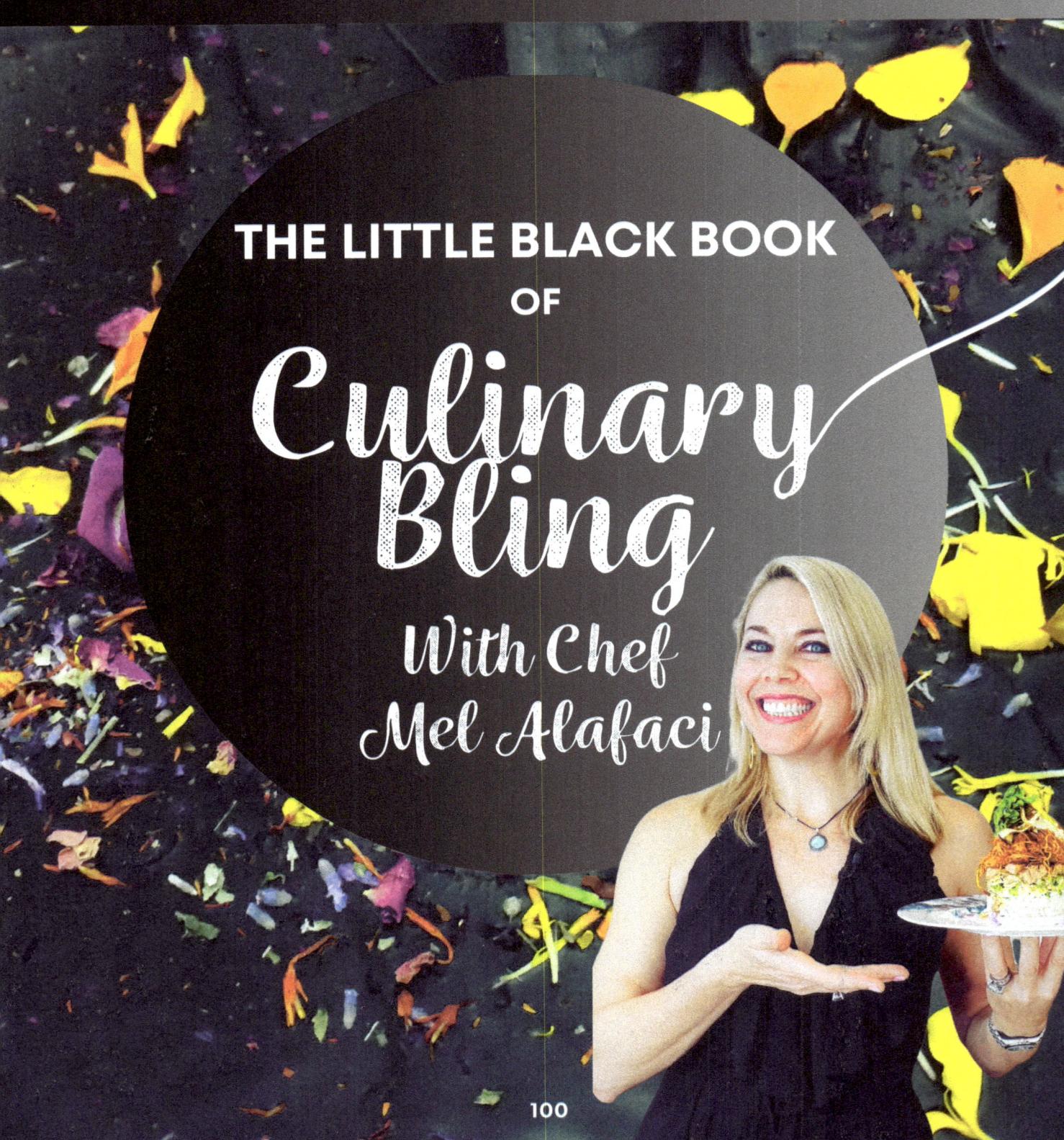

THE LITTLE BLACK BOOK OF
Culinary Bling
With Chef Mel Alafaci

Foreword

The Little Black Book of Culinary Bling is not just another recipe book.
A recipe book is a particular set of recipes and ingredients; whereas this book is about taking everyday meals you are already cooking and transforming them into amazing, colourful and exciting dishes.

It's a book about my long journey shared with thousands of amazing people, and that sparkle in their eyes when I show them how they, too, can create picture-perfect meals.
It's my passion to teach YOU how to transform all your meals with quick, easy and effective tricks to get personality on your plate.

A round of applause is possible with every single meal that you prepare - and so is living happily ever after in the kitchen.

Ultimately, it's how I became known as the Queen of Culinary Bling!

CONTENTS

103
Culinary Lingo
It's all about the description

104
Culinary Weapons
The tools of the trade

105
Culinary Bling
Adding interest to your plate

109
Culinary Trinkets
Adding charm and accessories to your food

112
Culinary Spray Tans & Salts
Adding colour and flavour

113
Culinary Flavour Dusts
Adding personality to your meal

114
Culinary High Heels
Adding height to your meal

Culinary Lingo

It's all about the description!

The art of Culinary Bling doesn't stop with the food and the bling - you must talk up your finished masterpieces.
There's a straightforward formula for creating excitement for your menu.

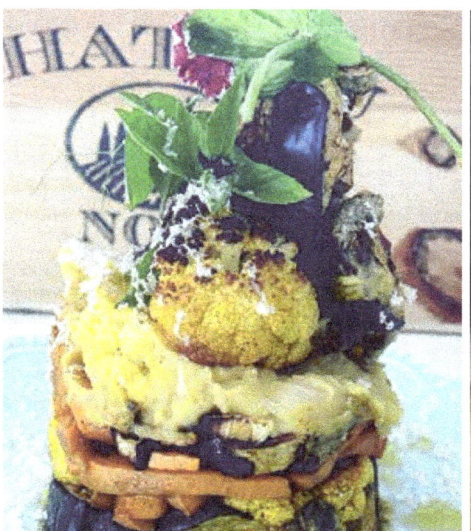
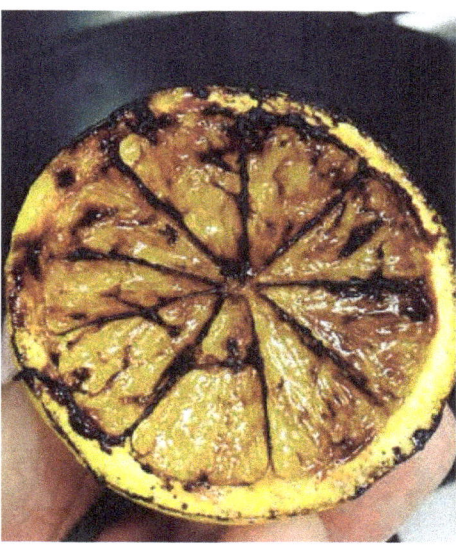

STEP 1: NAMING

Use chatty, cheffy words - fragranced, scented, infused.
It's not mac n cheese - it's cheese-infused pasta.
It's not crushed meringue; it's sweet, air-dried egg dust.
You're telling everyone what's in your dish and having some fun with it at the same time.

STEP 2: WHAT IS YOUR HERO?

Find the point of difference in your meal and highlight it.
Is it a roast chicken with stuffing? No! It's a ras el hanout scented chicken with sweet potato and speck stuffing - whose mouth doesn't water at that?

STEP 3: IT'S ALL ABOUT YOUR PLATING

Now that you've created excitement in your menu, and highlighted your hero, you can't just dump it on the plate. Think about your presentation - does it need height?
A dust? A cheffy schmear? Finish off with a bang.

STEP 4: TO DECORATE OR TO GARNISH?

And now for that final bit of information that will set you apart from the rest...
Knowing the difference between garnishing and decorating.
Garnishing is for savoury and decorating is for sweet and 'never the two shall meet'. So you can't decorate a chicken unless you put earrings on him while he's still alive!
Just remember, everything on the plate MUST be edible and must complement the dish. For example, only the petals of an edible flower can go on the plate, not the entire flower and the flavours must match.

Culinary Weapons

The tools of the trade that don't cost thousands.
You don't need much equipment to make all your presentation dreams come true, here are the basics for your bag of tricks:

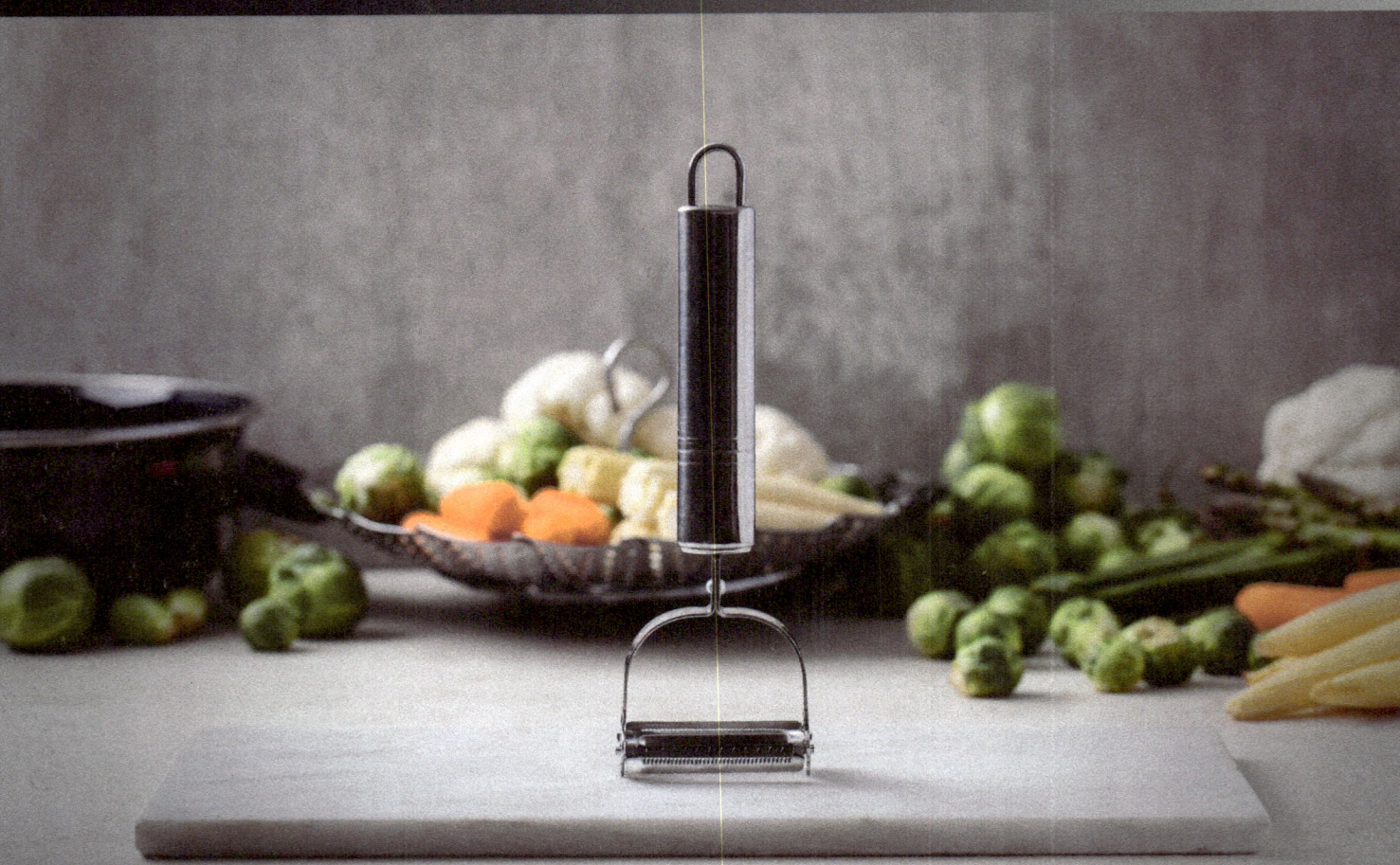

"Y" shaped peeler
Julienne peeler
Sharp knives
Squeezy bottles for drizzling
Sexy plates, bowls and Chinese spoons for presenting
Strainers
Stacking rings
Mortar and pestle
Blow Torch
Stick blender or food processor
Kitchen Aid or similar, with a balloon whisk, dough hook and batter paddle

Culinary Bling
Adding interest to your plate

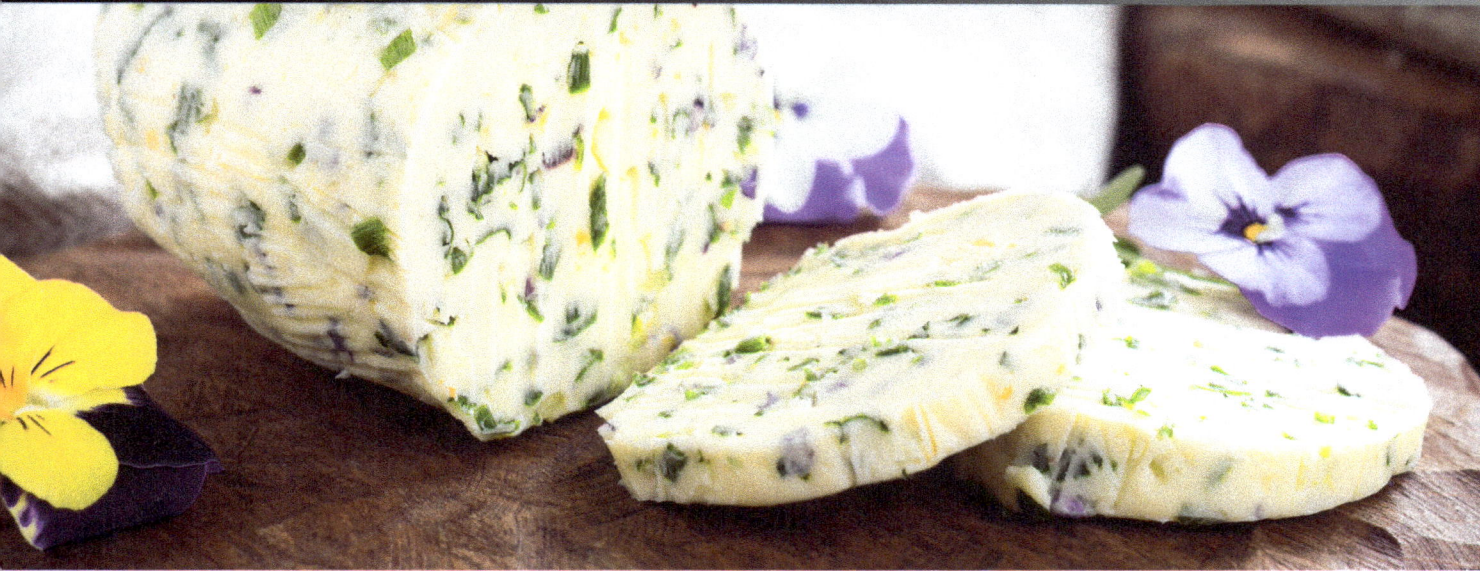

WHAT IS CULINARY BLING?

Culinary Bling is what you add to your food to create interest.
A splash of colour - taking the ordinary to the extraordinary.

Examples are:
Black flake salt
Nuts and berries
Balsamic Reductions
Herbs and spices
Scented oils
Micro herbs
Edible petals
Sprouts

EDIBLE PETALS AND FLOWERS

Petals and flowers add instant colour and personality to your plate.
You can have your own Culinary Bling garden! But it's important to know your edibles from your inedible.
First rule - don't poison the guests! You can also buy these already dried which is very handy.

The following flowers are beautiful and edible:

Violets   Carnations
Mallow   Dianthus
Pansies   Cornflower
Hibiscus   Gladiolus
Marigolds   Safflower
Lavender   Borage
Roses   Dandelion
Nasturtium

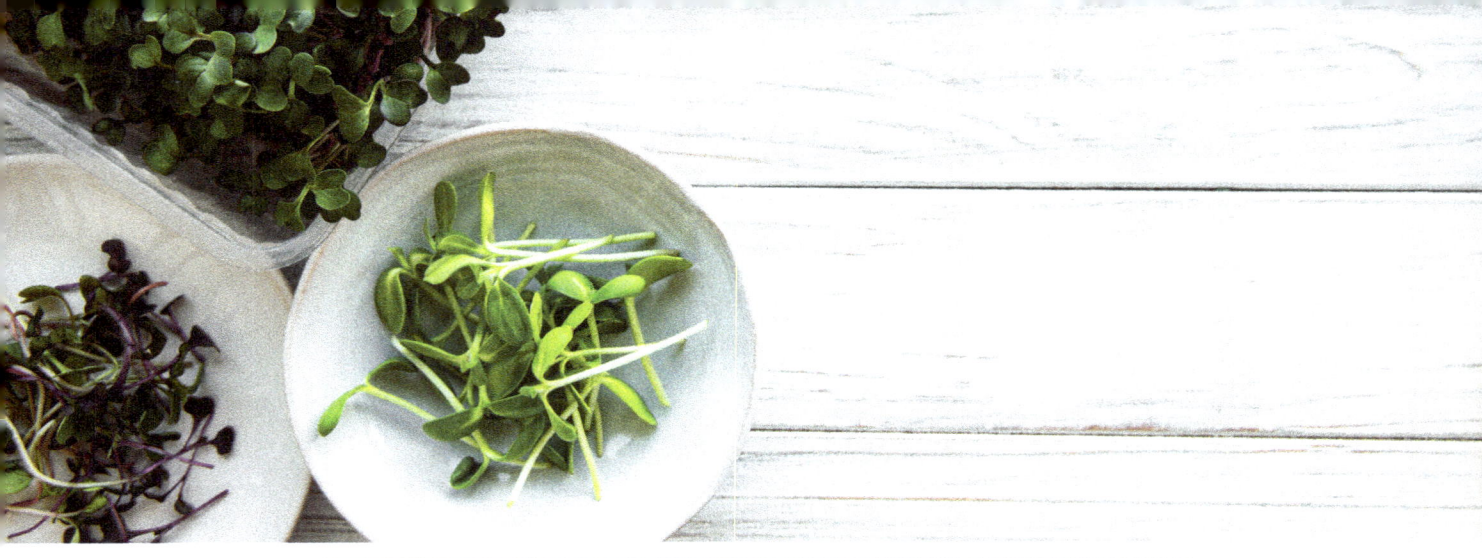

HERBS AND MICRO HERBS

Herbs and micro herbs add vibrant detail, flavour and colour to a plate.
Grow your own or speak to your local fruit and veg supplier to get some in stock for you for that special occasion. The best thing about these is that you can plant them afterwards and keep harvesting them.
Choose herbs and flowers that match your dish, micro herbs add that restaurant detail and sophistication to an everyday dish.
Got a green thumb? You can grow your own from seeds. It's always handy to have either dried edible petals or a bag of Bling handy for those days when you just don't have time.

SPROUTS

You can't get easier or cheaper than sprouts.
There's a variety available at your local supermarket or you could grow your own.
Use them to add colour, texture, height and flavour and vitality to a meal.
Best of all - sprouts have a long shelf life.

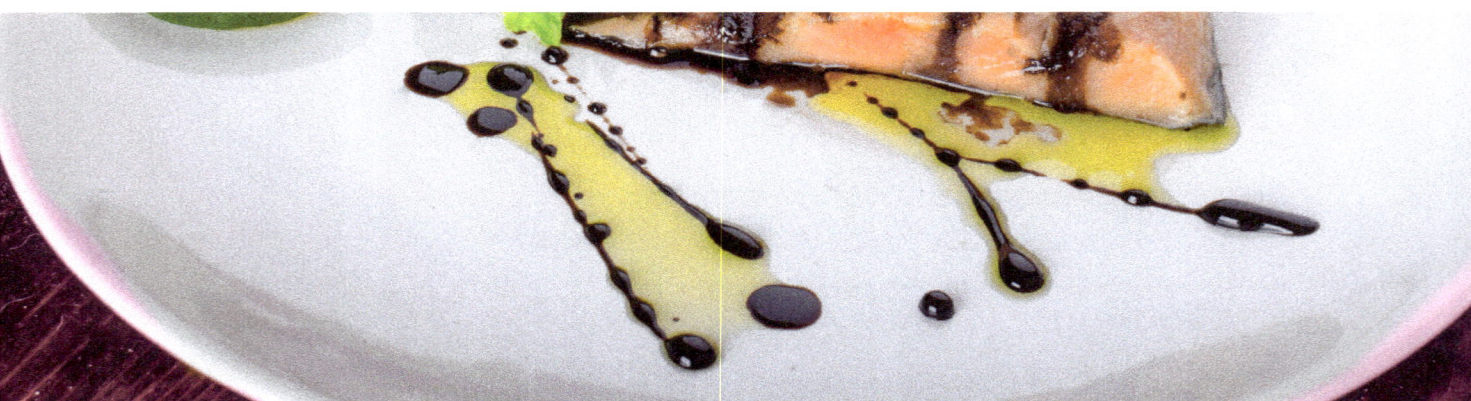

SCENTED OILS AND DRIZZLES

You can grab some balsamic reduction from your local supermarket or deli. There are different types and qualities, but even the most basic will add fabulous colour and personality to many dishes.
Be sure not to use too much, a light drizzle is much more effective than a giant, messy puddle.
Best of all, they generally come in an easy-to-use squeezy bottle.
I also love truffle, lemon, blood orange or basil olive oils.

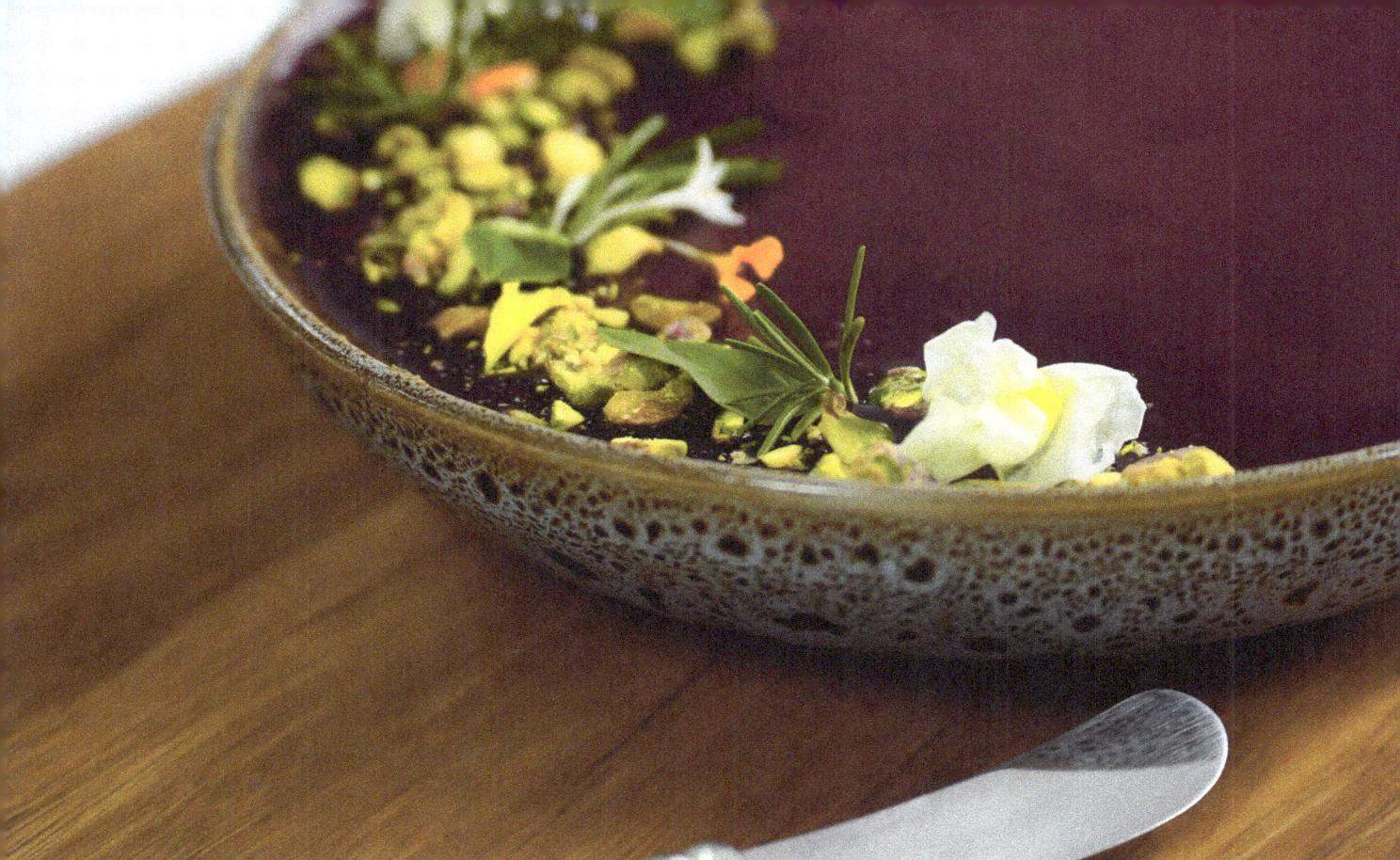

JELLIES

Jellies are creative and very easy to make. Leaf gelatine is now readily available at local supermarkets and is much better quality than the powdered kind. You can let your creative juices flow when adding jelly to a dish! My basic recipe is adding 250ml warm/hot liquid to 2 sheets of soaked leaves. Then you just need to add your flavour!
Add Shiraz, strawberry and balsamic for a fantastic jelly for chicken liver pate!
You can literally make any jelly to match your dish.

SWEET PASTES AND DRIZZLES

Chocolate is everyone's first choice for a dessert paste or drizzle. But you don't have to settle for a regular ganache. You can enhance good quality chocolate with vanilla bean paste, liqueurs, cream, rose water or other flavours. A basic chocolate drizzle can be made by melting equal parts chocolate with cream - add a shot of espresso for an easy and delicious paste or drizzle.

EDIBLE ASH

You can create edible ash by oven-roasting herbs of your choice until they are literally back and burnt. Once burnt and dry, place them in a mortar and pestle and pound them until you create a fine ash.
Why not bling up some whipped butter with turmeric, edible petals, Nigella seeds, and chilli, then wrap it in grease-proof paper before squaring it off in a sushi mat and rolling it in an edible ash? Slice with a hot knife and serve.
What sounds more impressive - plain old steak or steak with herb-infused butter finished in edible ash?

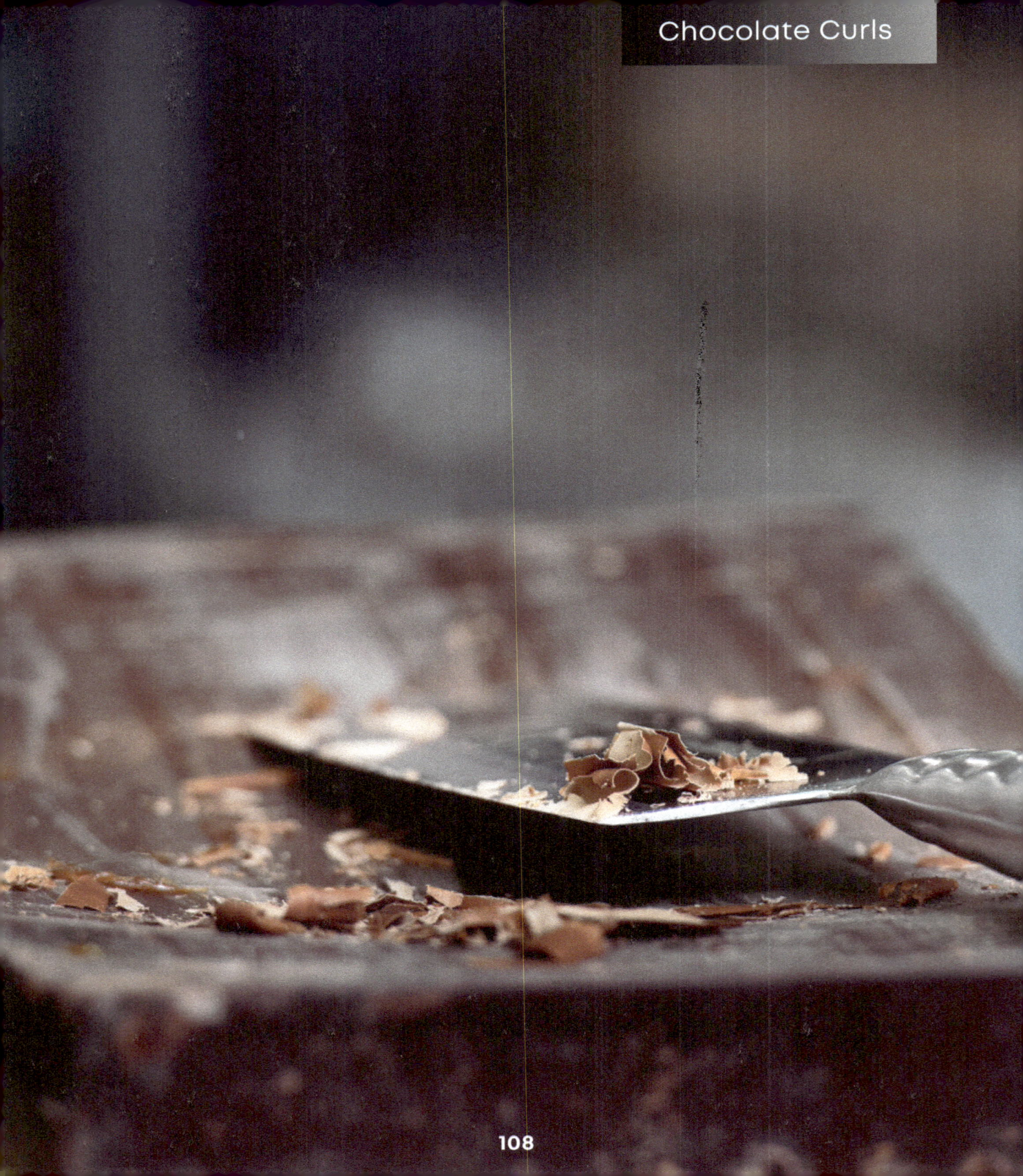
Chocolate Curls

Culinary Trinkets
Adding charm and accessories to your food

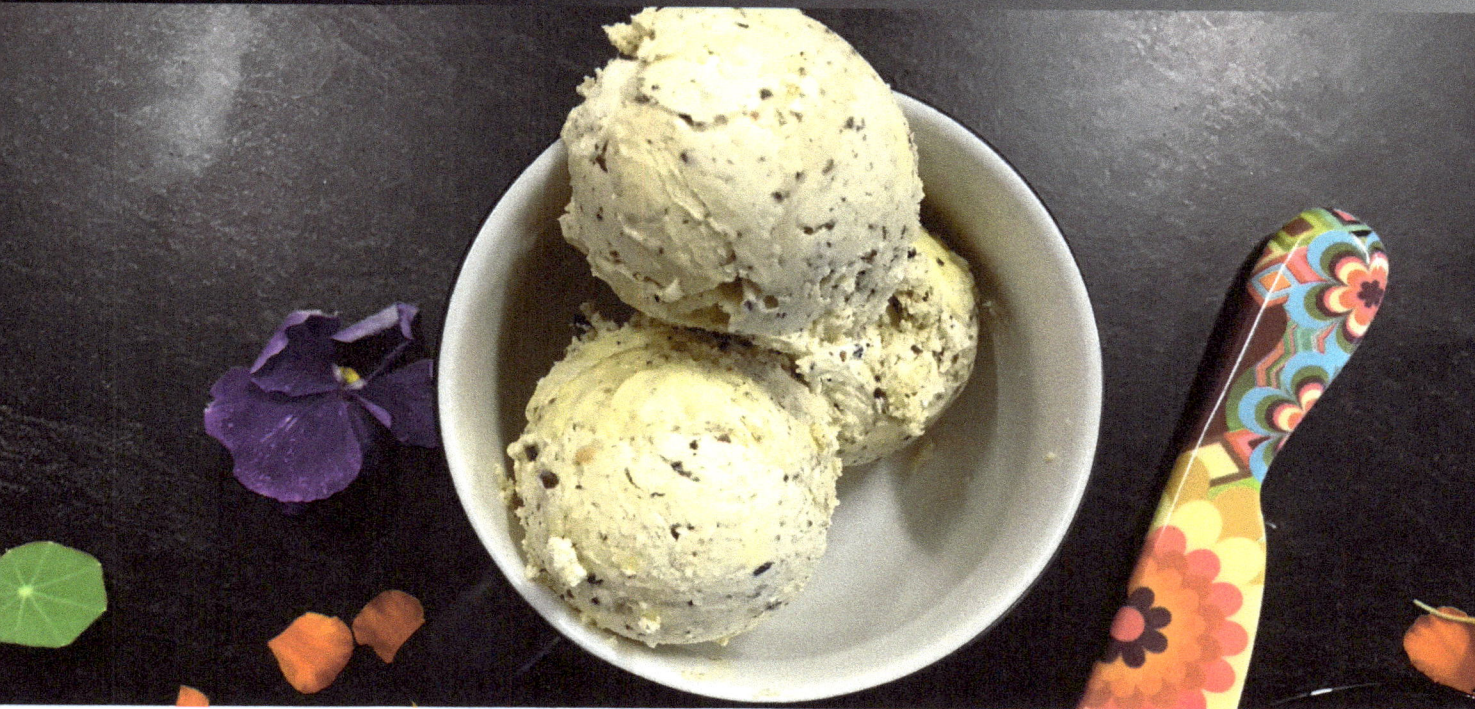

BLINGED GOATS CHEESE BALLS

Add some charm to your next cheese platter with some blinged-up goats cheese balls! The perfect accessory to many a dish.
Place edible petals, black seeds and micro herbs into a bowl. Roll goats cheese into balls, then roll the balls through the petal and seed bling! The bling will stick to the wet cheese.
Try it with cream cheese, Danish feta or even butter.

PROSCIUTTO BARK AND PECORINO SNOW

Sometimes, a dish just needs some charm.
For example, my famous Speck and Sweet Potato ravioli with burnt butter. I blinged it up with some prosciutto bark and Pecorino snow.
Roast some prosciutto on some grease-proof paper for 5 - 8 minutes until it's dried out - then break into pieces. Then create your Pecorino snow by using a zester (it's still just grated cheese, but Pecorino snow or fuzz sounds much more expensive and fun!)

SWEET TRINKETS AND CHOCOLATE BARK

There is something better than chocolate - and that's my blinged-up chocolate bark.
Melt 2 cups of good quality chocolate and add 2 tbsp of roasted pistachios, chopped Turkish delight and roasted, chopped almonds. Spread (paint) this mix onto a greased baking sheet about A4 size. Top with some Persian Fairy Floss and leave it to set.
Once set, break into shards and use the bark to add charm to your next dessert!

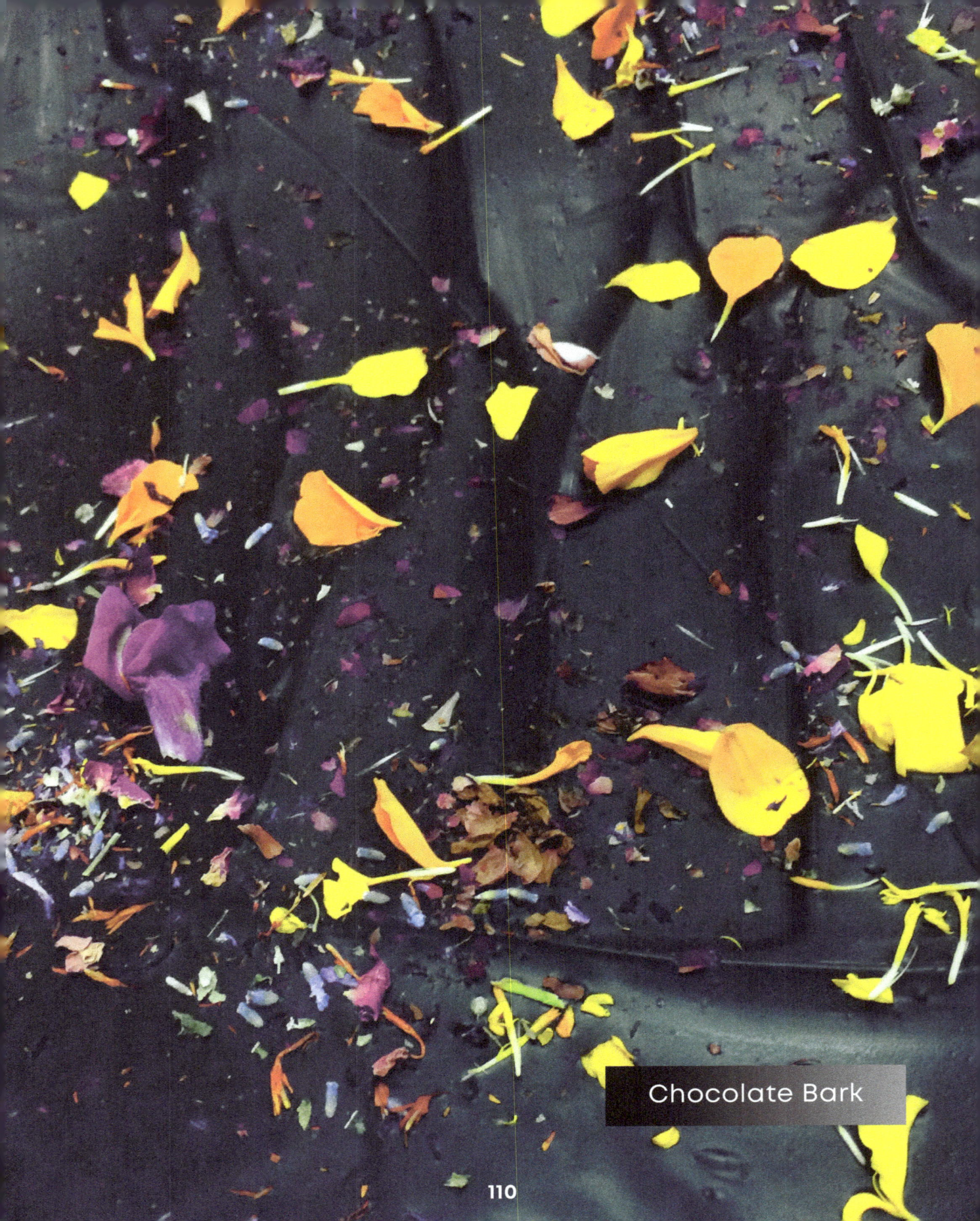

Chocolate Bark

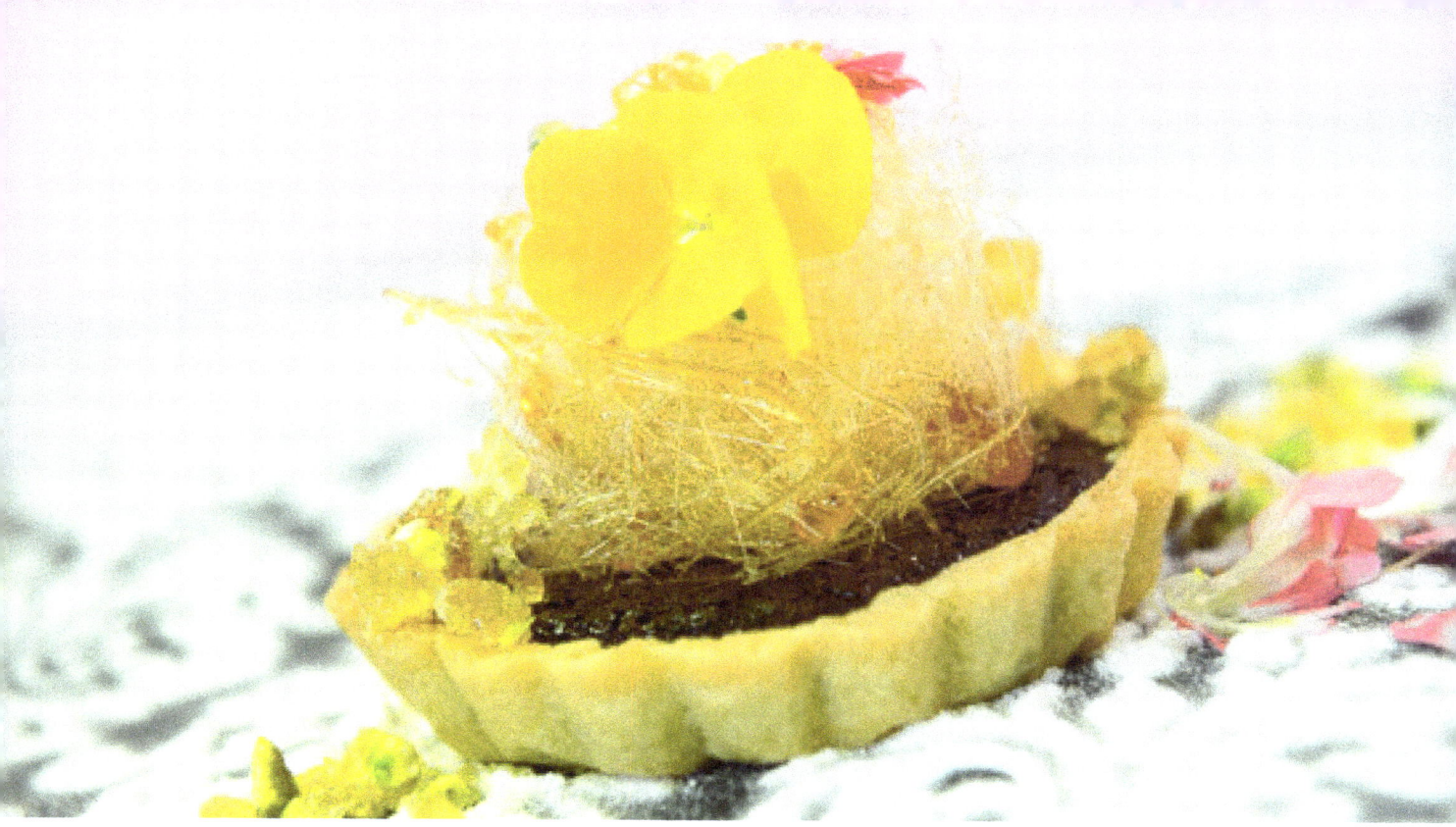

CHOCOLATE BARK FOR SAILS AND SHAPES

Melting chocolate and then painting it with a spatula onto greased paper will all you to be really creative with the bark it makes to decorate desserts - add some fruit, petals or dessert dust.

SPUN SUGAR AND SHARDS OF SUGAR GLASS

Sugar work is easy once you know how.
Simply place 1 cup of water and 1/2 cup of sugar into a saucepan and dissolve the sugar in the water.
Bring to a hot, fast boil and leave for 8 - 15 minutes until it turns a beautiful, deep caramel colour.
Be careful; this is really dangerous at this stage.
Grease a counter with cooking spray, remove the saucepan from the heat, and then, using two forks, flick the hot caramel over the bench to create long strands.
To make glass, simply pour it onto a greased baking sheet and allow it to set before breaking into shards.
Break it into lovely jagged shards or cut neatly into shapes with a hot knife.
It will keep in the fridge or freezer for months.

PERSIAN FAIRY FLOSS

The name alone makes it sound divine! Buy this delightful floss from various delis and fine food shops; it adds glamour and sophistication to any dessert.
Be sure to keep it in an airtight container or the freezer.
Adding a lemon or lime wedge to a plate is sooooo 70's.
Bling up your halved lemons or limes with some Nigella seeds and rose petals and caramelize them face down in a "swear word" hot pan and add sex appeal to your meal.
Add some "zebra stripes" to your vegetables to give them personality, and add pizazz to your plate.
Grease and heat a griddle pan or BBQ, and then griddle the vegetables hot and fast - don't turn them too much, or you'll smudge your stripes.

Spray Tans & Salts

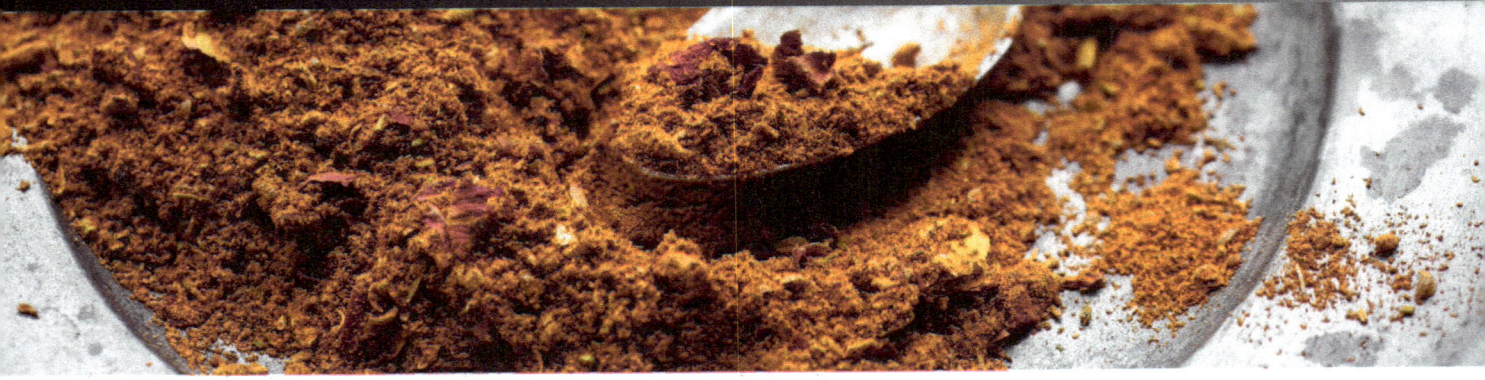

RAS EL HANOUT SPICE MIX

I know this is a massive investment, but once you have this made up, you will use it in so many different dishes! There are so many varieties of ras el hanout you will eventually end up with your own unique blend, just like I did! Make a double or triple batch; you can store it in the fridge or freezer.
Make sure your spices are fresh, or better yet, buy whole spices, pan roast, or oven roast them up and then use your spice grinder to get them into a powder! But ground spices are good enough, so have fun spicing up your life.

2 teaspoons cardamom
2 teaspoons nutmeg
2 teaspoons ground coriander
2 teaspoons ground cumin
2 teaspoons ground ginger
3 teaspoons turmeric ground
2 teaspoons ground cinnamon
3 teaspoons paprika
2 teaspoons ground black pepper
1 teaspoon pimento/allspice
½ teaspoon cloves ground
2 pinches saffron threads (optional)

BEETROOT, PINK PEPPERCORN & TURMERIC SPRAY TAN

1 small beetroot
1/4 cup salt
1 tbsp. pink peppercorns
2 tbsp. turmeric powder

Blend in a food processor and then use sparingly as a rub on lamb, chicken or beef.
Use as you would normal salt. You could also use this as a fun pinching salt on the table.

FENNEL, CELERY AND CHILLI SALT

1 small fennel
¼ cup salt
1 tbsp chopped celery leaves
1 tbsp chillies

Blend in a food processor and then use sparingly as a rub on lamb, chicken or beef - use as you would normal salt. Try your own special mix to match your dish.

TURMERIC AND RAS EL HANOUT SPRAY TAN

1 tablespoon ras el hanout
3 teaspoons oil or water
3 tablespoons turmeric powder
1 teaspoon cumin powder

Mix to a paste and then use sparingly as a rub on lamb, chicken or beef - use as you would normally salt. You can use a pastry brush to brush onto your dish.

Culinary Flavour Dusts

Adding personality to your meal. Dusting is not just for cleaning.
Creating personality on your plate with a sweet or savoury dust is simple. Ice cream is fabulous, but dusted ice cream is divine.

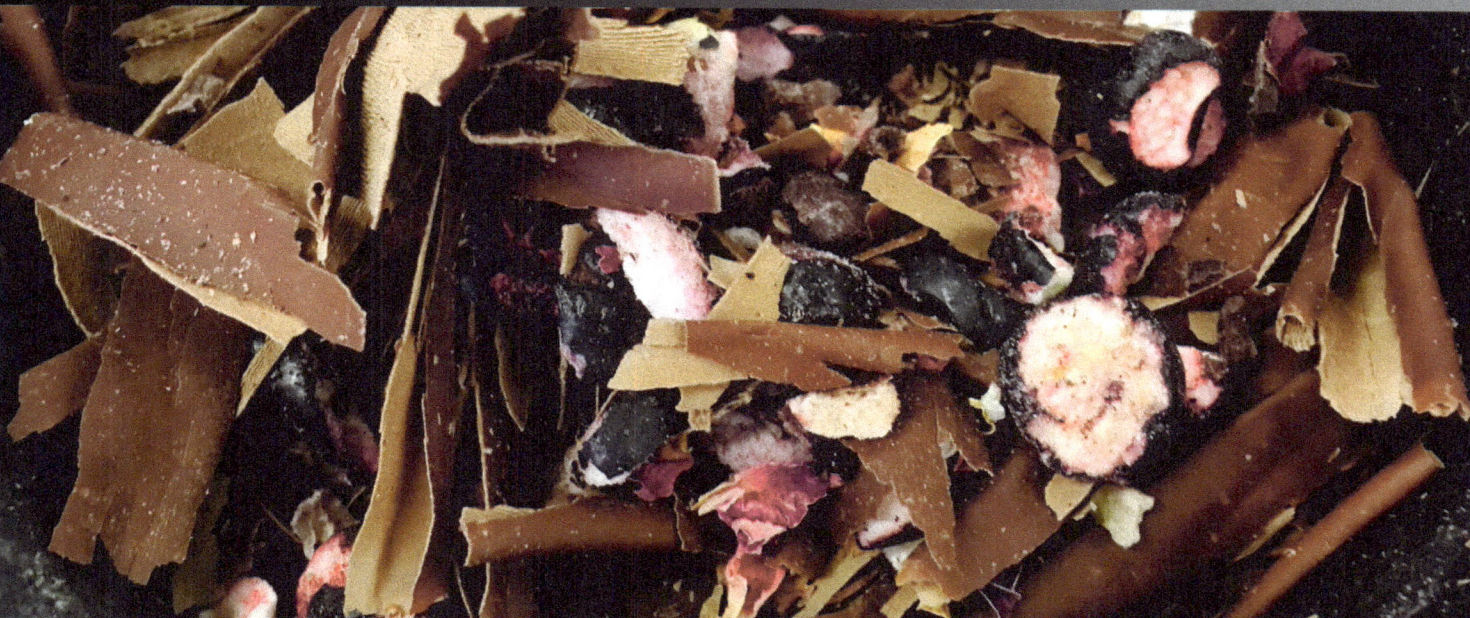

MAKE SOME SIMPLE DESSERT DUST TO ADD CHARM TO YOUR ICE CREAM

1/2 cup chopped meringue
1/2 cup honeycomb
1/2 cup cookie crumbs
1 tsp assorted edible petals
Roll the ice cream ball in the dust and serve and impress.

SWEET AND SAVOURY DUSTS
Simply bash or process into crumbs

SAVOURY

Pistachio, cumin, petals & black salt
Roasted almonds, caraway, Nigella seeds & turmeric
Roasted peanut, Asian shallots and dehydrated chilli
Dehydrated vegetables like beetroot and mushrooms, sweet potato.
Wasabi peas, chiffonade of nori, Asian shallots and black sesame seeds
Use ingredients that match your dish.

SWEET

Almond, praline & petals
Pistachio, meringues & Persian floss
Pistachio, honeycomb & halva gravel
Dehydrated berries, chocolate cookies & petals

Culinary High Heels

Adding height to your meal & getting height on your plate

Culinary high heels - it even sounds glamorous.

Remember that Culinary Bling isn't just about what you add to a dish or how you describe it. We eat with our eyes first, and that's where culinary high heels come in handy.
Using height adds interest and glamour to a dish; there are many ingredients you can use to bring your plate to dizzying heights! It's not just about propping everything up, you can also get height from angles; for example, use crispy salmon skin placed at an angle to add some height. Use roasted Prosciutto, Parmesan crisps, shaved vegetable chips and more.

Remember, just like real heels; it must match and complement the dish.
Want to add height to a dessert? Use a shard of sugar glass or spun sugar or even a chocolate sail.

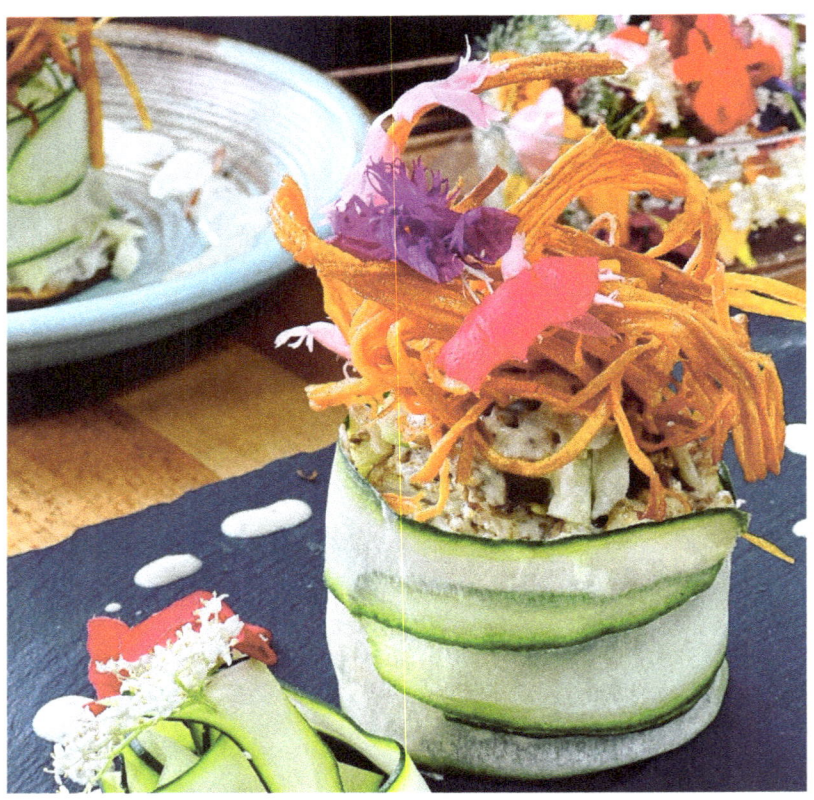

VEGETABLE STACKS

A stacking ring is a fabulous way to present your vegetable accompaniments in a neat, high tower on your plate.
You can buy stacking rings from your kitchen shop or make your own by cutting a clean dishwashing liquid bottle into two stacking rings.
All you have to do is press the vegetables into the ring with the back of a tablespoon and then lift it away.
Make your stack extra special by wrapping it in zebra-striped zucchini or roasted capsicum.

NOTES

Meet Chef Mel
THE HAPPY CHEF

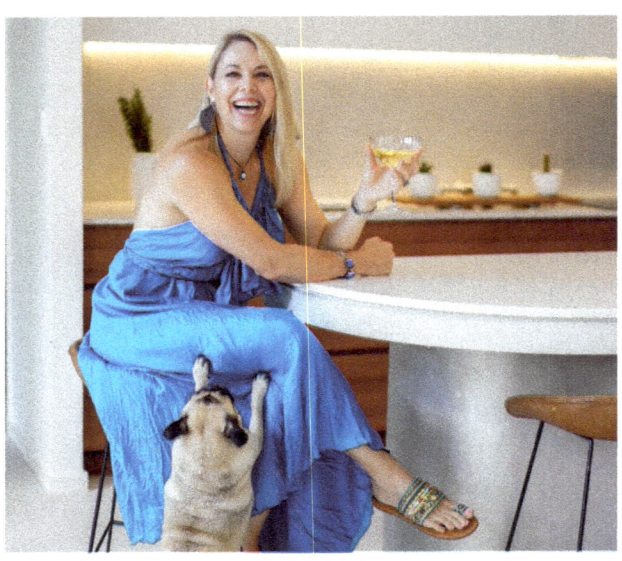

PASSIONATE FOODIE, AUTHOR, ENTREPRENEUR, COOKING SCHOOL TEACHER, ATHLETE, CULTURAL GASTRONOMER AND CHEF

With a smile that can light up a room, she has been dubbed "The Happy Chef" by her students; Chef Mel is brilliant at making everyday dishes dazzling. Her clever approach to cooking and teaching focuses on making recipes easy to understand, with time spent on excellent presentation skills.

The enthusiastic, entertaining, award-winning African-Australian chef and cooking school owner says that with a bit of know-how, anyone can plate up spectacular spreads like those you would expect to see in five-star restaurants. Her intoxicating enthusiasm, authenticity and culinary lingo will have you hungry to flex your muscles in the kitchen.

She promises that this book will teach you some seriously cheffy skills so that you will be so much more confident and happy in your kitchen.

She can't wait to help you become the foodie you have always wanted to be!

Get ready to make delicious discoveries!

www.ingramcontent.com/pod-product-compliance
Lightning Source LLC
Chambersburg PA
CBHW061802290426
44109CB00030B/2922